O F S

Life of the Clinician

Life of the Clinician

Michael J. Lepore, M.D.

THE UNIVERSITY OF ROCHESTER PRESS

First published 2002
by the University of Rochester Press

The University of Rochester Press
668 Mount Hope Avenue, Rochester, NY 14620, USA
www.urpress.com
and Boydell & Brewer, Ltd.
P.O. Box 9, Woodbridge, Suffolk 1P12 3DF, UK

Library of Congress Cataloging-in-Publication Data

Lepore, Michael J.
    The life of the clinician : the autobiography of Michael Lepore / Michael
J. Lepore.
        p. cm.
    ISBN 1-58046-116-6 (alk. paper)
        1. Lepore, Michael J. 2. Gastroenterologists--United States--Biography.
I. Title.

RC802 .L47 2002
616.3'3'0092--dc21
[B]

                                                               2002016173

British Library Cataloging-in-Publication
A catalogue record for this item is available from the British Library

Designed and typeset by Christine Menendez
Printed in the United States of America
This publication is printed on acid-free paper.

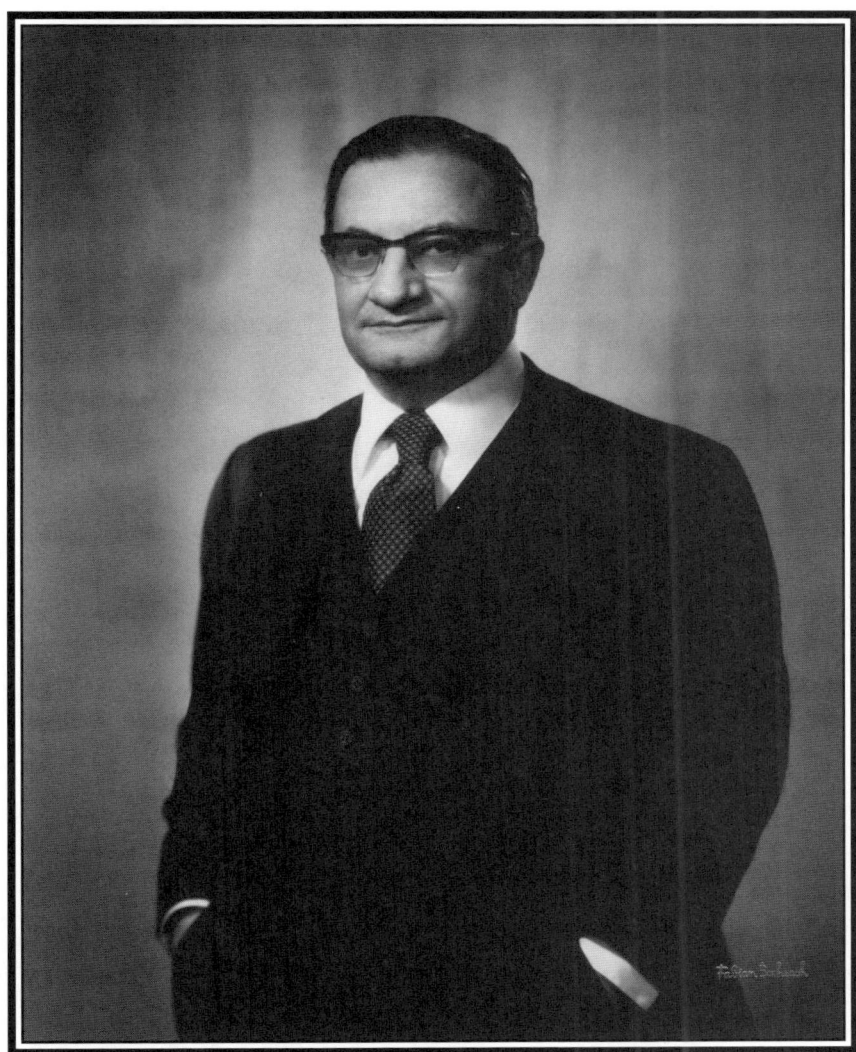

Dr. Michael J. Lepore
1910-2000

Contents

Illustrations

Preface

THIS IS A STORY of a son of Southern Italian immigrants from La Basilicata, Provincia di Potenza, Villaggio di Genzano e Muro Lucano. Born on 8 May 1910 in humble circumstances in a tenement in what was then Harlem's Little Italy and delivered into this world by the customary "Levatrice" or midwife, this young fellow was the third child of Giuseppe and Filomena Lepore whose family would increase to eight children, one of whom died in infancy. From this modest beginning, somehow there emerged a leader in American medicine, a teacher, an Oslerian clinician and diagnostician, a gastroenterologist, personal physician to many interesting and some famous persons - including a former President of the United States - and a pioneer in teaching medicine through the new medium of television.

We spoke Italian at home. I went to school to become an American and not to tell my teachers what should be taught. I attended New York City public schools and received an excellent education. The only books I read were those in use in school. There were no books at home and it would be several years before I learned to use the neighborhood libraries. My mother, who had a good education for her day, subscribed to and read *Il Progresso,* the Italian newspaper published by Generoso Pope. My father could barely sign his name and was essentially illiterate. Despite this, he became a successful small businessman who provided well for his family.

My original stimulus for writing this memoir came simply from my desire to leave for my immediate family a written record of an interesting life, illustrating how fortunate I was to be born in America and able to take advantage of the marvelous opportunities it opened to me. I have been blessed to have lived and practiced medicine and been a healer of the sick in what most of us believe has been the Golden Era of Clinical Medicine. My teachers and role models were almost all pupils of Sir William Osler, the greatest physician of modern times. To them I owe a tremendous debt that I can never repay.

To my immediate family I express my gratitude for their important contributions to my career, both economic and spiritual. To my beloved late wife, Ardean, I pay a special tribute for all she did for me epitomized in the book chapter "My One and Only Wife."

As a teacher of medical students, house staff, Fellows and other colleagues at Rochester, Duke, Yale, Columbia-Presbyterian Medical Center,

NYU, Roosevelt Hospital and St. Vincent's Medical Center of New York City, I remember them as part of my extended family and follow their careers with great interest and pride. I hope this memoir may be a reminder of the great days we spent together exploring the known and the unknown. Special and fond memories go to my colleagues and staff of my military service in WW II (1942-1946) at Army and Navy General Hospital, Hot Springs, Arkansas, Valley Forge General Hospital at Phoenixville, Pennsylvania, and overseas on Tinian with the Atom Bomb across the road from my hospital, on adjacent Saipan, and finally as professional Consultant to Tripler General Hospital on Oahu.

As I became immersed in writing this memoir, I was impressed by comments made by the gifted author, Gay Talese, in a New York Times interview with Shirley Horner on Sunday, 9 February 1992, regarding his best-selling book, *Unto the Sons,* a story of the Italian-American experience of his family. Talese said "The story of telling about the Italian-American is long overdue - It is an extraordinary story of ordinary people. But how many authors with Italian surnames are there? Why haven't the offspring of other tailors (his father was a tailor), plumbers, butchers and carpenters risen to the challenge?" My name ends in a vowel and my father was an iceman, an important occupation for Italians of that era. This comment of Talese spurred me on to write this memoir.

As I became involved in this venture, the threat of enormous changes in the American Health Care Delivery System was promoted by an incoming new President leading the Democratic Party. The major premise of the Clinton Plan was that our "Health Care Delivery System was broken and needed to be completely revised." Briefly, the Clinton Plan was, I believe, designed to destroy the personal private-practice fee-for-service system that has served American so well and to replace it with an enormous new bureaucracy, requiring massive government subsidies, and rationing and price controls, imperiling freedom of choice, impairing the quality of medical care, and interfering with the most intimate of personal relationships that the American people have enjoyed with their physicians. Predictions have been made that the private practice of medicine and the solo fee-for-service system are doomed and will be eliminated. Eight-five percent of Americans are more than satisfied with the present Health Care Delivery System. Should we destroy the present system in order to provide the remaining fifteen percent with better health care? Why not try to fix what is broken in incremental steps rather than sacrifice the entire system? At a time when Communism has failed so miserably to provide for its people, should America, the most successful democracy in the world, become a socialist state? "Not if I can help it," is the reply of the average American citizen. I do not believe that the personal private practice and fee-for-service system of medical practice is doomed. I believe that given a level playing field, it will not only survive, it will continue to thrive in America. I have always given more that I have taken from my profession. I was born in a generation of doctors who took care of the poor and the elderly by not charging them and I had plenty of company in my heyday.

I do not believe that Socialized Medicine is the treatment that will cure what is sick in the American system of health care. I prefer an incremental approach preserving the good features of the existing system and fixing the broken parts.

My hope is that those who read this memoir, especially the bright youngsters, will find in it the charm and appeal of the Way of Life chosen by the writer that brought to him and his family and patients, pleasure, success and fulfillment. I know I have often chosen the road less traveled and embraced Thoreau's maxim, "If a man does not keep pace with his companions, perhaps it is because he hears a different drummer. Let him step to the music which he hears, however measured or far away." My plea to our young people entering the study of medicine is to maintain its freedom and independence and refuse to be intimidated by those who would impose upon our great profession restraints and bureaucratic controls that would not for a minute be tolerated by any of the other professions, especially the law.

It was Albert Schweitzer who said at a commencement that he could not predict the future of the graduates except to say that those who learned to serve would achieve happiness. I HAVE LEARNED TO SERVE, and my hope is that those who follow me will be able to say the same.

I close this prologue with a biblical admonition:

> "Your God will bless you in everything that you do or undertake.
> The poor will always be with you in the land and for that reason
> I command you to be open-handed with your countrymen, both
> poor and distressed, in your own land."[1]

---

1. Deuteromony, 15:11. God's laws delivered by Moses.

Chapter 1

Early Days

I WAS BORN IN A FLAT IN HARLEM'S LITTLE ITALY on 115th Street in Manhattan where I was delivered by a midwife, as were all of my siblings. My arrival was greeted with jubilation and prayers of thanks to Our Lady of Mount Carmel whose church was nearby where my parents, immigrants from southern Italy, were communicants as were most of our neighbors. I was the third child born to Giuseppe and Filomena Lepore. The first born, also a son, died an infant, of something called "summer complaint," a diarrheal disease. In the tradition of Italian families, the first son had been named Michele for his paternal grandfather. The baby was buried by his grieving parents in a little plot in a cemetery in Brooklyn. The second child was a girl, Carmela. With my arrival my parents were faced with a dilemma. Should they name me Michael (Michele) and risk tempting fate (La Maluria) to strike me down as it had my little brother?

Religious belief overcame superstition with my arrival on St. Michael's Day, Sunday, May 8, 1910, and I was promptly named Michael in honor of my paternal grandfather. As luck would have it, I became ill during the summer of 1910 with a diarrheal disease similar to my deceased brother's and appeared headed for the same cemetery. My father, being a man of action, decided to send his wife and two children to Italy to live with the Lepore grandparents in Genzano, La Basilicata, Provincia di Potenza. There I regained my health and remained until I was three years old and thriving, at which time my father called us back to America. In retrospect, it is likely that I had lactase deficiency with milk intolerance. My mother was unable to breast-feed me and I had been placed on cow's milk formula resulting in severe diarrhea. In Italy I was passed around to ample-bosomed relatives and peasant women nursing their own children but willing and able to donate their surplus to my upbringing. Years later, I was still greeted by some of the same volunteer wet-nurses with a garlicky kiss on the cheek, a hug and "Benedette Sono Le Stizzi di Latto Che Io Dato" (Blessed are the drops of milk I gave you). I was similarly indebted to a fine collection of healthy goats on my grandfather's farm that contributed their milk not only to their kids but also to maintain my own nutrition when the wet nurses could not keep up with my demands. Probably for some genetic reason goat's milk did not upset me while cow's milk acted like a laxative.

I am not quite certain why my parents left Italy for America. Poverty was not the reason, for both my father and mother came from comfortable farm families that owned their land, tilled it, and did not want for the basic amenities of life. Neither were religious persecution or political upheaval motivating causes. At a time when villagers almost always married into families from the same village, my father defied custom when he, a native of Genzano, courted and married Filomena Melucci of nearby Muro Lucano, the daughter of a prosperous landowner and lessor of large tracts of grazing land for substantial herds of sheep. My mother was well educated for that day and served as her father's bookkeeper, a fact that caused him some distress when he lost her through marriage, especially to a "Forestiero" from another town, even though it was only a few miles away. My father would always be known as "Beppo il Genzanese" to his adjoining neighbors who were the Murese of Muro Lucano.

After my parents were married in the village church of Muro Lucano, they decided to emigrate to America where a number of their *paesani* had gone and sent back glowing reports of life in the New World. The decision could not have been an easy one for them. As it turned out, my father was the only one of five brothers who chose to leave Italy and my mother was the sole member of her immediate family to come to America. The experience was especially wrenching for my father who kept close ties with his family for the rest of his life, through correspondence and occasional personal visits via transatlantic liners. As best I can recall, my mother, whose own mother had died at an early age, seemed less attached to her family or so it seemed to me later when I was more alert to these matters. She never returned to Italy after the episode of 1910–1913.

On our return trip from Italy in 1913, the voyage was rough with mother seasick from the docks of Naples to those of New York harbor. I ran about the boat having a great time eating almost anything I could get my hands on or scrounge from friendly passengers. We traveled in second class thereby avoiding the humiliation and degradation of steerage and Ellis Island.

When we docked in New York, we were met by a rosy-jawed, black-haired stocky man with a large mustache, my father, who swept me up in his arms. Years later he told me on numerous occasions that the first thing I asked for was "Chocolatte." My father asked "Where did you learn about Chocolatte?" I answered, "From tata Michele," my grandfather. "That's what I thought" said my father and he soon purchased some chocolate for me. Grandfather Lepore had spoiled me in many ways. He was a very warm and gentle man, soft-spoken and kind. He was a successful farmer and with five sons he had quite a menage. My maternal grandfather Francisco Melucci was described as a rather austere widower who made a comfortable living by leasing large tracts of land for raising sheep. The wool from his herds was much sought after and he in turn had great respect for the sheep that produced it and the shepherds that managed the herds. He would visit the Lepores when he could and maintained cordial relations with them.

Grandfather Lepore had quite a sense of humor and could not resist a practical joke. One of these was to teach me what to say when he asked me certain questions. He would ask me, when my maternal grandfather was present, "Michele how are you going to watch sheep when you grow up?" My answer was always the same—"Appese"—that is strung or slaughtered. This would infuriate grandfather Melucci who thought that being a shepherd was a wonderful way of life. A live sheep meant more to him than a dead one.

I was a very lively and active boy who enjoyed play and company. My first school was nearby in Harlem, a public school. My mother was quite surprised when I brought home the first prize for being at the top of the class—a large bouquet of black-eyed Susans. My mother and her *paesani* disliked parochial schools and most of the Genzanese and Murese attended public schools in those days. For reasons unclear to me at the time, my mother disliked Harlem and was eager to move her growing family away from conditions that she felt were not good for raising young children. She also disliked the petty gossip, jealousies, and arguments abounding in the ingrown atmosphere of *paesani* who carried the feuds, prejudices, and rivalries of the old country into the daily life of a new world.

Pushcarts lining the streets sold food and one had to be quick and keen to discern poor produce and poor goods while at the same time protecting the pocketbook in more ways than one. I recall mother telling me this story of one of her shopping expeditions. My father had come home from work to find her appearing glum and in tears. His first fear was that bad news had arrived from Italy. She denied this. Finally she confessed that she had lost a ten dollar bill—lots of money in that day, while selecting fruit from a pushcart. Obviously someone had picked her pocket. Instead of being upset at this loss, my father said "forget it, there's more where that came from" and immediately replaced the loss without any fanfare. On another occasion when father had come from work she noticed that a large button had been torn from his brand new pea jacket and she asked how this had happened as she prepared to repair the damage. After some prodding the truth came out. Some weeks before, having tried several enterprises and having decided that he would never work for another person, my father had purchased a small business, for several hundred dollars, selling ice, coal and wood from a basement cellar. He was his own boss, so he thought. Gossip among the *paesani* was that Beppo il Genzanese had been suckered into paying out his hard earned cash by a rogue German bully who made it a practice to "sell" his business for cash to a gullible Italian, then coming back in a few weeks or months to reclaim the business without paying for it. The rogue was known as a tough street brawler of considerable strength and was feared by the *paesani*. Well, sure enough he tried to play the same trick on my father but he met with more than his match. My father was a very strong man, built like a football line-backer, who was not given to violence unless really provoked. He proceeded to take this rogue apart in a violent struggle that left his attacker beaten and subdued and tore father's pea jacket. There was never any more difficulty among the Italians caused by this rascal and the message was out to lay off Giuseppe Lepore and his *paesani*.

The emergence of my father as an iceman, lifting 300 pound cakes of ice as if they were egg crates, came as a great surprise to his father and family in Italy who shuddered to think that one of their prized members who had no real need to perform hard manual labor was now making his living the hard way in the New World.

One of the things my father had learned to do well on the farm in Italy was to break horses. He had a real talent for this despite the fact that he once fractured his femur while breaking in an especially wild horse.

My father started in the ice business in a cellar location. Later he acquired a pushcart to peddle ice to his various customers. Then the time came for him to purchase a horse and wagon. I recall as a small boy of six or seven years, accompanying my father to the horse auctions held at Fort Lee at the foot of 125th Street on the Hudson River. I liked to do this because father had promised me that someday he would buy me a pony. On this particular day he was looking for a strong, young horse for his ice wagon. One special horse caught his eye. He was a handsome chestnut stallion named John with a little fire in his eye and quite spirited. Most of the prospective buyers who looked at him shied away because they did not feel he was adequately broken. In retrospect, the horse may well have been a Morgan. Pop liked him immediately for his style, conformation, spirit, and his size—not too big for pulling ice wagons on the streets of New York and not too small to pull heavy loads from scratch. These were key considerations in those days and only an experienced horseman could make the necessary judgment. Percherons and Clydesdales looked good but they were much too big for the ice business and did not do well on the cobblestone streets of New York. Besides that, their food consumption tended to price them out of the market. My father was an excellent judge of horseflesh and I had never known him to make a poor choice. He also was very kind to his animals, fed them well and made sure that they were well shod and groomed. I recall accompanying my father on walks to our stable on 166th Street near Amsterdam Avenue where he would inspect each stall, check the feed to be sure that it was of high quality, the straw clean and the state of the horses' shoes good. In the process he would have a brief chat with the stable hand, making certain he was sober, not smoking, and taking good care of our most valuable properties, the horses that pulled Lepore Ice and Sun Maid Laundry wagons starting before dawn each weekday.

In later years my father would tell me that he had never seen a horse he could not train. So taken was he with "John," which he pronounced "Gian," that he paid the princely sum of seven hundred and fifty dollars in cash for him and took him away to our stable. The *paesani* witnessing this event soon labeled it "Beppo il Genzanese's Folly" and predicted that the horse would drag him into the river and kill him. John nearly did this the very first time out, heading out in a gallop for the East River. Somehow my dad was able to control him but not until they were near the water's edge.

John became one of our family; he was an intelligent, remarkable, almost human being. He knew the ice route by heart and knew when and where to stop or go. We had him for nearly 15 years and he was the leader of a stable my father was to acquire for delivering ice to retail and wholesale customers in the area known in those days as Washington Heights, where the bright yellow wagons of Lepore & Company had a tight monopoly on the wholesale and retail trade. On hot August days the neighborhood kids would jump onto the back of our wagons to retrieve broken slivers of ice to cool themselves off. I shall never forget the wonderful trips in that ice wagon with reliable, strong, and steady John pulling the heavy load up the steep hill at 158th Street heading for Broadway on the way to our customers in the apartment houses and stores in Washington Heights. Neither can I ever forget the sadness when I accompanied my father to our stable one evening when we were summoned because our beloved John, now 20 years old, could no longer get up because of a broken back. A policeman was called to mercifully dispose of John with a pistol shot. Dad and I shed tears all the way home as if we had lost a member of our family. And indeed we had!

The ice business attracted my father for a variety of reasons. First of all he felt he could be his own boss, responsible only to his customers. Second, it was a cash business and did not require an extensive inventory or expensive equipment. All that was needed was a hatchet, an ice pick, ice tongs and a strong back. The ice had to be sold as quickly as possible especially in hot weather. The wood and coal would keep and could take up the slack in winter when there was less demand for ice. In Washington Heights most of our customers lived in apartments that did not require wood or coal so our business was almost entirely with ice. The rental for the cellar storage space and refrigerator was minimal and the overhead was nil.

At the turn of the century, the ice business in America was undergoing some drastic changes. There were few ice plants for making artificial ice. Most of the ice was the natural form harvested each winter on the Hudson River or in Maine and New Hampshire and even in Wisconsin.

A recent article in the *New York Times* describes with nostalgia the era of the natural ice barges on the Hudson. "On the Staten Island side of the [Arthur] Kill, now crowded with tankers and container-ships that shun the city in favor of Newark and Elizabeth, a ship-breakers' yard had become the final resting place of scores of abandoned harbor craft. These wood and steel fossils awaiting final dissection offer clues to the past and hints of the future. A visitor wandering among the old hulks, as a *Times* photographer did recently, can find a wooden-hulled steam towboat that once plied the Hudson trailing as many as 50 ice barges. A family lived on every barge; some children could say they had never set foot ashore during the first 10 years of their lives. When Spring opened the upper Hudson to navigation, the flotillas of barges brought ice, cut from northern lakes, to the metropolis that until the early 1920s lacked any other widely available refrigerant."[1]

Another aspect of the ice business that had eluded me, was discussed in an article that appeared in *American Heritage* magazine, July-August 1991, pp. 71–76, by Susan N. Bean entitled, "Cold Mine," the fascinating story of how ice from America was first shipped to Calcutta, India, in 1833. Bean said "although surprising when first encountered, the ice trade was a mainstay of New England's nine-teenth-century commerce. The name most closely associated with it is Frederic Tudor, a Boston merchant who pioneered the transport of ice to the tropics in 1806. Tudor managed to keep far enough ahead of his imitators to become known as the Ice King.

---

1. Roger Starr, "Reading of Harbor Waves," New York Times, February 9, 1992.

"Beginning in the mid-nineteenth century, the trade he founded continued to grow until the 1880s—Tudor's first shipment of ice to the tropics went to Martinique (in 1805). The 130-ton cargo was harvested from a family pond in Saugus. The venture was not a financial success. Tudor had to solve problems of inefficiency in harvesting, of loss in transit and in storage. He also had to develop a market in Martinique. Tudor himself demonstrated how his product could be used to make ice cream. He promoted the use of iceboxes for keeping food fresh and fostered the medical application of ice in reducing fevers. He sold his ice cheaply to encourage customers and build his market, and he secured monopolies to ensure that market—by 1825, two decades of technological and marketing improvements had made Tudor's ice business profitable, but it was ten more years before he achieved his goal of providing New England ice to the world." In April, 1833, with two partners, Samuel Rogers and Samuel Austin, Jr., "he equipped a ship to transport ice to Calcutta, India, a feat never before attempted." By May 12, 1833, Tudor wrote in his diary "Sailed this day the ship Tuscany, Capt. Littlefield, for Calcutta with 180 tons of ice—an experiment I have been desirous of making for 20 years." The commander of the Tuscany, Clement Littlefield, recorded in his log: "Took in a cargo of ice for Calcutta and sailed the 12th of May being the first ice that ever crossed the equator. I arrived in Calcutta Sept. 10th with one hundred tons of ice witch [sic] astonished the natives." Within three days of the arrival of the Tuscany, the British residents raised money to build an icehouse to preserve the commodity. "In the years that followed, Tudor weathered every challenge to the trade he invented. Because of Tudor a British resident of Calcutta wrote, "I will not talk of nectar of elysium, but I will say that if there be a luxury here—I would point to the contents of our icehouse—The arrival of our English mail is not more anxiously expected than that of an American ice ship." "Because of Tudor," Thoreau would write, in *Walden*, that "the inhabitants of Madras and Bombay and Calcutta drink at my well. The pure Walden water is mingled with the sacred waters of the Ganges."

With the growth of the large cities, water pollution gradually made the natural ice unsightly and unsafe for human consumption. Mild weather would reduce the harvest from rivers, lakes, and ponds and wild fluctuations in the selling price limited the growth of this industry. However, increasing demands for ice were spurred by the need for year-round refrigeration for meats, vegetables, milk, ice cream, cold drinks, and fermenting beer. Inventors pursued the quest for ice-making machines, and starting with the mid-nineteenth century, they partially succeeded. Soon the output of artificial ice plants far exceeded that from natural sources. By 1920, the Census Bureau estimated 1800 plants produced 30,000,000 tons of which 25,000,000 was sold to the public. Approximately 160,000 people were employed in the production and distribution of ice. Total investment in the ice manufacturing business was about $450,000,000. In the same era 15,000,000 tons of natural ice were harvested. Total investment in this category was estimated at $194,000,000. the combined investment for natural and manufactured ice was about $644,000,000. The total industry ranked ninth in amount of investments among America's commercial enterprises. The "last gasp" for the natural ice industry was World War I—when the war ended, so did the patriotic reasons for perpetuating the natural ice business. The production of "plant ice" gained such inroads on the natural ice harvest that by 1925 little remained of the industry. Giant ice houses stood vacant along the Hudson, Kennebec, and other northern rivers and lakes. These were symbols of an industry that in a matter of decades experienced rapid growth and increasing importance for the American Economy, followed by unprecedented obsolescence.[2]

When my father became an iceman circa 1910, he was selling natural ice and I recall that one of the reasons he changed ice plants several years later was because the artificially made ice was cleaner, crystal clear, and easier to cut and shape for sale to his customers. His customers also told him that they preferred the plant ice to the natural ice.

Let us return to New York City at the turn of the century. It did not take long for the Italian immigrants to flock to the ice business. The work was hard and you had to have a strong body, and be willing to get up at 4 A.M. to hitch up the horses and get on line at the ice plants. This was one business that the New York Italians controlled from A to Z. Americans and other ethnic groups, the Irish, Jews, and Germans, avoided the ice business because it was menial and heavy work, leaving a vacuum that immigrant Italians were eager to fill.

My father imported quite a few young men from the old *paese* in Italy, paying their voyage from the old country and lending them money to get started. For some reason, I can find little or no public record of the contributions of Italian immigrants of New York City to the ice business. Perhaps it is because they kept to themselves, were law-abiding, sober, industrious, and good neighbors, features that would be passed on to their children and promote their successful

---

2. Joseph C. Jones Jr., *American Iceman* (Humble, Texas: Jobeco Books, 1984), p. 159.

assimilation into the mainstream of American life. While the activities of the Mafiosi, *Mano nero* (Black Hand), and the *Camorra* made head-lines and created an unfortunate and inaccurate image of the Italians, it would soon become clear that the majority of Italians were good, decent, hardworking people who would make enormous contribu-tions to their adopted country. Any story about the Italian-Americans in America that fails to mention the ice business must be regarded as flawed and incomplete.

The icemen and their families became prosperous, some quite wealthy and influential in their communities and church. Financial security made it possible for them to encourage their children to obtain the education they themselves had lacked. An era of prosperi-ty, security, and good-will was developing and the future appeared quite rosy.

The social life of the Italian immigrants consisted in the main of family parties and functions, weddings, baptisms, christenings, funer-als, and the like. The *paesani* from each village tended to socialize among themselves. They formed societies for mutual aid e.g.Societa di Mutuo Soccorso di Genzano. By paying monthly dues, funds were available to help their sick members, to bury those who died, and to provide a form of life insurance. A doctor was given a retainer to tend the sick.

All of this was done without any form of bureaucracy or govern-ment intervention. If a child had achieved a scholastic honor or had been graduated from elementary or high school, a party was usually held in a ballroom where good food and pastries were abundant and the red wine flowed generously. It was not very fancy but it was a happy life for these hardworking, honest families who asked very lit-tle for their share of the good things in life.

World War I inflicted its toll upon the Lepore family in Italy and taught us in America to fear the delivery of the black-bordered letters informing us of losses and injuries. One of my father's brothers was killed in combat on the Austrian front early in that war and another was captured by the Austrians and held prisoner for three years.

For the families of those involved in the ice business, the future seemed assured and for some there appeared to be no end to the good things of prosperity and financial independence. Little did they know that before long another scientific invention of the industrial age would throw the ice business into a tailspin. The invention was mechanical refrigeration, the gas or electric "ice box," that would put the icemen out of business.

Chapter 2

ᵔᵕᵔ

Washington Heights

MOTHER PERSISTED IN TRYING TO MOVE US AWAY from Harlem to the northern area of Manhattan. In a community called Fort George, there was a group of *paesani* who welcomed more of the same, but mother did not approve. Getting a place to live for a large family, still growing and especially one of Italian origin, was not easy. We were called, usually behind our backs, Wops or Guineas. I remember that my mother had to lie about the number of children she had in order for us to be accepted as tenants. No landlord welcomed a large family, especially Italians. At one time we shared with Godparents (*compari*) a small private house on Audubon Avenue near what became the Columbia-Presbyterian Medical Center. I remember attending P.S. 169, which was across the street, and receiving the first prize for scholarship, a knitted silk silver necktie for which I had little or no use but to assure my family that I was doing well in school. I was also "skipped' ahead one or two grades. I recall that mother would deck me out to the nines with Buster Brown collar and meticulously laundered clothes on school days. What she did not seem to appreciate was that while this attire looked nice enough it invited all sorts of jibes, occasional birdcalls and Bronx cheers, and led to fist fights that I enjoyed but sure messed up my clothes. I soon became quite adept at using my fists to the dismay of my would-be tormentors.

It was when we were living in the house on Audubon Avenue that Mr. and Mrs. Wicks, who lived in an adjacent apartment building, offered to take my sister and me to church on Sundays. My mother agreed at first, but became concerned when she learned there were no statues in this church and our prayers and hymns seemed so different from those she had learned in Italy. What had happened was that the Wicks were Presbyterian and we were going to the local Presbyterian Church. My mother quickly put an end to this and arranged for us to attend St. Rose of Lima Roman Catholic Church on 165th Street where the entire family worshipped. But I still remember *Rock of Ages* and *Brighten the Corner Where You Are* from my brief experience as a Presbyterian.

As I indicated, our ice business was centered on Washington Heights and was quite profitable. My father could handle people very well and he was well liked and a good business man. He was also a generous man. He would frequently pay passage for young men to come to America from our small towns in Italy. I recall meeting many of them at Ellis Island with their primitive luggage and packages reeking of olive oil, garlic, and provolone. Mother would put them up in our house until lodging elsewhere could be arranged. Father put them to work learning the ice business not as serf labor but ultimately as part of the management and partnership. When he felt they were ready, he lent them money to purchase a share of the business and never once did he charge them any interest nor did he demand collateral to secure the loan. All of these men prospered. My father and mother arranged many of their marriages. To my knowledge there was never a divorce among the twenty or more men we brought over from Italy. There was an almost filial relationship between them and my father. When you speak of an extended family, there it was!

We needed a large apartment for the seven children and two adults constituting our nuclear family, but where could we find one and who would take in nine Italians at one swoop? Luck came our way when the superintendent of one of the apartment houses in Washington Heights, whose ice requirements were controlled and served by Lepore & Company, decided that he did not want to live in the large basement apartment allocated to him at 615 West 162nd Street. He had arranged to move into a smaller and nicer apartment with a view on an upper floor of this six-story elevator apartment house. He liked my father and a deal was struck whereby our family would occupy the commodious basement apartment. We lived there for many years and enjoyed its comforts, security, and excellent utilities.

While we were living in Washington Heights, my father was approached in a basement one day by a well-groomed man wearing a derby hat and a Chesterfield coat who wanted to discuss some business matters with him. My father called him "Mr. Rockachild" (a contraction of Rockefeller and Rothschild), but I later learned that he was a Rothschild who had risked considerable sums in building a new ice-plant on Edgecombe Avenue nearby.

He was very eager to obtain father's promise to send his wagons to buy ice from his ice plant. My father had promised Mr. "Rockachild" that his wagons would be there but he could not and would not sign any written contract. This might have jeopardized his relationship with his existing ice supplier, the Sheffield Milk Company, with its ice plant at Fort Lee at the western foot of 125th Street on the Hudson River. Mr. Rothschild would have preferred a written commitment but realized that he was dealing with a man whose word was his bond. When the Rothschild plant opened up, true to my father's word the Lepore wagons were there and the Rothschild investment was secure and continued to prosper. Mr. Rothschild remembered this and for the rest of his remaining short life he never forgot the Lepores. He did many favors for us including getting two of my sisters positions in the Chelsea Exchange Bank on 42nd Street. The last favor was an offer to arrange a scholarship at Harvard for me when I was ready to go to college. The offer was made by Mr. Lapidus (for years I thought his name was La Peters), who was Mr. Rothschild's secretary and factotum. I still remember the day this happened; the day of the total eclipse of 1925. When I told my mother of the offer, she became very upset and with some reason, for although I was in my senior year in De Witt Clinton High School I was only fifteen. She had never heard of Harvard and saw no reason for my going away from home. I quickly realized that going away to college was simply out of the question; so we turned down Mr. Rothschild's generous offer. However, I told my parents that when I finished college I must go to medical school out of town and live on the campus, and they agreed, perhaps being guided by an old Italian proverb that by that time "another Pope would be born." "Ci Nascia un altro Papa."

When I was ten years old, I told my parents that I wanted to be a doctor because I wanted to help sick people. There were few role models among the Italians. Dr. Antonio Stella, a native of our village, was a greatly admired diagnostician and practitioner and I hoped to follow in his footsteps. My mother feared that working with my father in the ice business and pulling dumbwaiter ropes might injure my hands for the delicate work of a doctor.

She arranged for me to see our family doctor of that period, Dr. Julius Miller, to settle the matter. Dr. Miller examined me briefly and told my parents that hard manual work could help strengthen my hands and would not interfere with my plans to be a doctor. He advised me to keep up the good work.

Washington Heights circa 1917 was a beautiful, diversified, safe, and interesting part of Manhattan. It overlooked Riverside Drive and the Hudson River, with a magnificent view of the Palisades and ferry boats plying their trade long before the George Washington Bridge was built. Its people were law-abiding, decent, middle class, and well behaved, mostly native-born, and church-goers. At 168th Street, there were still remnants of the old farms. On the southwest corner of 168th Street and Broadway there was a large fenced-in empty lot covered with cinders, the former site of the Highlander's baseball park. When the lease ran out in 1912, the Highlanders, who became the New York Yankees, shifted their base to the Polo Grounds on the

Harlem River Drive below Coogan's Bluff, where they shared the stadium with the New York Giants until the "House that Ruth Built"—the Yankee Stadium—arose across the Harlem River in 1923.

Many years later, when I was a resident in medicine at Duke University Hospital and helped with the care of our baseball coach, Jack Coombs, the famous Philadelphia Athletics pitcher, he regaled me with many tales of baseball games played in the Highlander ballpark. Jack, who always referred to his great manager "Mr. Mack" (Connie Mack) with considerable respect, told me that one day he was being battered quite hard by the home team, the Highlanders, for no good reason. "Mr. Mack" came out of the dugout and asked Jack what was wrong, and the reply was "Nothing." "These birds seem to know exactly what and where I am going to throw the next pitch." Mr. Mack smelled a rat and sure enough turned up a rogue in the centerfield bleachers who had set up a Morse code contact with the dugout and with the aid of field glasses was systematically stealing the catcher's signals to Jack Coombs. This incident became part of baseball's history when it led to a ban on stealing signals within the ballpark, chortled Jack as he told me the story with obvious gusto even after many years had elapsed. Jack Coombs was the greatest southpaw pitcher of his day and for years held the record for consecutively pitched scoreless innings in World Series play. He made baseball at Duke the most popular sport on campus. He and his wife were great favorites of the students who became their "family" for they were childless.

During the First World War, I recall hearing Billie Sunday preaching under a large tan canvas tent on the Highlander ballpark lot. He was noted for his "silvery throat" advertising Luden's Yellow Menthol cough drops of that day. We kids went there to get the free samples of Luden's cough drops packaged in tiny boxes of two, not to listen to his preaching.

During WW I the same large plot was used as a storage depot by the 102nd Engineers whose armory was across the street. In 1918, after the armistice, I remember going to the armory to purchase Army surplus boxes filled with enormous jars of apple butter, a popular wartime spread.

I remember with pleasure tobogganing down Fort Washington Avenue starting at 168th Street where Harkness Pavilion and the Milstein Building now stand, and thundering down the hill, turning sharply to the right at 165th Street and flying down past the Deaf and Dumb Institute to Riverside Drive, turning right again and cruising for another mile. There was no automobile traffic and very little pedestrian activity except for the tobogganers returning to the top of the hill for another exhilarating ride.

Washington Heights in those days, in stark contrast to its present-day appearance, was full of pleasant and wholesome activities, a far cry from today's almost incredible decay, stench, immorality, filth, poverty, and criminal activity earning it the dubious distinction of being the modern Crack Capital of the nation. As a youngster I played stickball and handball against the wall on these streets and used the empty lots for baseball and football. Basketball was not so popular in those days.

Youngsters who had allowances saved them, or they saved their earnings from part-time work, to finance their athletic clubs and the purchase of gloves, uniforms, bats, balls, and other paraphernalia for their game. There were no little leagues. We did it all ourselves. Parents knew what was going on and they left us pretty much to our own devices and did not interfere. The teams representing these clubs were important for the development of the kids. Through our games we learned to compete fairly and aggressively, to win or lose without alienation. We ran our clubs along democratic lines and learned to respect one another's beliefs. The section we lived in had quite a mixture of various ethnic groups. Broadway was the dividing line. West of it toward Riverside Drive were modern six-story elevator apartment houses inhabited in the earlier years by a majority of WASPS of good circumstances who were slowly and steadily replaced by European Jews who were affluent and able to afford maids, some having cars, occasionally with a chauffeur. The Fox Audubon Theater at 165th Street and Broadway was noted for its vaudeville, its movies, silent at first and then with sound and later yet with color. Those who could afford it made a weekly visit to the Audubon. Above it, for more mature and venturesome types was the Audubon Ballroom where the gay blades and dames held forth. At the bend of 159th Street and Fort Washington Avenue a theater called the Costello, named for a popular movie star of the day, was a neighborhood gathering place on Saturday nights. Later on, Loew's Theater was built on nearby Broadway and I well remember in the thirties seeing *Gone with the Wind* for the first time in a full house, despite what seemed in those depression days an exorbitant admission charge.

Broadway in those days was immaculately clean, the stores were well kept, family-owned and run, and had a sense of style. There were no honky-tonks, graffiti, fast-food outlets, pizza or taco, smells of frying foods, blaring noise, and unkempt and disorderly people wandering about the streets. East of Broadway were modest small homes and tenements inhabited by low-income, middle-class people. When you reached Edgecombe Avenue there was an excellent public library that I used a great deal because there were no books in our home. An enclave of blacks and Jumel Mansion reminded us of the past.

Virtually all of these ethnic groups lived quietly and in harmony with their neighbors. Crime was minimal. There were no race riots. During Prohibition the usual "blind pigs" were there catering to the neighborhood needs. Policemen patrolled the beat on foot, appropriating their share of the fruit but enforcing law and order in a friendly and effective manner.

When we moved to 162nd Street I had to change schools again, going to P.S. 46 near Edgecombe Avenue and 159th Street. This was either the third or fourth school I had to attend in about five years and I took it pretty much in stride. It meant that I had to deal with new teachers, new methods of education, and the competition for superiority and survival among a new group of students. This did not bother me. I rather liked it. To this day, change is a challenge for me, not a threat.

One of my first experiences at P.S. 46 was an encounter with a first-class bully who was pummeling the hell out of a little red-headed kid on the sidewalk in front of the school. It looked so unfair that without any hesitation I waded into the fray, socked the bully several times and removed him from on top of the little chap he was beating. The little fellow got up and then charged his tormentor and together we drove him off. We then introduced ourselves, my little friend saying he was William Warren.

From this brief but hectic encounter, there developed a strong and lasting friendship. Bill Warren and I were destined to become a Damon-and-Pythias pair.

Bill Warren and his family lived on the sixth floor of a handsome elevator building on the southwest corner of 165th Street and Broadway commanding an excellent view of almost all of Washington Heights and the Palisades. The family consisted of his grandmother, Mrs. Elwood Kirby Warren, the widow of the former manager of Steeplechase Park, her bachelor brother, uncle Bill Hankinson, and one of her two sons, uncle Sam Warren. Bill was being raised by his grandmother and his elderly uncles through the tragedy of his birth. His father, Harry L. Warren, while a medical student at New York Bellevue Hospital Medical School, had fallen in love with a beautiful young nurse whom he married. When Bill was born, his mother died in childbirth. His father became so depressed that he quit medical school, turned the infant over to his mother, and left New York. For several years I am told he could not bear the sight of his little son and made infrequent holiday visits, usually laden down with expensive gifts. As the hurt healed with the passage of time, he made a new life for himself, remarried, raised another family and became the successful and prosperous president of a major oil company in Pennsylvania. One present he gave Bill was a handsome pure-bred Boston Bull

Terrier, who was promptly dubbed King Tut after the Egyptian monarch whose tomb had just been discovered. Tut became the team mascot and spent a lot of time with us. As Bill and I became close friends, a relationship encouraged by his grandmother who had taken an instant liking to me, I spent more and more time in the Warren household and would eat supper there more often than in my own house. Bill, in turn, would occasionally share our Italian bread, pasta, sausage, and meatballs that he seemed to enjoy more than I. Mrs. Warren had been a schoolteacher and she spent considerable time helping us with our lessons. As the widow of the former manager of Steeplechase Park, she held a permanent legal free pass to all of its amusements and also for free rides on the Hudson River boats that sailed from pier-side Manhattan down the bay to Steeplechase Park. Quite regularly she would take us on the ferry rides, insisting that we complete some reading and study (so that she might get a little rest for herself from the rigorous antics of two healthy young boys on a boat). If we passed a brief examination at the end of the sail, we were treated to several hours of rides on the merry-go-round, the whip, the roller coaster and other games and activities of the amusement park. The box lunches she prepared were delicious and never seemed adequate for our healthy appetites. She was an excellent cook and I can still smell the delicious aroma of the batches of cookies she used to bake for us. The ride back was always quiet and subdued at the end of another great day.

Bill and I enjoyed all sorts of sports. Baseball was the main one that took up most of our time. Bill was on the frail side and I was quite husky for my age. Since my father thought hard physical work was better for me than playing, I was required to help him with work delivering ice on the dumbwaiters to our customers. I did this every Saturday morning while school was in session and every day except Sunday during vacation. This involved lifting and carrying heavy pieces of ice and pulling dumbwaiters up to the various floors of the six-story apartments occupied by our customers. As a result of the physical activity I developed a pretty good set of muscles that served me well on the ball field and as an amateur boxer. I was a star pitcher of our club, the Washington Heights Indians, and used to carry a newspaper clipping saying I had set a record by striking out seventeen players in a seven-inning game. I was well known for my fast ball and what we called a "drop" and a good curve ball. Whenever we played ball, I always insisted that Bill Warren play shortstop as a condition for my participation. I was known in the neighborhood as Bill's chum and no one dared harm Bill while I was around or available. In those days, our only weapons in our fights were our fists and we abided by

Marquis of Queensberry rules. We fought bare-fisted without gloves. The tough Irish kids who lived on the east side of Broadway soon learned to lay off the Jewish boys who belonged to the Washington Heights Indians. The message was that the "Eyetalian" iceman's boy, Mike, was a terror with his fists and was best left alone.

In the Warren household I learned to appreciate the use of good silver and dinnerware and perfected my table manners. This information I brought home to my brother and my sisters. As the eldest son, as I grew up I assumed the role of mentor and teacher, correcting their speech, manners, and general behavior.

Since Italian was the language used by our parents, we reverted to it at the dinner table. In turn it was my job to help my parents to cope with the English language and customs.

As a result of my personal experience I have no use for so-called bilingual education. I think it is a political ploy to keep foreigners and their children within a self-imposed ghetto so they will always be at the beck-and-call of some tinhorn ward-heeler. My generation went to school to become Americans in a free society with opportunity to move up the ladder. We asked for no special favors because of our Italian heritage. We earned our keep the old-fashioned way through integrity, self discipline, and hard work.

Washington Heights in those days had quite an influx of baseball players from both leagues, the American and the National, so we young fellows got to know members of the New York Yankees and Giants close up. The most famous one was Babe Ruth who lived for a while in an apartment on 160th Street between Fort Washington Avenue and Riverside Drive on the south side of the street. I know this because the Babe was one of my customers. When the Yankees were on the road, the first Mrs. Ruth, a diminutive woman, could not lift the fifty-pound piece of ice from the dumbwaiter. I would pull the dumbwaiter rope until it reached the sixth floor, tie it to the wall and race to the elevator to get to the floor, take the piece of ice out and put it in the icebox. When the Babe was home, I could recognize his voice saying, "OK kiddo" as he himself handled the ice. We would occasionally see the Babe walk near his apartment. If we were playing stickball in the street he would sometimes stop to watch. In his brown cap and light brown camel hair coat, he was inimitable and he always had a kind saying for the kids. On my tenth birthday, the Warrens, Uncle Sam and Bill, took me to my first major-league baseball game at the Polo Grounds. We went there hoping to see Babe Ruth hit one of his famous home runs, but it was not to be, because the visitors' pitcher that day was the Big Train, Walter Johnson of the Washington Senators, whose fast ball could barely be seen. We had no way to accurately measure the rate of speed in those days but it must have been over 95 miles an hour. The Babe failed to hit a homer that day and struck out three times but in the process put on a show I have never forgotten. Watching Babe Ruth strike out was an experience in itself. He would whirl around the strike and cross his rather thin legs. You could almost hear the swish in the stands. The foul balls he hit seemed to just miss being homers and his fly balls hung up in the sky so high and for so long that we wondered how any fielder could possibly catch them.

One of the greatest lessons I learned from growing up in Washington Heights was to respect people of all races and creeds. I learned a great deal about WASPS and Americans from the Warrens and they something of Catholicism and Italians from me. My Jewish friends were close to me and there seemed to be no conflict in our relations attributable to our different religions.

As I drive to work each morning traveling on the upper level of the George Washington Bridge and down the ramp to the West Side Highway, usually bumper to bumper, I look to my left and I see the lovely apartment we occupied as office and home just before WW II at 200 Haven Avenue. A little farther south is the Columbia-Presbyterian Medical Center and Harkness Pavilion, now considerably expanded and undergoing renovation including an overhead crossway over Fort Washington Avenue linking the new Milstein Hospital with old Harkness Pavilion. I have fond memories of my early days in this section as a child and teenager and later as a practicing physician. In my own way I have a feeling about this neighborhood similar to that of a family practitioner passing by his small town where he was born and raised. I know these houses. I walked up their steps to serve the sick who called for help. For my patients I was their 911. I was also their key to access to the Medical Center.

It was a beautiful world and time to live in and in later years I would look back upon Washington Heights in my childhood with considerable nostalgia and affection. I find it almost incredible to believe what I see, hear, read, and smell of Washington Heights as it exists today. It hurts and almost moves me to tears for the loss of a past that should have been preserved for future generations. Why did this happen? Could this disaster have been prevented?

In the spring of 1991 I saw an article in the *New York Times* real-estate section on a place called Fort Washington. It is located just north of 181st Street on the border of Washington Heights, west of Broadway between the George Washington Bridge and the Inwood section. This remained a middle-class, safe, stable community despite the deterioration south, north, and east of its location. Most of the stability is attributed to Hudson View Gardens, a 353-unit cooperative built in 1925. Owning property is perhaps the best way to get people to protect it and preserve it, and this development is excellent proof of this real-estate axiom. "Co-ops account for more than half of the community's housing units. A 1000-square-foot, two-bedroom apartment on the bluff with a river view sells for $126,000 to $150,000—most rental units are either co-op sublets or have stabilized lease. Rents on stabilized units average about $1000 a month" (*New York Times*, 1991).

With the construction of the subway A train in 1935, the area became a popular bedroom community for Manhattanites who could afford it. I well remember when Dr. Charles Paterno, in 1939, tore down his castle on the hill and built the Castle Village Apartments in Fort Washington, in the middle of the worst economic depression this country has ever seen. Some who witnessed the grand scale of the development were inclined to call it "Paterno's Folly," but they were wrong. The apartments were spacious and well constructed. The amenities were first rate, including a 7.5-acre private park and underground parking and excellent security. The rents were high for the era, the occupants carefully screened to keep out undesirables. The development consisted of five towers of 13 to 15 stories on a cliff overlooking the Hudson River for its 1170 tenants. As a young physician practicing in Washington Heights, I made occasional house calls to patients in Castle Village and recall the opulence of the apartments with their dramatic view of the Hudson River.

The amazing thing is that in spite of the decay, moral, physical, and economic, of adjacent Washington Heights, Fort Washington has maintained its ambiance, style, good manners, and prosperous appearance. A woman resident of 23 years in Castle Village is quoted in a recent interview by the *New York Times*: "This is the Sutton Place of Washington Heights." There is no "Berlin-style Wall" or gate separating Fort George with its Hudson View Gardens and Castle Village from Washington Heights. Why did we fail so miserably in Washington Heights and succeed so well in Fort Washington?

It is apparent from this narrative that baseball was a very important part of our young lives during my early days in Washington Heights. It kept us out of mischief and busy with healthy pursuits and channeled our energy into positive activities. A recent series of articles in the *New York Times* by Sara Rimer has focused on a hopeful development in that decaying community now flooded with Dominicans, many of whom are looking to baseball as their possible escape from life on the crime-ridden streets now taken over by crack addicts, dealers, hookers, and criminals. Some Dominicans have become outstanding stars with major league teams. They have assumed heroic stature in the Dominican colony in Washington Heights as well as their native land and the youngsters seek to emulate them. The center of the baseball action in New York City is in the George Washington High School on a hill at Audubon Avenue and 192nd Street, the alma mater of Henry Kissinger. There, a dedicated baseball coach, Steve Mandl, is responsible for a renaissance. George Washington, one of 94 New York City public high school baseball teams, has won the Manhattan division baseball Championship for the past seven seasons. The 20 ball players on the varsity team are all Dominican.

In June 1991 one of them, Manny Ramirez, rated the best high school player in New York, was drafted by a major league ball club, the Cleveland Indians, and given a $250,000 bonus plus a good contract. He is on his way up and the idol of the Dominican enclave in Washington Heights. He has found his way out of it.

Let us return to Washington Heights and its problems. Some skeptics may question whether the production of a few baseball stars can do anything to stem the tide of the drug culture and its by-products. Perhaps this is true, but it is apparent that the many millions of dollars already poured into the battle have accomplished very little. Merely saying "No" has not solved the problem, but if it were part of an educational program reinforced by pressure from admired peers working in a common cause, it might just work. My patient and friend, former president Herbert C. Hoover, was a great humanitarian who loved children. He was an avid baseball fan, a Yankee fan, in their glory days, who knew each player's name and the numbers on his back. President Hoover felt that baseball was a great sport, through which youngsters learned the importance of team effort, self-discipline, fair play, and abiding by the rules of the game. The Boys' Clubs that he supported, and for which he raised large sums of money, focused their attention on baseball. President Hoover loved to boast that his San Francisco Boys' Club had produced many major-league baseball stars from humble beginnings, including Hall of Famer Joe DiMaggio and his brothers, Dominick and Vincent, as well as Don Larsen who pitched that perfect World Series no-hitter. The Chief, as he was called by his intimate friends, once told me that if he could raise the money to build another boys' club in Harlem, youth crime in that area would be drastically reduced. One day in 1961, on one of my daily visits, Mr. Hoover said to me that he was not a person of enormous wealth but he knew how to raise money for worthy causes. He then showed me a check for $750,000 sent to him by an admirer for support of the Boys' Club of America. I know there is more where that check came from. What we need is someone like President Hoover to lead the crusade. Perhaps the Milbank family, great friends of the former president, might be willing to lead the charge.

The importance of baseball in Washington Heights should not be judged solely by the number of major-league players produced. The sport is part of the lifeblood of the Dominicans both here and in their country. Here in Washington Heights there are many Little League teams supported and encouraged by their parents, families, and friends. Children in the most vulnerable period of their lives are exposed to positive and constructive ways to play, persevere, practice, and interact with their peers, their parents, and, hopefully, good role models. It is wonderful that the Dominicans are doing all of this on their own, but I would also hope that others might pitch in. If President Hoover were alive, I am certain he would have a Boys' Club in Washington Heights and I would be among the first to ask him to arrange it. Admittedly, this would be only a small start but it would be in the right direction at a time when all else has failed. It is said by some that the newer crop of rich individuals in our society is less inclined than its predecessors to help the poor and the minorities, the attitude being "I've worked for mine. Let them work for theirs" or "Let the government take care of them." Yet the government's record in this era leaves much to be desired, no matter which party is in power. Is it not high time for voluntary efforts to be made when others have failed? Why don't we initiate a renaissance of the Boys' Clubs or perhaps Children's Clubs in the affected inner cities? Let us keep the government bureaucrats and politicians out of them. Let the people pour forth their time, effort, commitment, and concern for the children of our inner cities. Let the more prosperous and successful, of their own volition, help to fund these activities.

Chapter 3

Speyer School for Gifted Children

I HAVE ALREADY MENTIONED MY EARLY DAYS in the elementary schools of New York City. When I enrolled in P.S. 46 in Manhattan because our apartment on 162nd Street was in that school's district, I was faced with a brand new environment and new teachers. This was a challenge that did not faze me one bit, but I soon ran into a problem. The head boy in my first class was a chap named, Edward Minor, who had been the local teacher's pet. Mrs. Hamill, who was in charge of that class, had a method of rewarding outstanding performance by assigning the number-one seat in the class to the best scholar. It was not long before I was challenging Minor and soon I was assigned to the catbird seat ahead of him. Then we had a small disaster. When I was called upon for recitation Master Minor moved the pages of my book so that I lost my place. Mrs. Hamill demoted me to the second seat and moved my rival to the number-one spot. We were not supposed to fight in class, so I swallowed my anger for the moment. When school was out, on my way home I just happened to run into Master Minor and I proceeded to give him "what for" with a real good pasting. He ran home and told his mother who happened to be a good friend of our teacher to whom she complained vigorously demanding that I be punished. I don't think her son told her exactly why I had shellacked him. The next thing I knew Mrs. Hamill requested that I bring my father to school or lacking that, ask my mother to come to see her. Since neither of my parents spoke English, and since they were fully occupied with their family responsibilities and making a living, an invitation to come to school was a serious threat to me. By this time I had gotten to know Bill Warren's grandmother quite well and after telling her about my predicament she agreed to come to school to have a talk with Mrs. Hamill and she did this in place of my parents. When Mrs. Hamill heard the whole story, I was reinstated to the first seat and stayed there without further challenge or mischief.

While at P.S. 46, I was discovered to have an excellent soprano voice and was called upon frequently to solo in assembly. Life at P.S. 46 went along quite well until one day the school was asked to nominate its best students for consideration for transfer to a new experimental Junior High School for gifted children named the Speyer School, after the millionaire philanthropist, James Speyer, who was subsidizing it. This school sought to have us complete three years work in two under the tutelage of a superb faculty recruited from Columbia University Teacher's College. The experiment was rare for its time, involving small classes, extracurricular activities, early introduction to foreign languages and a degree of self-government most unusual in the public school of that day. There was no tuition and the selections process paid no heed to ethnic origin, race, religion, or color. You simply had to be judged to be gifted, at the top of the class, and worthy of inclusion in the program. The only restriction was that you be a boy. No girls were permitted. I am not certain why this was the case, but it was not unusual in the New York City school system of that era. Coeducation had not come of age. Some of those offered admission feared the change and turned it down because they were more comfortable with the existing schools. Traveling by subway was necessary because the school was located two miles south of P.S. 46. Some parents had reservations about letting a child of ten ride alone on the subway. Instead of coming home for lunch, we had to carry our lunch in a brown paper bag or in a special box. I was so enthusiastic about this move that I persuaded my parents to give their permission. I felt badly about leaving Bill Warren, who was not offered this opportunity, but I knew that we would remain good friends and neighbors.

Speyer School was a marvelous idea and a great place for a young fellow to attend. It was in a small building on 124th Street between Amsterdam Avenue and Broadway. The faculty was outstanding in its experience and flexibility, and clearly challenged by this novel experiment in teaching a selected small group of gifted students. We served as guinea pigs for many innovations. French was the one foreign language taught, for the nation was not yet over the discrimination against German and Italian due to World War I.

Madame Langtry was my French teacher and she used the phonetic method of teaching this language. We learned in part by singing songs in French. Classroom conversations in her classes were conducted in French. We learned to appreciate the lovely sounds of this great language and the enthusiasm with which it was being taught. Madame Langtry almost made a Frenchman of me. I still remember in the final term of our two years the visit to the Speyer School by a committee of the Alliance Française that spent a good deal of time in our classroom listening and whispering among themselves as we went through a class demonstration. At the end, Madame Langtry announced with some emotion that the little Italian kid from Washington Heights had won a city-wide Alliance Française Medal for proficiency in French, thereby bringing honor to Speyer School. The phrase "honor to Speyer School" had been ingrained in us from the first day we were admitted and virtually every one of us sought to live up to this motto. In a way, many years later I would be reminded that Speyer was a poor man's prep school, its motto not unlike that of Groton's "Obedience to the Unenforceable."[1] There were other activities at Speyer School besides the routine topics of instruction. Each student was expected to qualify in a variety of sports activities, with the best candidates awarded small silver or bronze medals for completing what was the equivalent of a child's decathlon. I still remember the wiry bandy-legged teacher of athletics, Mr. Levy, who got the most out of every student, even those disinclined toward exercise. Once weekly we traveled as a class to the Metropolitan Museum of Art for a lecture and demonstration. To this day I recall almost verbatim some of these sessions describing the characteristics of a Holbein, Titian, Rubens, Winslow Homer, Turner, and other classics. Visits to the Museum of Natural History were equally remarkable but failed to reach the heights of the Museum of Art.

The small classes at Speyer led to cohesiveness and a warm spirit of collaboration without unhealthy competition. We were periodically given special intelligence tests in an attempt to document our progress or failures. School assemblies were occasions we attended without fail and enjoyed because of the singing and renewal of the spirit of the school.

Our music department in collaboration with P.S. 143, a nearby co-ed school, put on quite a professional performance of *The Student Prince*. I started as the star but my voice changed in the middle of rehearsal and I was then cast as Enterich the villain instead. My croaking speaking voice was quite suited for the part and when the time came to perform in public my family and the audience laughed and enjoyed my struggle.

Each class at Speyer had its own democratic method of governance and freedom of expression monitored by its gifted teachers. I remember that the teachers seemed to be enjoying the experience at least as much as the students and sometimes even more.

When I graduated from Speyer School in 1923 with honors in French and the Alliance Française Medal, this was a fine excuse for the "Societa di Mutuo Soccorso di Genzano di La Basilicata," our *paesani*, to put on a fine party with good food, soda, ice cream, wine, music, and grand company in a hired hall. There was a good deal of

---

1. Stephen Birmingham, *The Right People* (Boston-Toronto: Little Brown and Company, 1968), pp. 330–331.

speechmaking in praise of the first of this generation of Italo-Americans to graduate from anything and to win a medal. In honor of this occasion I was given a gold Waltham watch with an appropriate inscription engraved on its back. Congressman Fiorello LaGuardia came to the party and made encouraging comments in his squeaky Italian. I became an admirer of Mr. LaGuardia, who was called the Little Flower, and have remained one ever since. From this point on, I was a marked youngster among the *paesani* and all sorts of good things were expected of me. I could not let them down.

Following my graduation in 1923 from Speyer School, I elected to enter the junior year at De Witt Clinton High School, then located on 59th Street and Tenth Avenue, across the street from the Columbia University College of Physicians and Surgeons and its affiliated hospitals. I chose this school because it was said to have the best academic program in all of New York. George Washington High School in Washington Heights was quite new, its reputation not exceptional. The High School of Commerce was for those contemplating careers in business. Stuyvesant High School was for those heading for engineering. There really was not too much choice.

When I started at De Witt Clinton, the entire affair struck me as a disaster. The classes were tremendous, the curriculum crowded, and worst of all because of overcrowding the school was run on two sessions, a morning session and an afternoon session, with many of the teachers doing double duty. There was little or no personal contact with the teachers, and after the remarkable experience at Speyer the letdown was simply dreadful.

I tried to adjust to the best of my ability but the system seemed at first impossible for me to accept. There was no one I could turn to for advice and there were no other options. With time, I began to find my place, but it was far from easy. One of the bright spots was Clinton's emphasis on certain extra-curricular activities. I tried out for the baseball team and survived one cut. I was really too short for varsity athletics. I found satisfaction in contributing my services to the G.O. (General Organization) Store where I learned a great deal about running a fairly large business and handling large sums of money. I especially liked selling and buying athletic goods for all sports. This was under the supervision of Dr. Julius Freynick, an English teacher who became a warm friend. By my senior year I was made captain of the G.O. Store Squad and elected to Arista, the High School Honor Society. The courses in French were excellent and I found that the start I was given at Speyer School was far superior to the teaching of this subject at Clinton. English was well taught and at times, inspirational. The sciences were adequate for that day but pedestrian and uninspired. I remember with respect Dr. Paul, the scholarly principal, and "Doc" Guernsey, who seemed closest to the student body and was universally beloved. One person who was there that I wish I had gotten to know better was Dr. Leonard Covello, teacher of Italian, who rose to considerable eminence in the New York City high school system and was a great proponent of Italian-American causes. Perhaps the reason I failed to join Dr Covello's group was that I did not want to be tied down to my Italian heritage. I was attending school to become an American, the sooner the better.

I graduated from Clinton in January 1926, an awkward date because most of the universities were not accepting students in the middle of the year. I had wished to go to college outside of New York, but despite the offer by Mr. Rothschild of a scholarship to Harvard, my family said no to this proposal. A close-knit Italian family now leaning heavily on the eldest son for various duties looked with horror at the prospect of a fifteen-year-old boy going to a strange city with no relatives or friends to lean upon.

By 1926, my parents had purchased a brand-new, well-built, brick house in the Wakefield section of the Bronx, then a quiet suburban neighborhood with empty lots, grass, trees, and many small gardens. Because of its proximity, willingness to accept new students at mid-year, and its excellent scholastic reputation, I applied for admission to New York University at University Heights in the Bronx and was promptly accepted. I would be the first in my family to obtain a college education.

Chapter 4

New York University at University Heights

NEW YORK UNIVERSITY at University Heights in the Bronx in January 1926 was not a very impressive sight. There had been a mixture of snow, sleet, and rain, turning the paths into mud puddles that were traversed only by walking atop wooden walkways built of slats of lumber. The buildings were modest. The students appeared businesslike as they hurried from one class to another. The faculty was kindly as well as scholarly. I soon found that the atmosphere was extremely competitive, especially among the premedical students who seemed greatly preoccupied by their grade standing. I was only fifteen years old when I enrolled. Most of the students were eighteen.

Since I lived at home and commuted each day to classes, there was very little semblance of any college life or social activity for me. The greatest excitement in those days centered on NYU's great football team under the renowned coach, Chick Meehan. This team had achieved national eminence at its pinnacle until Al Lassman, tackle and captain and a potential heavyweight boxing champion, had the grave misfortune to suffer a skull fracture in the game with the formidable Carnegie Tech team, resulting in permanent brain injury and hemiplegia. From this point on it was all downhill for NYU and major football. Al Lassman was one of our great heroes and I still recall how sadly we watched this magnificent human being reduced to the life of a permanent cripple. We thought it was an awful price to pay for supremacy in a sport. Still, if it had not happened then, and had he gone on to become a professional boxer, sooner or later brain injury may or may not have occurred. Who would ever forget the scene at Ohio Field, our home ground, when Frank X. Briante almost single-handedly in our backfield was trying to defend against the overpowering offensive of a virtually unheard of Davis and Elkins squad from West Virginia whose brawn made the NYU team seem almost midgets. Basketball at NYU under Howard Cann was a great sport in those days while running for track coach Von Elling was well worth the effort.

The faculty was competent and some of it was outstanding. The science courses were well taught and demanding. Unfortunately, there were too many didactic lectures and masses of data that required memorization. The laboratory courses were crowded but we did get to know some of the instructors pretty well. I recall that in Comparative Anatomy I would spend more time with my specimens than the other students and I resented having to get out of the laboratory at a fixed hour before I could complete my work. During this course, I made friends with one of the instructors, Dr. Ross Nigrelli, who took me aside one day and said that he had been watching my work and hoped that when the time came for me to go to medical school, I might try for Johns Hopkins, where he thought a student with my bent of mind would have a better opportunity to develop than in the existing New York City medical schools. This was an interesting remark that came at just the right time in my life, for I was glad to know that there were medical schools where the emphasis was not merely on grades and rote memory but on other qualities that might just be more important. My generation of idealistic youngsters was fired up by the recent publication of Sinclair Lewis' *Arrowsmith* and I wanted to hear more about research and the discovery of new remedies and cures for illness. My mind was made up. I was going outside of New York City for my medical education, come hell or high water.

Years later when I was practicing as a specialist in internal medicine on Park Avenue and at Harkness Pavilion, Dr. Ross Nigrelli, my former teacher, became my patient and friend. By this time he had achieved well-deserved acclaim and fame as a marine biologist and director of the Osborn Laboratory of Marine Sciences and Director of the New York Aquarium. I learned from him interesting things about liver cancer in trout. On one occasion I gave him some advice on how to treat a seal who had developed intestinal obstruction after swallowing a plastic toy tossed to him by a visitor at the Aquarium. Dr. Nigrelli was the expert often consulted when red algae polluted waters off the coast. His latest hobby was searching for potential sources of new antibiotics in the coastal waters at Bimini in the Bahamian Islands. He was also the inspiration for the young woman who wrote the best-selling *Lady with a Spear*, a tale of snorkeling on Saipan.

A number of other well-respected members of the biology and chemistry departments were effective teachers, but the atmosphere was too charged with competition for grades and petty jealousy among the premedical students, who were busily swallowing and regurgitating so-called "facts" that, unfortunately, might no longer be true in five years or less.

I found myself turned off by these grade-grubbers, who were almost all trying to get into medical school, usually NYU, or what they called "Bella Vue," with only three years of college, and avoiding any courses other than science and avoiding the humanities like the plague, especially those making heavy scholarly demands. Without any formal advice on these matters, I decided to stay in college for my B.S. degree before going to medical school and to take additional courses in the humanities because I genuinely enjoyed them. I continued with French all through college, studying under the talented and friendly Professor Henri Olinger, who encouraged me to take French as my minor while biology remained my major. When you have learned to read Victor Hugo, Molière, or Balzac in French, how can you possibly accept any substitute for the original? Professor Orestes Bontempo, who taught Italian, was also a campus leader in cultural activities. Through his efforts concerts were arranged at NYU by Eugene Ormandy, long before he became famous, and guest performances by Ernest Goosens, Lilly Pons, and Reinwald Weirenrath. A welcome surprise was the arrival on campus of Professor Eric Ponder, who taught the course in physiology. He was a product of the Edinburgh University School of Medicine and a superb, articulate, and beautifully organized speaker. He was already the author of a good text and a recognized expert in hemolysis of red cells. He so challenged me that I undertook with his support a study of hemolysis of red cells using various solutions of saponin and sodium taurocholate. Nothing earthshaking came of this, but I learned to organize a protocol to test a hypothesis, keep accurate records, and use equipment such as the Ostwald Viscosimeter, pipettes, and stopwatches. Ponder made physiology come alive for me in 1928 and I shall never forget him.

During my senior year I was elected vice president of the Draper Chemical Society. I also participated in intramural athletics, baseball, and football and, of all things, had a role in the Varsity Show of that year, which involved rehearsals in downtown New York City. The supervisor, a Mr. Daniels, was a successful director who held forth in a night club and speakeasy where Texas Guinan, a popular entertainer of the day, was appearing.

The senior year was dominated by concern over getting into medical school, filing applications, and obtaining letters of reference and interviews. I learned about a new medical school in Rochester, New York, called by its proponents the Johns Hopkins of New York. I was very pleased to receive an invitation from Dean George Hoyt Whipple to come to Rochester for an interview.

Chapter 5

To Each His Farthest Star–A Medical Student at Rochester: 1929–1934

Bliss was it in that dawn to be alive
but to be young was very heaven

William Wordsworth
The Prelude, Book XI.

L ET ME TELL YOU WHAT IT WAS LIKE to be a student in this new medical school at Rochester in the early days. In the spring of 1929 I was invited to appear in Rochester for my interview for admission to the medical school. At eighteen years of age, except for my childhood voyage to Italy, this was my first long trip away from my home in New York City and I was not too well informed about the procedure to follow. The train fare was quite high and I found that the bus fare was about half the price, so I took the bus. The ride was long and boring, involving many local stops bearing the names of communities like Painted Post, Binghamton, Utica, Syracuse, etc., which were to become quite familiar to me in the future. As I recall it, the trip took over thirteen hours and I arrived in Rochester after midnight without a hotel reservation. A chap I had met on the bus suggested we try the YMCA, but we found they had no space available. I then went to a cheap hotel, the Ford, where for one dollar a night I had a clean room, a metal locker, and a toilet, as well as a shower at the end of the hall. I slept soundly, had breakfast, and then took the trolley car out to the medical school on Crittenden Boulevard. One of the things I remember about the trolley was a sign, "Suppose Nobody Cared," which was my first introduction to something called the Community Chest. It gave me a warm feeling to know that here was a city where people did care. When I arrived at the medical school I entered the Strong Memorial Hospital lobby, which was well furnished and had an air of quiet elegance and comfort. I was directed to the Dean's office to the rear of the hospital where, much to my surprise, a charming and very attractive young woman, Miss Hilda De Brine, secretary to Dr. Whipple, greeted me by name and asked me to take a seat in the office until Dr. Whipple could see me. Accustomed to the quick shuffle and impersonal attitudes of New York City, I was almost overwhelmed by the courteous, reassuring reception. The interview with Dean Whipple was to prove a milestone in my life. He sought to put me at ease by asking some general questions. He had noticed that I had played baseball and had coached the St. Aloysius Boys' Club team and we talked a little about this. Years later I would learn that he had been a great athlete at Yale, the top gymnast and star pitcher and infielder on the varsity baseball team. At Johns Hopkins he pitched against the Baltimore Orioles and was offered a contract with them but turned it down for better things.

He asked me about a research project I was doing with Dr. Eric Ponder at NYU on hemolysis of red cells. Other questions followed, and, while tense, I enjoyed every minute of my discussion with the dean. In retrospect, the thing that really stood out for me during this interview was that Dean Whipple spent all of the time finding out what *I* was doing, and not what my father was doing for a living. When the interview was over, I was asked to see Dr. Corner, professor of anatomy, Dr. Bloor, professor of biochemistry, and several other members of the teaching staff, and I was assigned to Louis Zeidberg, an NYU graduate, who was then a sophomore medical student. Lou, a total stranger, was gracious and hospitable. He took me to lunch in the student cafeteria and introduced me to a number of other students who were friendly and communicative.

My interview with Dr. George Washington Corner was stimulating. He was very youthful and his eyes sparkled as he talked, and I gathered that he greatly enjoyed his work. Corner had spotted in my transcript that I had received A's in Physiology, but had a C in Comparative Anatomy, and he asked me why this had happened. It was a moment of truth for me and I looked at him, gulped, and said that I disliked rote memory, and that was the way the course was being taught, whereas physiology under Ponder was a joyful experience. Ponder, a graduate of Edinburgh, should really have been teaching in a medical school. He lit a fire under me and I shall forever be in his debt for stimulating my interest in physiology. This answer, accompanied by some rather pithy comments about the professor teaching comparative anatomy, did not seem to upset Dr. Corner and I sensed the interview had gone well.

When I returned home, I told my parents and family that Rochester was the only place I wanted to go to medical school. I had been treated like a real human being and accorded every courtesy and individual attention. My parents found it very hard to understand why I wanted to go to medical school outside of New York City, but they felt that since I had acceded to their wishes by going to college in New York City, the choice of a medical school was up to me.

When my letter of acceptance, signed by Dean Whipple, arrived at my home I proceeded to shout with joy and soon had the whole family in a frenzy. No one but a medical student can really appreciate what it means to gain acceptance to his number-one school. I could hardly wait until the fall of 1929, when I again arrived in Rochester now as a medical student holding a B.S. degree from New York University. While walking down Main Street, I spotted John Rooney, a familiar face, who had worked as a bookkeeper during the summer at the Knickerbocker Ice Plant in Pelham, New York, where I would drive a truck to pick up a load of 300-pound cakes of ice for sale and delivery on my father's ice route in Tuckahoe, New York. John was a hefty-looking six-foot-tall, black-haired Irishman who did paperwork, while I, weighing all of 130 pounds, lifted the 300-pound blocks of ice onto my truck for delivery. We said hello to each other, and John asked me what the devil I was doing in Rochester. I answered that I was about to start medical school, and he admitted to being in the same predicament. Before this, neither one of us knew that the other was a college student or a premedical student. We were merely hacking ice to buy bread for our families.

The next step was to find a place to live while going to school. In 1929, the River Campus had not been built and there were no medical school dormitories. Most of the medical students rented rooms in the modest, private homes lining Crittenden Boulevard facing the medical school. The homeowners were glad to have us and were pleased to rent rooms to us for four dollars a week, including linens. Meals could be obtained at Strong Memorial Hospital, but many of us preferred, to Dean Whipple's consternation, inferior food prepared at an institution on the corner dubbed the "greasy spoon." I had never smelled a skunk before going to Rochester, but I soon became quite familiar with the smell which assailed my nostrils frequently when I made my way to the greasy spoon for supper. The skunk and her family had apparently taken up permanent quarters under the restaurant.

The house I lived in during my first two years at Rochester was on Crittenden Boulevard, owned by a quiet, unobtrusive, childless couple. Larry Mucci, an Amherst graduate, had one room and I had the other. Larry and I became close friends and shared many activities.

The fall of the year is the finest season in Rochester. The air is crisp and clear, the foliage is in bloom and beginning to turn to the reds, yellows and bronzes that are the glory of this region. People walk quickly, their conversations are brisk, and action and work are the order of the day. The chatter of students is heard up and down

Crittenden Boulevard, usually from the sidewalk. There are few porches on these houses, and even they are seldom occupied. The medical students are busy with their work and studies, and time for play is limited, at least during the first semester. The students are dead serious about their work and, despite frequent reassurances by faculty and friends, they wonder whether they will really make it. Automobiles are few and far between so far as the students are concerned. The main desire of some students is to acquire a girl friend with a car. Some even aspire to one who has a job that might provide as easily for two as for one. At night the lights are on in all of the rooms with students attempting to grind away, mastering the intricacies of anatomy. The smell of the anatomy room clings to them, serving to identify the freshmen from the upper classmen. Once you have smelled it, you can never forget it. Radios are few and far between, the era being that of crystal detectors. Our sophomore friend, Mike Carpinella, who lived in an attic room, had a radio, and Larry and I would hurry there almost every evening to hear the most popular program of the day—*Amos and Andy*. We nick-named our associates according to the characters in this show, the Kingfish being a favorite. All of us acquired the Amos-and-Andy vocabulary and lingo, which then were part of the American way of life. An announcer and singer named "Mac" McComber entertained over station WHAM and had no qualms about audibly clearing his throat and hawking while in the midst of a song. Rudy Vallee was in his prime and almost all of us tried to imitate his nasal baritone rendition of *The Maine Stein Song*.

Money was scarce and with the stock-market crash and ensuing depression it would become the bane of our existence. The lack of money for anything but the bare essentials was not all bad, for students had less for play, amusement, and extracurricular affairs. The school was relatively isolated at the edge of the city and there were not too many distractions in the immediate vicinity. Prohibition was the law of the land and while the more adventuresome could easily find the blind pigs, they cost money to frequent and to get to. The Rochester Maenerchor still had good beer but you had to be introduced by a member and it took money to get into town. The movie houses were good, even the beautiful Eastman Theatre was used for movies and most of us would go to the movies on the weekend, taking the trolley into town. When we wanted to eat spaghetti, we would call Joe's on North Street just before starting out, and he would start things going. We would hire a cab, which was cheaper for four or five than the trolley fare. On arriving at this plain restaurant we were served a portion of excellent spaghetti *al dente* with delicious tomato sauce all for thirty-five cents. Those who asked for black coffee were served red wine in coffee mugs at extra cost. There was no spaghetti like it in Rochester and I doubt there is any restaurant now in Rochester serving such delicious pasta. Sometimes we would go into town in a car owned by one of our schoolmates. It is very curious that the car owners of that day seldom emerged as solid contributors to our alumni fund as they got older. Did they spend it all in the early days? Or were they from the beginning takers rather than givers?

The winters in Rochester were severe and prolonged. When the snows came the horse-drawn sidewalk plows would start to work early on, the clop, clop, clop of the horse making a distinctive sound on the sidewalks. Soon the snow would be piled high on both sides of the streets. The trolley cars would keep going up and down Crittenden Boulevard, virtually the sole method of transportation for hardy souls venturing out into the weather. Large snow plows kept busy clearing the main streets. Walking down Crittenden Boulevard to the hospital and school on a blustery winter day required warm clothes and guts. Many a day I thought my ears would drop off on the way down to the hospital to take care of a delivery to the tune of an age-old medical student's refrain, "Why, oh why, do babies always have to be born in the middle of the night?" Worse luck yet, was to be called during the night after having been out on a rare late binge. As students we were required to do the blood counts and urine examinations on our own patients. I well recall the night a slightly hung-over classmate stuck his own finger rather than his patient's with his lancet, and to complete the performance, proceeded to suck up his own blood with his pipette for a count, until we advised him of his error. When the snow reached levels of the second story of our rooming houses, there was nothing to do but to stay in our rooms, carrying on endless bull sessions that are an important part of growing up and of the education of the young physician.

Almost no one in our class was married and, except for occasional dates, most of our time was spent with our classmates, studying, bulling, working, reading, playing, or, rarely, plain loafing. Contributing to all of this was the relative isolation of the medical school and hospital from the rest of the city, the scarcity of easy transportation, almost no cars, the lack of money except for the basic essentials, and the paucity of distractions from our work as students of medicine. I suppose some would criticize this system but there is no question that the medical student of that day spent infinitely more time with his studies than the present generation. There was no television to watch and social affairs were relatively infrequent.

The competition among the students was seldom expressed in grades, for these were never published. Still, each student knew who was good and who was stupid. We soon learned that a Phi Beta Kappa key or an Ivy League degree was not an open sesame to success in medical school. The top students were quickly identified as were the lowest ones, but for the group in between it was hard to know who was doing better or worse and perhaps it was just as well. Many of us had come to Rochester seeking to escape the highly competitive, grade-grubbing existence then and now in vogue in most institutions educating premedical students. Rochester was an enormous relief for us, although in the beginning there was much uneasiness because we couldn't tell whether we were doing poorly or well. Exams were few and far between. Attendance was never formally taken and there were no external pressures to produce tangible results. On the other hand, we soon learned that the faculty outnumbered us, there being 22 students in the first-year class and only 42 in my own class in 1929. The faculty knew us intimately, perhaps too much so. It had been much easier in college to merely take an exam at the middle or end of a course. Now you had to produce every day under the eagle eye of an instructor who said little but noticed a great deal. On the whole, rather than an easier system to live with, it soon became apparent to us that the Rochester system was tougher and more demanding than the structured, visible, lock-step, regimented approach to education in vogue in our undergraduate schools. More than anything else, we were impressed by the Rochester motto that the scientific spirit was more important than the acquisition of information by rote. The motto, at first unfamiliar, soon became the bellwether of the school. We quickly learned that our professors sought to teach us to observe, record, criticize, and interpret facts and to use them in a rational approach to solving problems. They seemed more interested in *how* we went about analyzing a problem than in whether we had the right answer. This became a butt for jokes among the students who marvelled that one could be wrong and at the same time successful. In essence we were being treated as graduate students. High on the list of our role models was integrity and total honesty, and no student could fail to be impressed by these traits in all of the senior professors and the juniors who served under them. Didactic lectures were few and far between. Elective time was ample. Class attendance was never taken. The honor code was strictly observed and monitored by the students themselves.

From the very first day, the stimulus to use the medical library played a major role in the education of every student. The library, apple of George Whipple's eye, was from its beginning a marvelous place—quiet, private, and well stocked, thanks to George Washington Corner. Corner was the first professor we met and he was a joy to behold. Enthusiastic, warm, and exciting, a truly charismatic figure, his youthful bounce stirred all of us and made us want to rise to the standards he set. I shall never forget his peering over my shoulder while I was looking at the circulation in a frog lung under my microscope. "Lepore, who was Malpighi?" Good heavens, I thought, here I am having trouble identifying what is going on under the microscope and he asks me about some Italian I never heard of. He relieved my suspense by saying that Malpighi, the great sixteenth-century anatomist, was the first to describe the capillaries, the connecting links between the arteries and veins, a fact that had eluded the great Harvey. Dr. Corner aroused in me, as he did in others, an interest and reverence for the past, the history of medicine, that has never left me. He taught the history of medicine in his everyday contacts by his example, by his quotations, and by his encouragement of every student to remember his heritage. It was he who stimulated me to present a paper before the Medical History Society at Rochester (now appropriately called the George W. Corner History of Medicine Society) in 1931. I submitted the title, *Molière, the Cervantes of French Medicine,* and regaled the audience with Molière's diatribes against the doctors. Dr. Stanhope Bayne-Jones, our professor of bacteriology, commented favorably on the lecture and hoped I would publish it, which I failed to do because I did not feel that it was sufficiently original. I shall never forget running into Dr. Corner in the hall one day when he showed me a letter and said "Lepore, we have caught a fish! Harvey Cushing has written asking me why Molière was the Cervantes of French medicine." Some years later, in fact in 1935, I was to tell this story to Dr. Cushing at Yale, where Dr. Bayne-Jones had become the dean and I was the American College of Physicians Research Fellow under Dr. John P. Peters.

Other activities that occupied us at Rochester were the monthly scientific meetings held in the evening in the main auditorium of the medical school. Here it was that the most promising new research projects were presented for review and criticism. The discussions were at times quite heated and served to introduce us early in our careers to the type of give-and-take and honest criticism that is the hallmark of our profession. I vividly recall one evening when Dr. Konrad Birkhaug, a brilliant but somewhat controversial bacteriologist, presented his findings on the erysipelas antitoxin that he had developed by injecting bacteria into a donkey's bloodstream. The whole school knew the story that Birkhaug, while at Johns Hopkins, had started the project with a co-worker, Dr. Harold Amoss, who was later to become professor of medicine at Duke. Apparently, when Birkhaug left for Rochester, without saying anything to Amoss, he shipped his donkey to Rochester to use in the erysipelas research. When Amoss discovered his loss, he was enraged and went about the hallowed Hopkins halls crying out that Birkhaug had stolen his ass and gone to Rochester. The evening of the presentation of the erysipelas antitoxin work saw a full auditorium and a feeling of tension in the audience that all hell might break loose. Birkhaug's presentation seemed smooth and persuasive except to the brilliant young professor of medicine, Dr. William S. McCann, who got up to express his disbelief and challenged Birkhaug's results in no uncertain terms. In fact, I seem to recall that Dr. McCann's final words were that the antitoxin was about as effective as pouring water on the wall—only I don't believe he said water, but referred to a renal excretory product. Birkhaug's reply was equally strong and we medical students wondered what would happen next. At this juncture, Dean Whipple, sitting in the front row, got up and said, "Gentlemen, I believe this evening's performance has shed more heat than light on this subject and I believe we had best terminate this discussion." This was for many of us the first, but certainly not the last, demonstration of how tough doctors can be in evaluating research work.

I would hate to mislead you by inferring that all of our activities at Rochester were saintly and devoted to purely scientific pursuits. Bill Tierney, Larry Mucci, and a chap named Stewart who subsequently dropped out, joined me in a singing quartet, harmonizing on old songs and making wonderful sounds. Bill Tierney was a big, overweight, pleasant fellow who had a really good voice with a wide range and had sung with the Rochester Glee Club. It was easy for the rest of us to adapt our less capable voices to Bill's and we made some pretty good sounding music. We soon found that the best place for rehearsal was the toilet in the student locker room, which, being tiled to the ceiling, had excellent acoustics. With the medical students' classical capacity for appropriate nicknames, we were quickly dubbed the Craphouse Quartet. Not only did we enjoy the singing and harmonizing, we also entertained the patients in Strong Memorial on numerous summer evenings by singing below their windows.

Another sport we indulged in, especially on winter nights when we were confined to our quarters, was vying for the blue-flame award for flatulence. Our food, for financial reasons, was apt to be rather high in starches, and baked beans were a popular item. One of our more gifted students had discovered that some individuals could blast out gas by rectum which would, on occasion, burn briskly when a light was applied, singeing the seat of the pants. The best performers were given the order of the blue flame, signifying that a considerable amount of methane gas was being generated in the colon. This simple experiment was to attract my interest later in life when I became involved in gastroenterology.

Each year, the staff house residents would have a ribald and bawdy party during which the teaching staff was taken over the jumps with no holds barred. The dean attended these sessions and seemed to enjoy what was going on. I especially recall one raunchy performance when the master of ceremonies asked the audience, "Who knows the most about brewing here?" Up rose a chap resembling Konrad Birkhaug (the bacteriologist and bachelor who had quite a reputation for being something of a ladies' man), and mimicking his Norwegian accent, said "I do." Up rose Andy Marchetti, a soft-spoken Virginian, impersonating Birkhaug's chief, Dr. Stanhope Bayne-Jones, saying "Why Konrad Beerkeg, you little shit, do you mean to tell me you know more about brewing than I do?" Birkhaug replied "brewing? I thought you said screwing!"

It was also at one of these staff-house sessions when I was a Physiology Fellow that I just missed being given a prestigious award. Our rooms in the staff house had no toilets, only a wash bowl. Having to get out of bed to go down the hall to the can could get to be a great nuisance on a cold winter night, so many of us would urinate into the sink. Unfortunately, the sinks were set at a uniform height which was too high for the shorter men. To solve the dilemma, one of the residents with some talent in carpentry had built a small wooden platform which could help a short man to reach the sink to relieve himself. This platform was presented each year with great fanfare, at the annual meeting of the house staff, to the shortest man on the house staff. The year I lived in these quarters, I just missed getting this award because one of the surgical residents was two inches shorter than I.

It must be recalled that those were the days of the great experiment with prohibition, and we young people rebelled against it, much as the current generation has opposed other restraints. We thought it was great fun to drink and to blow off steam. One of the indoor sports at Rochester, which some of our hardier souls indulged in, was stealing the laboratory alcohol and using it for cocktails. This was considered great fun until a mean and sadistic physician hospital-administrator, whose name I won't mention, got the bright idea of putting some croton oil into the ethanol supply. This clever trick nearly ruined our house staff one weekend when they were having an innocent house party.

On another occasion, my roommate, Larry Mucci, had obtained some gin from a bootlegger on Lake Ontario who vouched for its purity, saying he had smuggled it across the lake from Toronto. Mucci proceeded to have a few drinks, went to bed, and all seemed peaceful until I woke up to a commotion. Instead of his usual snoring, he was wheezing loudly, covered with hives and obviously quite sick. We had to take him to the Emergency Room at Strong Memorial where he was given adrenalin until the attack came under control. The intern was never told what we suspected. Larry was very allergic to peppermint and oil of wintergreen which had been surreptitiously added to the gin by the bootlegger to improve its flavor. Our official story was that he had gotten sick from the damned powdered eggs served in the hospital cafeteria. The next day when Larry dragged himself back to the school cafeteria, he was held up as a prime example of how sick the cafeteria food could make you and he emerged from the incident as somewhat of a folk hero in our fight against cafeteria food.

Medical students' bull sessions are no different from those of other young people, only they may be more fecal and more anatomic. The subject of women and woman-chasing was always popular and there were always the swordsmen boasting of their adventures, somehow escaping disaster and always emerging victorious from their encounters. I remember one of my classmates, who was carrying on a liaison with a probable nymphomaniac, being warned by a married surgeon to stop sleeping with her because excessive sexual activity would surely drain his energy from his main task of succeeding in his studies. This was offered as rather fatherly advice to my friend, who promptly disregarded it. By and large, however, the liaisons of that day were less obvious and less common than those of today and, on the whole, were more discreetly conducted.

Jim Bouton, in his 1970 book on baseball players (*Ball Four*) pointed out their juvenile actions and their addictions to voyeurism, especially peeping into hotel windows to observe the nudity and sexual antics of their neighbors. Medical students are very similar. In one house on Raleigh Street we had a pre-arranged signal to tip us off that the rather promiscuous young woman next door was entertaining a boy friend in her boudoir without deigning to lower the window blind. The key words were, "its raining," which could bring the entire house pell-mell into the room with the views. It served to break up the monotony of some of our days.

To return to the educational program of the medical school, Dr. Corner's course in anatomy was followed by physiology under Wallace O. Fenn and Edward F. Adolph. This was a very challenging experience, stressing concepts of muscle-nerve physiology and fluid balance. The experiments were difficult and they often failed to give predictable results, but we learned by doing and experienced the frustrations and tensions that every honest experimenter goes through. The equipment was, by today's standards, quite primitive but the best of its day. Smoking drums became a real art in the department of physiology of those days, a far cry from smoking of marijuana of the 1960s. By the time we were midway in the course, physiology had hooked some of us. When Dr. Adolph offered me a student fellowship in physiology to study the phenomena of fluid balance, I accepted with alacrity. This meant that I would drop out of the class of 1933 and finish with 1934, thereby delaying my graduation. I explained to my parents that it was an honor to be offered a student fellowship, and I thought it would help me to become a better doctor and equip me to make new discoveries in medicine. The student fellowship was the great innovation in medical education, started in California by Dean Whipple and transplanted to Rochester where it was to flourish and become an essential part of the educational experience in the new medical school. This fellowship paid exactly $18.75 per month, and provided room and board in the staff house where, as a young student, I became friendly with an older generation of physicians who were serving their residencies and internships in the various departments. Dr. Whipple, having himself been a great athlete, encouraged us all to participate in some form of physical activity. Each class, the faculty, the employees, and the house staff had a baseball team. Since I had some experience in playing baseball, I played third base on the house staff team, which had as its star pitcher Dr. Andrew Marchetti, resident in obstetrics and gynecology. We would cheer "Marc" along with appropriate comments such as "nice delivery, Marc," music to the ears of any obstetrician. Dr. Marchetti and I became warm friends, a relationship that was to continue when he became an important staff member of the New York Lying-In Hospital of Cornell University Medical School and took care of many of my early patients and also members of my family. I had played hardball for years and never been injured despite some close calls. The game we played in Rochester was so-called softball which called for a smaller diamond and a larger ball and no gloves. I found the ball to be quite difficult to handle, especially when it was hit hard down the third base line where I usually played. Our league softball games were played during the noon lunch hour on a diamond on the medical school grounds just outside Dean Whipple's office windows. He enjoyed watching us cavort and encouraged the sport as good wholesome fun. I had the misfortune to fracture my ankle in a slide into third base and spent the first six weeks of my physiology fellowship hopping around on crutches.

My preceptor for the fellowship year was Dr. Edward F. Adolph, who was then a young man in his early thirties. He was interested in water balance and fluid exchange and was already one of the great leaders in this field. Since I was his only fellow that year, I was the beneficiary of an extraordinarily personal teaching and learning experience. He had his Ph.D. from Harvard and had worked in the Kaiser Wilhelm Institute für Physiologie, and was beautifully trained in investigational techniques then in vogue on the continent. He was a quiet, taciturn man who taught by his example and by asking questions, rather than answering them. Each morning I would have a short session with him and more prolonged ones when necessary. He was always available and his door was always open.

At first my work as a fellow consisted of experiments which Dr. Adolph had designed, many of these being done on frogs or frog skins. I became convinced that the frog was a very difficult subject for water-balance study. As we went along, I shared experiments with my teacher during which we worked on anesthetized cats and dogs, continuing to probe phenomena of fluid and water balance. We conducted experiments on each other as well as on medical students who "volunteered" to serve as subjects. I still have the marks of a burn on my left arm induced by galvanic current given to blister the skin and to study the blister fluid content. One of my arm veins will never be the same after having been clobbered one day by my preceptor who was not too expert at vein sticking in those days. In addition to my research activities, I attended weekly afternoon departmental seminars in physiology where tea was served and I listened to presentations far over my head, but learned a great deal about the processes of studying a problem and the importance of clear and honest thinking and being able to take criticism without flinching. These seminars often had distinguished visitors from abroad as well as from other parts of America.

Dr. Wallace O. Fenn, chairman of the department, had a nose for ferreting out young people of promise and bringing them into our seminars. It was on just such an occasion that I met Lee DuBridge, then a young and promising physicist. An occurrence that has stayed with me took place during a seminar when I became so immersed in the subject that I nearly missed a reading that I needed to record, and ran down the hall to the laboratory. As I did this, a stopwatch fell from my pocket and clattered on to the floor and was badly damaged. Equipment was hard to come by, and I knew Dr. Adolph would be upset. I said nothing about the accident when I returned to the seminar and sweated it out overnight. The next morning, rather than evade the issue, I saw Dr. Adolph and told him that I had dropped the stopwatch and was very sorry. He said "I know. I heard it drop. Pretty clumsy of you, wasn't it?" That was the end of the incident, but I never forgot it. The lesson I had learned was to face the music and take the reprimand like a man. Any other way would have been totally out of keeping with Dr. Adolph's goals, and mine as well.

In addition to our seminars, the Fellows took an active role in teaching the first-year class of medical students. This was a very interesting experience. Both Dr. Fenn and Dr. Adolph felt that the participation of the Fellows was important because they could relate well to the medical students and provide input into the program which could be obtained in no other way. Since the student fellows would ultimately join the class they were teaching and become identified with it, it was important that a good relationship be established with the students, for the transition from teacher and grader to being one of the class might otherwise have been difficult. I would sit in on grading sessions with the professorial staff and find that they were uniformly fair in their appraisals. In fact, the student fellows were tougher on the students than the professors. I also learned that not infrequently the professors' appraisal of a candidate were at variance with my own and usually much more accurate.

My teaching assignments in physiology were often beyond my ken. Dr. Fenn assigned me to teach the physiology of the eye, and when I told him I knew nothing about it, he confessed his own ignorance, and advised me to do my best. It was not easy, but I somehow managed to prepare the essential material in a form which the medical students could understand and accept. As a reward for hard work, I was given a coveted assignment to teach the nursing students the physiology of blood pressure. This assignment paid a tidy fee which made it all the more attractive. I chose to demonstrate some aspects of blood pressure on an anesthetized cat with a carotid cannula attached to a water manometer. All went well with the demonstration until I injected adrenalin into the cat. The pressure rose to an extremely high level, spilling blood over the top of the manometer onto the ceiling, creating a rather gory mess. I felt very much like the Reverend Stephen Hales must have felt when he measured blood pressure in the village square by placing a goose quill into the carotid artery of a mare and measuring with a yardstick the height of the systolic thrust from the heart. Two young nurses fainted at the sight of my experiment, and I was advised not to use this dramatic method for teaching the nurses about blood pressure. In his calm, quizzical way, Dr. Fenn said it was a great demonstration but a little too vivid for impressionable teenagers.

The thrust of my research program in physiology gradually became apparent as an approach to the study of the Starling hypothesis of fluid exchange. The gist of the hypothesis is that the net transport of fluid through the capillary wall is dependent on the difference between the effective hydrostatic capillary pressure and the osmotic pressure exerted by the plasma proteins within the capillary. The key to the concept is that the capillary pressure pushing fluids out of the vascular system into the tissues is balanced by the opposite force, that of the plasma proteins, especially albumin, which act like a sponge to control the leakage of intravascular fluids from the blood vessels into the extravascular tissues. Were it not for this mechanism, the human being would leak his plasma volume out of his vessels and be in a state of shock and hypovolemia. Delicate balances between the "out" and the "in" forces served to regulate the ebb and flow of fluids, nutrients, and electrolytes into and out of the bloodstream, thereby maintaining the homeostasis of the body, something Starling called "the wisdom of the body." Dr. Adolph and I tested this hypothesis by concentrating at first on the hydrostatic pressure within the capillaries and we subsequently published a series of joint papers on fluid transport into tissues in a variety of experimental conditions including hemorrhage, infusions, and transfusions. The concentration was on mechanical factors, i.e., the pressure, within the arterial, and capillary, and venous systems.

It was at this juncture that I became convinced that the role of the plasma proteins in the Starling equilibrium had been inadequately studied and needed further investigation. I had spent a good deal of time in thinking this through and finally came up with a design for an experiment to test the hypothesis. I should add that one evening a week, as a Fellow, I allowed myself the luxury of what I called an "idea" night. I would relax in the solitude of my room, read my bible of that day—*Quantitative Clinical Chemistry*, Volume I: *Interpretations* by John P. Peters and Donald Van Slyke (Baltimore, The Williams & Wilkins Company 1931)—and dream up new experiments and evaluate current ones. Out of these self-imposed skull-sessions, some of my best thoughts would evolve. It was out of just such a session that the need for studying the role of the plasma proteins in fluid exchange became a number-one item on my list. I discussed this with Dr. Adolph who felt that I was at a stage in my fellowship when I should have an independent project to handle by myself. I decided to approach this problem by depleting the plasma proteins of dogs by a process called plasmapheresis, which was discovered by Morawitz in Heidelberg, and the process probably was brought to the attention of John Jacob Abel, professor of pharmacology at Hopkins, by his devoted student, George Whipple, who had worked with Morawitz during his *wanderjahr* in Germany in 1909. Abel published a paper on the plasmapheresis technique in 1914, in which he reported on the effects of removing blood from dogs, centrifuging it, and separating the red cells from the plasma, and then returning the red cells, suspended in Locke's solution, to the donor animal while discarding the plasma.[1] Abel's main emphasis in this paper was on the safety and ease with which this technique could be applied in removing large amounts of plasma. He saw in it a way to apply bloodletting to patients without depleting them of their red cells and white cells and endangering the oxygen-carrying capacity of their blood. In another paper, "Experimental and Chemical Studies of the Blood with an Appeal for More Extended Chemical Training for the Biological and Medical Investigator," he made this prophetic statement in 1915:

> It may yet be possible to attach an electrically controlled centrifugalizing apparatus directly to the blood vessels of an animal and tap off a desired quantity of the fluid part of the blood while directing the stream of corpuscles back into the body (vice versa), the whole apparatus being analogous in a way to the modern cream separator.[2]

He also conducted experiments designed to probe the limits to which plasmapheresis might be performed and to study pathological changes that might ensue when the procedure was carried to a life-threatening stage. He found that he could sharply reduce the circulating plasma proteins and derived evidence that there was a continual renewal of plasma proteins from a pool in the extravascular tissues. With excessive plasmapheresis, the blood pressure could not be sustained in some animals despite the replacement of plasma with Locke's solution which is isotonic but devoid of plasma proteins. Starling's hypothesis of fluid exchange had been published in 1896, but there is no mention of it in Abel's papers of 1914–15. Abel, fully informed of new developments overseas, could hardly have missed this publication of Starling's. We must assume that at that point in time, Abel did not appreciate the significant role of the plasma proteins in maintaining fluid equilibrium, a project awaiting the interest of other investigators not yet on the scene. Perhaps World War I interfered with communications.

---

1. J. J. Abel, L. G. Rowntree, and B. B. Turner, "Plasma Removal with Return of Corpuscles (Plasmapheresis)," *J Pharmacol Exp Ther* 5 (1913–1914), pp. 625–641.

2. J. J. Abel, "Experimental and Chemical Studies of the Blood with an Appeal for More Extended Chemical Training for the Biological and Medical Investigator," *Science* N.S. 42, no. 1074 (July 30, 1915), pp. 134–147.

The technique of plasmapheresis was to surface again in 1917, when Whipple's group in San Francisco pursued the question of whether antibodies formed against infectious organisms are identical with or related to the plasma proteins. The approach to this was to deplete the plasma proteins in dogs by repeated plasmapheresis. A good deal was learned about the regeneration of plasma proteins but nothing came of the antibody search, the tools of the day being rather inadequate to solve the problem.

Whipple and his group continued to use plasmapheresis to deplete plasma proteins, and established that rapid lowering of these essential colloids was lethal to the dogs, who developed shock. The shock could be reversed or prevented by infusing plasma proteins into the blood stream. The liver was shown to play a role in plasma protein formation. A simple technique of blood volume measurement using a dye shown subsequently to attach itself to the albumin molecule was developed in Whipple's laboratory, facilitating quantitative estimation of plasma protein changes. Again Whipple's attention was focused largely on regeneration of the plasma proteins except for a study of the "stabilizing" effects of these substances in the perfusion of living organs and tissues. No mention is made in any of those papers of the Starling hypothesis and its possible role in the shock-like state produced by rapid plasma protein depletion. By 1921, Whipple had left the field of plasma protein studies to pursue hemoglobin regeneration and other more pressing studies culminating in his Nobel Prize in 1934. He was not to return to the plasma proteins until a good many years later when one of his medical students at Rochester would play a key role in reviving his interest in them and in plasmapheresis. I was fortunate enough to be that medical student, and this is how the story goes.

When Dr. Adolph and I were testing the Starling hypothesis, as I have indicated, I became convinced that a great deal more needed to be known of the role of the plasma proteins in maintaining fluid balance. I decided to go ahead with plasmapheresis to deplete the plasma proteins in dogs. I felt that if Starling were right, I should be able to produce edema in the dog by depleting the plasma proteins without changing blood pressure or capillary pressure.

In 1930 the only published lead on this was a short report by Louis Leiter of the Rockefeller Institute on the production of edema in dogs by depleting the plasma proteins by plasmapheresis.[3] We felt that we should try to reproduce these results and confirm them by utilizing techniques of tissue-fluid analysis which we had developed.

I soon found out that plasmapheresing healthy dogs to reduce their plasma protein levels was not a simple task. I was working alone and had to make many trips to the animal house to bleed the dogs, return to the laboratory to centrifuge the blood, and then return to the animal house to replace the dogs' own red cells. Technical problems were common. I soon found, as others had, that veins thrombosed after frequent needling and it was often quite frustrating and at times dangerous for the animals to delay replacement of blood for too long. Leiter had resorted to cardiac puncture for bleeding, but I felt this was unduly hazardous and, indeed, he had some accidental deaths, as well as questions of whether cardiac injury might have been responsible for edema. I decided to use the femoral arteries which were easier to deal with in the dog. This was approached with some trepidation, because my clinical friends warned me that sticking an artery might be followed by gangrene of the extremities. In those days, no one put needles into arteries except for very real and urgent reasons. Nevertheless, I went ahead and encountered no problems with the arterial punctures in the dog and they became rather routine techniques in my work and facilitated bleeding and re-infusion of blood. The tissue water and chloride analyses I did myself and many of the biochemical studies were done by Augusta McCoord, a dedicated, competent, and able technician who was working for an advanced degree. I soon learned that healthy and well-nourished dogs, who were being well fed, were extremely difficult to deplete of plasma protein, whereas malnourished animals were easily made edematous and hypoproteinemic. The most striking example of this was my experience with two dogs who had been inadvertently locked up in a box car for over one month and had been given to the medical school for sacrifice experiments. They were both emaciated and the first was so weak, it had to be sacrificed and used as a control. The second was plasmapheresed and within several hours, developed edema and hypoproteinemia, whereas it usually took me some days before I could significantly deplete a normal dog's plasma proteins. Clearly, a reserve store of plasma-protein building blocks was possessed by normal animals and there was some evidence that a nutritious diet encouraged plasma-protein regeneration. My experiments, which included tissue water measurements as well as balance studies, confirmed that animals whose plasma proteins had been depleted by plasmapheresis and who had access to sufficient water and salt would consistently develop edema of their tissues. I presented my research

---

3. L. Leiter. "Experimental Nephrotic Edema," *Proc Soc Exper Biol Med* 26 (1928), p. 173.

findings at a seminar in the department of physiology and vital economics and, much to my surprise, Dean Whipple, who did not often come to these functions, was seated in the front. When I finished the presentation, the Dean rose to comment and for a man noted for his reserve, he was so rich in his praise of the work that I almost fell over.

At the end of my talk, I had explained that my fellowship year in physiology was now over and I hoped that the plasmapheresis work would continue. I thought the problem of the Starling hypothesis and edema formation had been settled by my work, but questions had arisen that would require further study. Among these were the role of diet in plasma-protein regeneration and the pursuit of protein factors that might enhance protein formation. This would require abundant resources and personnel of a scope impossible for us to command in the department of physiology. My suggestion was that Dean Whipple's department with its animal colony and its past interest in the plasma proteins once again enter this field of research. Dean Whipple invited me to see him about this matter and it was not long before he candidly discussed resuming the plasmapheresis research. As I recall it, he said he had discussed the matter in the past with Dr. Donald D. Van Slyke, a close friend at the Rockefeller Institute, and plans for pursuing the work had been outlined, but other research had higher priority. Now he was almost ready to start and he invited me to sit in on the planning sessions. I was, of course, deeply flattered and, more than that, quite excited about the new programs. The Dean was true to his word and I, in turn, learned very quickly how a really great investigator goes about planning his work. The Dean chose to focus his attention on factors having to do with the regeneration and origin of the plasma proteins. Years of work were to follow and many important contributions to knowledge were to emerge. I was privileged to sit in on some of the early planning sessions and was impressed by the freedom of exchange and by the respect accorded to even the most junior person.

In Dean Whipple's autobiographical sketch published in *Perspectives in Biology and Medicine* (vol. II, no. 3, Spring 1959, p. 266) he tells the story of Dr. Charles Hooper, one of his young research associates in California, who in 1918 had a liver extract that he wanted to test on patients with pernicious anemia:

> His extract was an alcoholic, fat-free preparation and was given subcutaneously to three pernicious anemia patients and there were remissions and improved hemoglobin levels. The clinicians laughed him out of the wards and told him these were spontaneous remissions and were of no significance. Hooper was a very

> shy, sensitive young man, and this unfortunate attitude of the clinicians caused him to quit this clinical work. It was most unfortunate, as his extract almost certainly contained the potent B12 factor from the liver and the clinical liver therapy might have been discovered in 1918. It is tragic that he made no published record of this material, its preparation, and its effect on clinical cases. The story illustrates an important principle that a junior worker should never be turned back by self-styled experts or critics. The critics should be helpful, and the junior should persist in spite of various thoughtless comments.

This was Dr. Whipple's creed and I know from personal experience as one of his students who worked in his department that he meant every word of it. Years later, I remember chatting with Dr. Whipple about the Nobel Prize and the role played by his coworker, Dr. Murphy, who earned a share of the prize by doing the reticulocyte and blood counts. Dean Whipple told me that Dr. Murphy earned every bit of his share because he was the one that had the evangelistic fervor to persuade his patients to eat the large amounts of liver needed each day to achieve remission of the disease. Clinicians before him had failed to persuade the patients to cooperate.

Among the highlights of my year out in physiology were visits we made to other medical schools in western New York state. A round-robin of regional meetings of the Society for Experimental Biology and Medicine (nicknamed the Meltzer Verein for its founder, Dr. Samuel Meltzer of the Rockefeller Institute) took us from Rochester to Buffalo and Syracuse. There we would present our early work for discussion and criticism before members of the physiology departments of these schools. I remember interacting at Buffalo with an extraordinary group of their young scientists that included a red-haired medical student, George Thorn, destined to become professor of medicine at Harvard, the Cori's, husband and wife, who in 1947 would soar to Nobel fame, and Frank Hartman and Katherine Brownell of adrenal physiology renown. The University of Buffalo School of Medicine did not have the high reputation it has since earned and it had little or no endowment. I remember saying to Dr. Adolph when we drove back to Rochester how impressed I was by the Buffalo group and amazed that they were doing such outstanding work in rather primitive surroundings. Little did I know that I had the privilege of observing and interacting with a group of the most talented investigators extant. I learned early on that in research, money, bricks, and mortar don't rule the roost.

Another milestone in that year was a trip to Montreal, Canada, to attend the International Congress of Physiology. The costs of attending this meeting were beyond our means, but Dr. Fenn arranged for each of us to receive a check for a one-way Pullman ticket to Montreal. How would we get back? One of the instructors in physiology, Al Hegnauer, had an ancient Hudson automobile that he was willing to drive to Montreal and back. By cashing our checks and pooling our allowances we created a common fund to see us through a week in Montreal. This was in 1931 when a haircut was 35 cents, a Coke was five cents, and a cigar was five cents. In Montreal we stayed in a modest but clean YMCA. The Congress was something I shall never forget. The city of Montreal regaled us with a banquet in an elegant setting atop Mount Royal with its large cross. I tasted Bordeaux Blanc wine for the first time and enjoyed a magnificent dinner. Even the speeches by the mayor and other dignitaries were stimulating. This is the only time I can recall that a city gave hundreds of visitors a free meal. It was a great start on a week I shall never forget. My knowledge of French helped me to get around in this bilingual city.

The meetings were full of new information and remarkable people. I saw most of the physiologists of that era socially and in action with Dr. Adolph helping me to identify them. The brisk and sometimes bruising arguments among the various scientists were exciting. Here I quickly became aware of AJ (Ajax) Carlson of Chicago, who rose to question many of the speakers. His questions were so pertinent and knowledgeable and at times devastating that I came away with the feeling that here was a major figure in America. Watching Carlson was like seeing Babe Ruth at bat. One session was devoted to mechanisms of dyspnea with Gesell of the University of Michigan pitted against Glenn Cullen of Vanderbilt University. It was heady wine, almost making you wish to become a physiologist. At the end of the week we headed for Rochester in our beat-up car. All went well until we were about 50 miles from Rochester when the motor conked out in a quiet village on a Sunday. We managed to find a mechanic who was able to repair the motor. After paying him there were merely a few pennies left in our fund. A tired lot of young physiologists arrived in Rochester without further delay, broke but happy, not an uncommon condition in those depression years.

As I look back on my year as a student research fellow in physiology I realize more than ever that it was a great milestone in my life. It was a most unusual opportunity to learn by being immersed in the day-to-day activities of a simply amazing department, small in size but high in quality. In 1930 the entire department of physiology at Rochester consisted of Professor and Chairman Dr. Wallace O. Fenn, Assistant Professor Dr. Edward Adolph, assistant professor Instructors Albert Hegnauer and Charles Wright, technicians Bill Latchford and Mr.

Nudo, and two student fellows, my friend John Jares and myself. It was a happy group and I do not recall any arguments or dissension.

In those days the student fellows were selected by the faculty, usually from the top-ranking group in the class. One did not apply for the fellowship; one was honored by being asked. In later years students could apply for a fellowship. While this was good for the students, I believe it served to diminish the lustre of the fellowship.

In 1958 Dr. Leonard F. Fenninger reported on the performance and careers of all graduates who had taken a one-year fellowship prior to 1953.[4] He concluded "that more than 12 percent of graduates who did not participate in the fellowship program had chosen careers in teaching and research on a full-time basis. In contrast, 2½ times as many (some 30 percent) of those who had participated in the fellowship program were engaged in full-time academic and research careers—the opportunity to participate in research early in their professional careers was an important factor in their scientific achievement."

In 1964 and 1972, the recorded holders of the fellowship were again reviewed by Stotz. In the 1964 study, at least 50 percent of the fellows chose full-time academic or research work and in 1972 the figure was 65 percent. Stotz concluded, "While it is recognized that some who start may not remain in academic medicine over the years, the impact of Rochester's year-out fellowship program on choice of careers seems unmistakable." Stotz, a Ph.D., concluded with this prescient comment: "Not to be overlooked in this prospectus, which emphasizes the influence of the year-out fellowship experience on the choice of an academic career, are the many year-out graduates who have not chosen an academic or research career. Presumably these were also aided by their year-out experience in making the choice to practice medicine rather than to engage in full-time academic work."[5]

A factor not mentioned by Stotz was the dramatic increase in full-time positions following WW II owing to enormous NIH grants for research, including salaries and indirect and direct costs. Another point I would make is that it may be a mistake to overemphasize the percentage of awardees going into academic full-time medicine and research.

---

4. "The Rochester Student Fellowship Program," *The Journal of Medical Education* 33, no. 3 (March 1958).

5. Elmer Stotz, *To Each His Farthest Star* (Rochester, N.Y.: University of Rochester Medical Center, 1975), p. 88.

A number of factors other than idealism may influence such decisions. To look upon the private practice of medicine as a less worthy endeavor than academic medicine serves to denigrate the way of life of those who have chosen this path to serve the public. There are many unsung heroes in this arena. The difficulty is in how to identify them and evaluate what they are doing. While we are justly proud of our academicians, we should not neglect our outstanding practitioners, clinicians, and voluntary part-time teachers. I believe our school should establish an award for the country's Alumnus-Clinician of the Year.

While we are on the topic of the year-out fellowships, I wish to touch upon a criticism of this program made in recent years by one of our most distinguished medical graduates, Dr. Arthur Kornberg, class of 1941 and Nobel Laureate (1959) for the enzymatic synthesis of DNA. I first became aware of his adverse comments regarding the selections of the year-out fellows in 1984 when I read a book by Allen B. Weisse, M.D. entitled, *Conversations in Medicine: The Story of Twentieth-Century American Medicine in the Words of Those Who Created It* (New York: New York University Press, 1984, pp. 375–399). I found the interviews and vignettes rather fascinating. The last person interviewed was Arthur Kornberg, who grew up in poverty in Brooklyn, the son of Jewish immigrants. Despite being a top scholar at the demanding College of the City of New York (CCNY), he was turned down in 1937 by every medical school to which he applied except Long Island College and Rochester. Especially galling to him was a rejection from the Columbia University College of Physicians and Surgeons, where an endowed scholarship for a City College graduate went begging for nine years because there were no "acceptable" candidates. He elected to go to Rochester where he received a full-tuition scholarship. However, he claims that anti-Semitism was rife at Rochester, and in Weisse's interview he declared that there was anti-Italian sentiment present as well. In support of his statement, he said that because of the anti-Semitism he was never offered a year-out student fellowship even though he stood at the top of his class.[6]

My own experience was that neither anti-Semitic nor anti-Italian prejudice existed at Rochester medical school. Much like Kornberg, I came from a modest background in the Bronx, the son of Italian

---

6. Arthur Kornberg, *For the Love of Enzymes* (Cambridge, Mass. and England: Harvard University Press, 1989), pp. 310–311.

immigrants who spoke Italian at home. I had seen and heard nothing at Rochester to support any claim that the faculty was anti-Italian or anti-Semitic. As an outstanding first-year student, I was offered and accepted a year-out fellowship in physiology where I spent a marvelous year and several summers followed by a summer in Dean Whipple's department working in the plasma protein project. At no time was I aware of anti-Italian bias or anti-Semitism. In fact I felt that our medical school was remarkably free of those trends.

It is true that in the late 1930s anti-Semitism was rife in America and abroad. Rochester had a large population of prosperous Germans working as skilled technicians, many of whom were indeed anti-Semitic. While growing up in Brooklyn, Kornberg may have been insulated from anti-Semitic remarks by living in a Jewish area, surrounded by Jewish friends with little or no contact with non-Jews. In his high school and at CCNY almost all of his fellow students were Jewish. The real world outside of these enclaves was different in the 1930s. Anti-Semitism was rampant. Alan M. Dershowitz, the controversial Harvard law professor, describes the scene with accuracy and verve in his recently published monograph, *Chutzpah*. It was the era of quotas for Jews, Italians, blacks, and women at the Ivy League Universities, including Harvard, Yale, Columbia, Princeton, Dartmouth, and others. The Wall Street law firms were sharply segregated, most of them anti-Semitic and anti-Italian. Not a very pretty sight for a Jewish youth from Brooklyn or an Italian from the Bronx. Yet, when I look back at my days at Rochester, starting in 1929, I was simply unaware of anti-Semitic or anti-Italian trends at the University of Rochester School of Medicine. In fact, I know that it was remarkably free of these sentiments. If ever there was a true meritocracy, it existed at Rochester in this brand-new medical school inspired by Abraham Flexner, a Jew, Mr. George Eastman, a Christian, John D. Rockefeller, a Baptist, and President Rush Rhees, a Baptist, and led by its Founding Father, Dean George Hoyt Whipple, a New Hampshire Yankee of the highest integrity and a born leader.

In October 1953 at an alumni reunion at Rochester, Dean Whipple, then 75 years young, joined a group of alumni for an informal lunch in the Strong Memorial Hospital cafeteria. One of us asked the Dean whether he had any secrets to pass on to us on how to select good candidates for admission to the medical school. His answer, as I recall it, was that "there were no secrets; the real purpose of the interview was to observe the person as a human being. His grades and letters of recommendation had already been reviewed but how did he measure up to our expectations? Would this man or woman make the kind of doctor you would want to have it you were sick? You men are all doctors in practice and every day you are called upon to make judgments like these; so it really should be quite simple."

Of course, it was not that simple. Dean Whipple was an excellent judge of "horseflesh" who made very few mistakes. How many Deans of medical schools do we know who personally interviewed all applicants? I am aware only of Dean Wilburt C. Davison of Duke, like Whipple, an Oslerian and Hopkins graduate.

George Whipple picked his faculty for his medical school with great care. He also knew that the ultimate success of his medical school would depend upon the quality of his students. His interviews were focused on evaluating leadership traits, stamina and good health, breadth of interests, hobbies, character, integrity, community activities, and the capacity for work. My belief is that he also had a plan for the school to accept only the best students, male or female, from across the country, a cross-section of America without regard to religion, color, or ethnic origin. For me, it is impossible to believe that this great man could stoop to anti-Semitism or anti-Italian sentiments in the performance of his duties as the Dean of a medical school he was destined to lead to greatness.

In the summer of 1931, through the good auspices of Dr. Adolph, arrangements had been made with Dr. Donald Van Slyke, the famous biochemist, for me to work at the Rockefeller Institute in his laboratory. I had never before visited the Rockefeller and it was quite an interesting experience for a young medical student. Some readers may recall that in 1925 Sinclair Lewis's *Arrowsmith* had fascinated a generation of college and medical students, and the movie version of it had stamped the picture of the entrance hall of the McGurk Institute on the minds of thousands of viewers. The McGurk Institute was said to be the Rockefeller, which Paul De Kruif, through Lewis, criticized for what he felt was its phony facade. As a result, many medical students, familiar with this portrayal, had reservations about the great Institute. I was one of these, and when I approached the entrance of the Rockefeller, these were the thoughts going through my mind. The clerk at the reception desk was courteous and called Dr. Van Slyke, who immediately came down to see me. Dr. Van Slyke was a warm, pleasant scientist who appeared quite upset at having forgotten that I was due to come to work in his laboratory. He said he had been unexpectedly advised by his doctor to take the summer off for his health. When he saw the disappointment on my face, he said not to worry, that I could work with one of his associates. He took me to a crowded, cluttered laboratory and introduced me to a bushy-haired young man, Irvine Page, who was busily engaged in biochemical studies. At this stage in his career, Page had not yet achieved the reputation which was to come to him in later years. With due respect for Page, I had arranged to work with Van Slyke and I had grave reservations over settling for a lesser light. Before leaving, Dr. Van Slyke asked me to go downstairs to see Dr. Rufus Cole, who was in charge of the Institute that summer. I recall Dr. Cole as a remote, rather cold individual who seemed quite upset that a mere medical student had been given permission to work at the Institute. He seemed displeased with Van Slyke and said he was always doing something unorthodox. By this time, I was really feeling very uncomfortable and insecure, and I began to appreciate some of the unpleasant things De Kruif had said about the Institute. Dr. Cole told me that he could not assume the responsibility for letting me work at the Rockefeller until he had discussed it with Dr. Simon Flexner, who was on vacation. He asked me to return one week later for the answer. I left with mixed feelings and some anger. It was no fault of mine that Dr. Van Slyke had failed to clear with the front office, and I wasn't too enthusiastic about working with Page, whose research project was not especially interesting to me. I decided to try my luck at the Babies' Hospital of the Columbia-Presbyterian Medical Center, where Dr. Ashley Weech was in charge while Dr. Rustin McIntosh was away. Weech had been working on plasma-protein depletion induced by feeding a low-protein diet to dogs. He was a charming, warm, and friendly man who treated me as an equal. He was greatly interested in my technique for conducting plasmapheresis and measuring blood volume, and he sensed that we might exchange information. He offered me a laboratory, two dogs, materials, equipment, and funds for the special low-protein diet which I would have to prepare myself, and the help of Gagarin, his laboratory assistant. Gagarin, a Russian nobleman, who had fallen on hard times, proved a competent assistant and a good friend. Before starting at the Babies' Hospital, I kept my appointment with Dr. Cole at the Rockefeller. I think he had cleared the way with Dr. Flexner, but I had decided to go with Weech and told him so. He seemed a little miffed that I would pass up an opportunity to work at the Rockefeller, but that wasn't the impression I was left with after our first interview. Later in the fall, when I saw Dr. Whipple, he was upset at the mixup at the Rockefeller and wished I had telephoned him about it, but I had hesitated to make an issue out of a small matter. Besides, the trip to Babies' Hospital by trolley car from the Bronx cost me only five cents each way, an important consideration in those depression days, quite a savings in time and money from the trip to the Rockefeller Institute. In any event, the summer at Babies' Hospital was very productive and I published a paper based upon work on nutritional edema in which I established that, within certain limits, the plasma proteins had a role in regulating plasma volume. Dr. Weech and I became good friends. I also made rounds with Dr. Robert F. Loeb, who was making major discoveries about Addison's Disease. I was greatly impressed by him as a teacher and investigator.

On my return to Rochester, in the fall of 1931, I joined the Class of '34 for some courses and continued to work in the department of physiology as well. One of my greatest experiences at Rochester was the course in pathology, which was under the direction of Dean Whipple. He took personal charge of it, and all of the class, in groups of four, did one autopsy with him and he reviewed the slides with us. We realized we had a brilliant teacher and were stimulated and challenged by his example. His CPCs (Clinical Pathologic Conferences) were crowded and he exhibited wisdom and great skill in pursuing the lessons to be learned from each case. He welcomed questions from the students but had a way of cutting off a foolish or attention-seeking question in midstream. His weekly quiz sessions were the talk of the school and something the students never missed. In anticipation, we would bone up on the topic of the day and be all set for his questions—or so we thought. An over-confident student was quickly brought down to earth after giving a long list of causes of a specific condition, finally running out of possibilities and having to face the Dean's query over his half-glasses—"and what else, Mr. So-and-So?" Another favorite question was how to diagnose leprosy. Almost no one guessed that a nasal smear for acid-fast bacilli was the correct answer. He was excellent at relating postmortem findings to pathophysiologic processes and he insisted that we approach pathology in this way. For us, pathology was a living science, physiologically and biochemically oriented and ideal preparation for the clinical years that lay ahead. Who among us would ever forget the first experiment in our pathology course when we studied the harmful effects of chloroform anesthesia on the dog's liver. For this, in groups of four, we anesthetized a dog for a brief period, let it recover, and four days later sacrificed the dog and studied its liver, finding striking changes caused by the chloroform. Needless to say, we would never use chloroform as an anesthetic.

Another highlight of the year was the course in bacteriology conducted by Dr. Stanhope Bayne-Jones and his associate, Konrad Birkhaug. This was beautifully organized and taught in person by these two outstanding educators. Dr. Bayne-Jones was the co-author of Hans Zinsser's textbook of bacteriology, which was the medical students' *vade mecum* of the day. In those early days the professors were omnipresent in the classrooms at the side of the students, asking questions, observing and intimately involved in the teaching program. One of the teaching exercises was the study of human sputum with various stains including the Ziehl-Nielsen for acid-fast (TB) organisms. The students were paired off and seated at their microscopes in alphabetical order and were instructed to examine each other's sputum. So it was during a routine class exercise in 1930 that a student named Willard Allen examined the sputum of a classmate, Lauren Ackerman, and spotted tubercle bacilli on the slide. He quietly summoned Dr. Bayne-Jones, who confirmed his findings and notified Ackerman that he had tuberculosis. In those pre-antibiotic days this meant at least a year in a tuberculosis sanitarium. While at Trudeau Sanitarium, Ackerman, to pass the time, requested the loan of pathology slides from Dean Whipple, who complied. From this beginning came the career of a man who became a world leader in surgical pathology and the author of the classic *Surgical Pathology*, first published in 1953 and now in its eighth edition. Dr. Williard Allen, who made the diagnosis of tuberculosis as a medical student, also helped Dr. George W. Corner to isolate progesterone, the corpus luteum hormone in 1929, and went on to become a distinguished professor and chairman of the department of obstetrics and gynecology at Washington University, St. Louis. Dr. Ackerman continued to teach into his eighty-eighth year, when he died of cancer on 27 July 1993.

My bacteriology course at Rochester in 1931 was the last conducted by Dr. Bayne-Jones, who accepted a position as chairman of bacteriology at Yale, where he soon succeeded Winternitz as Dean.

With the advent of WW II he became a consultant to the Army on preventive medicine and performed important duties leading to his promotion to brigadier general. Finally, after WW II he became the president of the Cornell University-New York Hospital Medical Center.

In 1949, he delivered a message, "The Hospital as a Center of Preventive Medicine," which became one of his most popular and influential, and, one might add, most prescient.[7]

"His audience (American College of Physicians) at the Waldorf-Astoria comprised four thousand specialists in internal medicine. He urged that the hospitals' inpatient services be viewed as a means to prevent as well as to cure illness. He wished to see diagnostic clinics expanded with the aim of forestalling illness. He suggested that consultation services for both doctors and patients in the community be

---

7. Stanhope-Bayne Jones, "The Hospital as a Center of Preventive Medicine," *Annals of Internal Medicine* 31 (July 1949), pp. 7–16.

enlarged. He favored the growth of group practice both inside and outside the hospital and he urged the development of home-care programs based in the hospital. He wanted education and training in preventive medicine and, of course, more research in the field. Perhaps idealistically, he hoped to combine personal attention to the patient with institutional growth and social medicine."[8]

When I was a medical student at Rochester there were two departments of physiology. The first one we encountered during the freshman year, and there we learned basic science stressing muscle-nerve physiology, the forte of Dr. Wallace O. Fenn, the chairman of the department and his one assistant professor, Dr. Edward F. Adolph, whose field of interest was water balance.

The Warburg apparatus was Dr. Fenn's symbol while Dr. Adolph's was the beam balance or weight scales and the graduated cylinder for measuring fluid intake and output. Both were men of high intelligence and excellent teachers. Even then, although they were in their early thirties, we quickly realized that we were being exposed to exceptional minds. At the same time we doubted that we could ever match them or live up to their expectations. They had been selected for their positions with great care by Dean George H. Whipple, who was bombarded with candidates proposed by Abraham Flexner, who favored O. F. Meyerhof of Germany, internationally famous and a Nobel laureate in 1922. Dr. Whipple had reservations about bringing in a foreigner with a language barrier to lead the teaching of physiology in his brand-new medical school. He felt that American physiology and basic science had come of age and he looked carefully for an American to head the department. On the way to this decision, he considered an Englishman, E. D. Adrian, destined to win a Nobel Prize in 1933, who turned down the position, as did A. V. Hill, who shared the 1922 Nobel Prize with Meyerhof. Hill recommended W. O. Fenn, only 31 years old, a Harvard Ph.D. who was working as a Fellow under Hill in Great Britain. Dean Whipple appointed Fenn as the first chairman of the department of physiology at Rochester. The choice was nothing short of brilliant. Fenn blossomed as a great star in the Rochester firmament, going from muscle-nerve physiology to respiratory physiology and life in space, becoming a world authority and winning the Feltrinelli prize as well as many other great honors.

---

8. Albert E. Cowdrey, *War and Healing; Stanhope Bayne-Jones and the Maturing of American Medicine* (Baton Rouge and London: Louisiana State University Press, 1992), p. 172.

His discovery of the Fenn effect in 1922 and 1923 "set a course for the study of the energetics of muscular contraction that has successfully taken us into the present and continues to point to the most promising direction for the future."[9] It was worthy of a Nobel Prize.

He was generally regarded as the greatest intellect of the key professors of the original faculty at our Medical School. Dr. Edward F. Adolph another Harvard Ph.D., also in his early thirties, kept pace with his chief and became world famous for his contributions to water and fluid balance. His work during WW II on man in the desert provided essential information on water balance that helped the British and American tanks under General Montgomery and General Patton to win many battles. Little did we know as medical students in the thirties that so much of the instruction that we were receiving that seemed rather esoteric and irrelevant would very soon become essential and very practical in the new medicine of the twentieth century.

Here I will digress to pay tribute to Dr. Adolph, whose first medical student research Fellow I was in 1930 at Rochester. Somehow, despite heavy demands made upon him, he found the time to write to me on a regular basis during my years of military service (1942–1946). His letters were always informative and interesting. In July 1945, Dr. Adolph wrote to me on Tinian, telling me something of his important wartime research on soldiers in the California desert, where he was head of a civilian unit from the department of physiology of the University of Rochester School of Medicine. He wrote:

> Dear Dr. Lepore:
>   Your address card recently arrived. I assume that you are on your way to overseas service. Perhaps you will welcome it after your long tour of home duty—At the moment I am getting my first summer vacation in three or four years. And it is pleasant. It is productive of reorientations which are needed more than ever with war jobs on our hands. My laboratory group has just finished preparing for publication a monograph on the Physiology of Man in the Desert. It represents our war work of 2½ years. Probably another 8 months will see it in print. I had to do most of the polishing myself but it is none the less a cooperative effort. At one time or another ten other men were associated in the work. I picture the army and war strategy in terms of our field experience of two and three years ago. Probably methods

---

9. Wallace O. Fenn (1893–1971) Obituary, *J. Gen. Physiology* 58 (1971), pp. 481–483.

are all different by now. Our field and laboratory efforts now go into the study of the effects of heat and of cold. As you sweat through the hot weather wherever you are, you can think of us trying to define the tolerance limits for men at diverse activities and trying to find out what working and sleeping in the heat does to a man. We have coordinated a somewhat national program of investigations on the subject. You would be intrigued by the plans for a long-term study of men under conditions of tropical settlement. But we still need some institution to finance the study. In the laboratory we are building a cold room and planning to put a calorimeter in it. Then we can find out, we hope, whether men acclimatize to cold or only think they do. Probably we will still be pegging away at that problem when you get back to civilian life.

The monograph, "Physiology of Man in the Desert," published in 1947 by Interscience Publishers, Inc., of New York and London, is now a classic in the field. My copy is a treasured memento of my revered Professor Edward F. Adolph. What Dr. Adolph failed to tell me was that he and an associate, conducting their experiments as civilians in the California desert, had an unpleasant experience when General George S. Patton, previously unaware of their existence, stumbled upon them and proceeded to chew them out for being unmilitary, failing to salute and out of uniform! The tank corpsmen and General Patton would forever be indebted to Adolph *et al.* for insisting that ample drinking water was as vital for them as was the gasoline for their tanks.

Let us now return to Rochester and the department of physiology circa 1929. Formal lectures were few and far between. Those given by Dr. Fenn were extraordinarily clear and instructive. He remained committed to the formal lecture as part of his teaching for the rest of his life. In his hands it was a superb part of the physiology program at Rochester. Perhaps the greatest strength in the program in physiology was its emphasis upon experiments on cats, dogs, frogs, and turtle hearts, and, last but not least, human experiments upon ourselves. These were not demonstrations performed by instructors in an amphitheater. They were experiments conducted by the students, under supervision, in groups of two or four. We learned the hard way how frustrating some of these ventures can be and how rewarding when they worked out. Above all, it was sound instruction in the way knowledge can be acquired. With the steady rise over the years in the size of classes at Rochester, due not only to increases in medical students but also large numbers of postgraduate students, this method of instruction was slowly replaced by neat and successfully performed demonstrations with the medical students becoming observers instead of participants. The instructors did all of the work. In my opinion something very important was lost in the process.

In the second year of medical school at Rochester, we took a second course in physiology focusing on mammalian work with dogs, cats, and ourselves. The course was called "Vital Economics." The department had been created and named in accordance with the 1915 bequest of Lewis P. Ross, a Rochester manufacturer and University trustee, who left his large residuary estate to finance teaching and research in physiology and nutrition. The bulk of the money was to be used to maintain a university department that would provide opportunities to pursue college teaching, scientific investigation, and extramural instruction in the fields of hygiene and human nutrition. This was, of course, before any thought had been given to creating a medical school at Rochester.[10]

In 1917, Dr. John R. Murlin, a distinguished physiologist and disciple of Graham Lusk of Cornell University Medical School, was appointed director of the newly created department of vital economics at Rochester with the title of professor of nutritional physiology. Since there was no medical school at the time, the appointment was to the undergraduate faculty. Hot on the trail of the antidiabetic hormone (insulin), Murlin and an associate, Benjamin Kramer, had published papers in 1913 and 1916 on the effects of pancreatic and duodenal extracts on the glycosuria and respiratory metabolism of depancreatized dogs. This work was interrupted when Dr. Murlin was called to Washington in 1916 for wartime service and was not resumed until his return to Rochester in the spring of 1919, when he took charge of his newly created department of vital economics housed in laboratory space in the Eastman Building of the Rochester campus.

Early in 1920 discussions were initiated by Abraham Flexner leading to the establishment of a new medical school at Rochester.[11] In 1925 the new medical school admitted its first class of twenty men and two women. With establishment of the medical school a dilemma arose that might have caused some awkward moments. What should be done about the department of vital economics and Dr. Murlin? The decision made by Dean Whipple was to move the department of vital economics into the new medical school, in an area

---

10. Arthur J. May, *A History of the University of Rochester, 1850–1962* (Princeton, N.J.: Princeton University Press, 1977), p. 199.

11. Michael J. Lepore, *Death of the Clinician: Requiem or Reveille?* (Springfield, Ill.: Charles C. Thomas, 1982), pp. 96–130.

adjoining but separate from Dr. Fenn's department of physiology. In effect, we had two departments of physiology. Basic physiology could be learned in the first year in Dr. Fenn's department and in the second year the vital economics department would focus upon mammalian physiology and nutrition. What might have been a problem was solved by this arrangement, due in a large measure to Dr. Murlin's tolerance and the exceptional diplomacy of Dr. Wallace O. Fenn.

When I started the course in vital economics, my classmate John Jares and I were paired off as partners in dog surgery. We were required by Dr. Murlin to develop a project that would be completed during that semester and written up as a sort of thesis. I had read in the French *Journal Compte Rendu de Physiologie* that a physiologist named B. A. Houssay in Argentina had removed the pituitary gland of frogs and found that the hypophysectomized frog was very sensitive to insulin and could easily be sent into hypoglycemic insulin shock by a dose the normal frog could tolerate without any adverse effects. In 1947 Houssay would share the Nobel Prize for this work on the role of the anterior pituitary in the metabolism of sugar. John Jares and I decided to hypophysectomize a dog to test whether Houssay's findings in the frog could be confirmed in the dog. Dr. Murlin approved of our protocol and supplied us with the dogs and equipment. Little did John and I know that we were stepping into a field very close to Dr. Murlin's heart—the insulin story. We knew nothing about his heartbreaking failure to be the first to prepare a safe extract of insulin despite many years of dedicated and intense research. Later in the year he would relate to our entire class the details of how he just missed discovering insulin.

We quickly found that performing hypophysectomy on the dog by the transbuccal approach (across the roof of the mouth) was not an easy procedure. Our equipment was primitive and we were especially handicapped by our inability to prevent or control hemorrhage. After several failures, John and I regrouped, held a long discussion and decided we needed some help. We got in touch with Dr. William P. Van Wagenen, the chief of neurosurgery and a former Harvey Cushing resident. He graciously agreed to help us and set aside one or two afternoons a week for this purpose. He also brought with him some excellent operating-room equipment, including better drills and methods for controlling hemorrhage. Under his guidance, we finally had two living hypophysectomized dogs. We then proceeded to confirm that the hypophysectomized dog was extremely sensitive to a dose of insulin that caused almost no change in the normal animal, confirming Houssay's findings in the frog. We wrote this up and submitted the report for the archives in the department of vital economics with the suggestion that further work be done with these animals.

The department of vital economics was well organized and efficiently administered. The staff was seasoned, intelligent, and enthusiastic. Nutrition was exceptionally well taught by Dr. Estelle Hawley, who soon had us looking at a slice of bread or a tomato or potato and rattling off their carbohydrate, protein, fat, and calorie count. She made it look simple, but it is indeed an art and one that is much neglected in our medical schools today, where nutrition education has no place in the curriculum while a great deal of other less useful information is being poured into the students. Dr. Ed Nassett was another favorite. He was especially strong in teaching us operative techniques on the dogs and cats. Dr. Murlin was concerned about vivisection and told the class that anyone of us who was cruel to a cat or dog did not deserve to be a doctor. In addition to the cats and dogs, we also performed experiments on ourselves. A key experiment was for each of us to eat a basal diet, collecting 24-hour urine specimens as a baseline. Then we would add to the basal diet (that we had to cook ourselves) a test food, and monitor the urinary output of a metabolic product of the ingested foodstuff. I chose to eat one-half pound of sliced liver each day and tested my urine for uric acid products. I thought I would never again want to eat liver after this exercise. I detected large amounts of urates in my urine samples but failed to study serum uric acid levels. In retrospect, most of us ate too much of the baseline control diet and then added the test food to the meals. Part of the problem was that the food was given to us without charge and we were living for the two weeks of the study "on the house" free of charge.

Dr. Murlin missed insulin, although he was very close to it. Had it not been for World War I government service and the lack of access to a medical school in Rochester during the most exciting era of insulin research, he might well have made the discovery that earned the Nobel Prize for the Toronto investigators led by Dr. Frederick Banting in 1924, two years before the medical school of the University of Rochester was opened. Dr. Murlin did not come out of this insulin research without at least one substantial discovery. In 1923 he and his collaborators discovered a glucogenic substance in an extract of pancreas that they named "glucagon," or mobilizer of glucose. While this was not as big as insulin, it was enough to ensure Dr. Murlin's fame, but a far cry from the discovery of insulin and a Nobel Prize. With Murlin's obligatory retirement on age, in 1945, the department of vital economics was absorbed by the department of physiology without fanfare. In the process, the teaching of nutrition at Rochester declined and no longer is this a showcase segment of the curriculum.

Dr. Arthur Kornberg, in his book *For the Love of Enzymes*, pays tribute to his education in nutrition at Rochester in the department of vital economics and bemoans the decline in nutrition teaching and research that has occurred in leading medical schools since then, saying it is a shambles. We are graduating doctors from our medical schools who are grossly ignorant in the field of human nutrition.

No wonder the field has been taken over by assorted quacks, hustlers, faddists, and entrepreneurs. Kornberg, in his trenchant prose, says: "Fashions in science are as influential and nearly as mercurial as styles in dress. Driven by the funding tastes of government agencies and major foundations, the stampede of scientists around the world to fashionable scientific activities leaves ghost towns in still fertile areas. Such was the fate of nutrition as a major scientific discipline when in the 1940s and 1950s biochemists were lured away by access to the molecular details of cellular operations. The word "nutrition" no longer appears on the lintel of the expanded biochemistry building of the University of Wisconsin, once the seat of world leadership in a proud science."[12] He continues: "Whither Human Nutrition? How can we cope with the numerous and complex problems and the extraordinary difficulty of doing controlled long-term dietary experiments on humans? Considering the importance of acquiring definitive dietary information for health and economic welfare, nutrition cannot be left to the art of medicine or the exploitation of hustlers. The only answer is science, hard science. Progress demands these actions (1) invest in the training and support of scientists to work in nutrition, (2) narrow the focus of experimental work to doable problems, urgent or not, (3) use a variety of animal models, (4) insulate research from broad social issues and (5) sustain the faith that persistent scientific effort eventually solves most problems, often in a surprisingly novel way."[13]

Kornberg is on the highest possible ground when he advocates measures to strengthen the scientific base of nutrition education in our medical schools. But there is yet another question that must be resolved. How do we make the teaching of nutrition an essential part of the curriculum in our medical schools? Why, as stated in a recent

---

12. Arthur Kornberg, *For the Love of Enzymes* (Cambridge Mass. and London, England: Harvard University Press, 1989), pp. 25–26.

13. Ibid., pp. 27–28.

14. Marian Burros, "Eating Well — No Wonder Doctors Know Little About Nutrition," *New York Times*, April 1, 1992, p. C 4.

article in the *New York Times*,[14] "do only about one-third of the 125 or so medical schools in the country require students to take courses in nutrition? And most of those courses are short. The one at Cornell is eight hours."

What can you learn about nutrition in eight hours? The answer may well be to restore the teaching of nutrition at Rochester to the high levels of the 1930s.

The junior year at Rochester was the toughest of all. You had to work like hell doing all sorts of blood counts, urine examinations, stool and sputum tests, work-ups, intravenouses, and acting as factotum for the house staff. The hours were horrendous, starting at 7:00 A.M. and ending at midnight—if we were lucky.

We were never through and there was little time for play or relaxation. New admissions had to be worked up and we had to be ready for presentation of our cases to key teaching attendings. If we did well, we felt good. If not, we were quite unhappy. The amount to be learned was overwhelming but we tried with varying degrees of success.

This was the year in medical school at Rochester that we had eagerly been awaiting. This was when we would, for the first time, really come to grips with patients and the people and problems that had attracted many of us to the study of medicine. Everything else was mere preparation. Many of us had chafed at having to wait so long to come to the patients, while others like me felt that the better our basic preparation, the better we would cope with the problems of clinical medicine. For the few who had some experience in research, the wards of our hospitals opened up new vistas into the sea of clinical investigation. No matter what our special interest might be, all of us were now assigned to duties clearly relevant to the work of a physician.

This was the moment we had spent years preparing for. Now we would see how well we could handle people, their problems, and their illnesses. The first thing we had to learn to do well was to take a good history. To this day, this remains the foundation stone of competent medical practice. You learn to talk with people, not to them. You learn to communicate and establish a dialogue. You learn to listen. You may learn that frightened and sick people may open up their hearts to an interested listener, and may tell a medical student more than they would tell someone higher on the totem pole. You also learn that some people, luckily a minority, look upon medical students as a nuisance and resent their intrusion into their privacy. We had a little more of this at Strong Memorial and Rochester Municipal Hospital in the early days because the town-and-gown struggle had led to the spreading of rumors by our competitors that the hospitals were staffed by medical students who would do nothing but experiment on patients. We were assigned to various services of the hospitals and given a number of patients whose blood counts and stool and urine examinations we had to perform ourselves. In fact, we functioned as another pair of hands and legs for the busy intern staff.

We accepted the apparent drudgery of the "routine" duties as part of what it takes to make a doctor and we dared not complain. By today's standards we were overloaded with patients and "scut work," but it didn't seem to bother us too much. Medicine is in many ways full of trade-offs; the more we did for the intern, the more time he had to teach us. A good intern was worth his weight in gold as a teacher at this stage in our careers, and we learned more from the interns than we did from some of the professors. The hours on ward service were horrendous, leaving little time for sleeping or eating, almost none for play. If we had spare time, it was spent in the library reading up on an "interesting case." Rounds with our professors were stimulating and exciting. Dr. McCann, our brilliant professor of medicine, was an artist at the bedside who made rare diagnoses seem easy. He had a way with patients, putting them at ease and performing his examinations with skill and gentleness. He never said anything to upset the patients and they enjoyed having him on teaching rounds. In addition to his teaching, Dr. McCann maintained a limited consulting practice and his experience in this area was transmitted to the students in very practical ways at the bedside. His noon clinics in the amphitheater were beautiful demonstrations of how to correlate basic data with clinical problems. He was, above all, an excellent teacher and speaker who made difficult problems seem easy. His chief associate, Dr. John S. Lawrence, was entirely different. He was a plodding, quiet, methodical person whose steady, slow relentless approach to a problem at the bedside, so different from Dr. McCann's, was equally good for the medical students. Our reaction was that if a plugger like John Lawrence could succeed in making diagnoses, then there must be hope for some of us with average capabilities and lacking McCann's brilliance. Rounds in obstetrics and gynecology with Karl Wilson and especially Robert Ritchie were the talk of the medical school. Ritchie, a McGill graduate, never published a paper, but he taught obstetrics and gynecology in a way we never forgot. He had the knack of telling stories you would always remember. He would usher us into a room and point to a woman with an obvious abdominal swelling, and start quizzing the group. Somewhere along the line, he would ask, "What is the most common tumor of the abdomen in a young woman?" The answer would vary from day to day. One day it would be pregnancy, another a distended bladder. If we forgot to mention the latter, he would not tell us this. He would say "You had better go down to Scrantom's (a pharmaceutical and medical supplies house in

Rochester) and buy a rubber necklace to put around your neck," the necklace being a catheter. On one occasion, a group of students was taking turns performing a pelvic examination on a patient who was under anesthesia preparatory to be being explored. Ritchie would always give us a misleading history as we warily approached this quiz session. On one occasion, one of the students achieved instant fame because of a slip in technique. Dr. Ritchie had taught us to always do a bimanual examination of the pelvis. The student proceeded with the examination and said that he felt a soft, six-centimeter mass. Ritchie interrupted him and asked, "With which hand do you feel the mass, doctor?" The student had his left hand in his pocket and not on the patient's abdomen. You can imagine how quickly he removed his left hand from his pocket and performed the examination as he had been taught. The rest of us never again made that mistake.

On another occasion in the gynecology outpatient clinic I was assigned to a patient who complained of left-lower-quadrant pain. After taking a thorough history, I proceeded with the general examination chaperoned by the student nurse. Then I asked for a pelvic-examination tray and proceeded to do a pelvic examination. I was quite certain I palpated an ovarian mass in the left adnexal region. At this juncture the attending gynecologist repeated the pelvic examination and said I was right. He recommended that she be admitted for operation. We explained this to the patient and she agreed. In the hospital, Dr. Karl Wilson, the chairman of the department, a kind and talented man, renowned as a teacher and widely known for his skill, met the patient for the first time, examined her and agreed that she should be operated upon. To everyone's surprise, she looked up at the professor and said she thought that her own doctor, "Dr. Lepore," was going to do the operation. Instead of laughing at this, Dr. Wilson quietly said that I would be in the operating room with him. When that day came, Dr. Wilson looked up at the small balcony and said, "Is Dr. Lepore there?" I answered "Yes sir." Dr. Wilson then said this patient wanted Dr. Lepore, to operate, "but I persuaded her that I would do it with you in attendance." This is a story that spread around the medical school like a brush fire. The lesson in it is that a great professor of obstetrics and gynecology would go to extremes to support the "doctor-patient" relationship of a medical student and his first gynecological patient.

Our professor of surgery, Dr. John Morton, impressed us all by his calmness and integrity. He was unshakable under fire, and in his quiet way instilled a respect in us for the work of the surgeon. He had a sound department of loyal and capable men who enjoyed having students around and spent a good deal of time with them. Pediatrics was well taught by Dr. S. W. Clausen and Dr. William Bradford, but for most of us it lacked the excitement and challenges of adult medicine. Psychiatry in those days was a very primitive specialty confined largely to institutionalized patients. This would change dramatically with the advent of Dr. John Romano after WW II as chairman of psychiatry. He revolutionized psychiatry not only at Rochester but across the country by placing it within the framework of the general hospital and clinics and introducing the concept of strong liaison programs with the major specialties. He brought psychiatry out of the closet of remote and separate institutions for the insane into the daylight of the wards and clinics and private rooms of our teaching hospitals. In my opinion, the appointment of this brilliant and dynamic scholar and humanist to Rochester was one of the best since that of our founding Dean, George Hoyt Whipple. Neurology was one of our best-taught subjects, the professor being a red-haired young man, Dr. Paul Garvey, who had the knack of instilling the fundamentals of solid clinical neurology into each of our minds. He published very little, but he knew clinical neurology and was a superb clinical teacher. Walking through the ward one day, a patient, in for some other complaints, made a flip remark about Dr. Garvey's red hair, and Garvey took one look at him and said, "He probably has a frontal-lobe tumor," which he did, to the utter consternation of those in charge of that patient. We emerged from the junior year as competent students who had developed good skills in history taking and physical examination, and we were real cracker-jacks at drawing blood, starting infusions, and doing blood counts and urine and stool examinations.

This is more than I can say for our modern counterparts who have been spared so much that they can do so little without an expensive technician or I.V. team at their side. Medicine remains a profession where doing is more important than reading about it. Decision-making, the actual experience in the laboratory, the actual feel of the abdomen, the smell of wards, the active exposure to people in distress, and the need to suffer with your patient, are the hallmarks of a good medical education. We got this and more during this wonderful tough third year at Rochester. We were never without our stethoscopes, knew how to use them, and were constantly improving our techniques of percussion, auscultation, and palpation. We had learned to lean very heavily upon our own senses and not to request excessive laboratory tests, x rays, etc. We were trained as clinicians, not technicians. Our role models preached this and practiced this. They inspired us to emulate them.

As I look back to those wonderful student years at Rochester, I realize how fortunate we were to have been among the last of the "Osler-trained" medical students of that era. Almost every one of my professors had been a student of Osler at Hopkins, and I know now that we were educated and trained by what Osler called "The Natural Method of Teaching the Subject of Medicine." In an essay published at the turn of the century, Osler said:

> I wish to tell a plain tale of the method of teaching medicine at the Johns Hopkins University. There is nothing very novel about it, except that in the third and fourth years the hospital is made the equivalent of the laboratories of the first and second and in it the student learns the practical art of medicine. This may be called the natural mode of teaching the subject. Ask a practitioner of twenty-years standing how he has become proficient in his art, he will reply, by constant contact with disease; and he will add that the medicine he learned in the school was totally different from the medicine he learned at the bedside. The graduate of a quarter of a century ago went out with little practical knowledge, which increased as his practice increased. In the natural method of teaching, the student begins with the patient, continues with the patient, and ends his studies with the patient, using books and lectures as tools, as means to an end.[15]

Osler, in his parting address at Johns Hopkins University on February 22, 1905, prior to moving to Oxford to be the regius professor of medicine, said:

> Personally, there is nothing in life in which I take greater pride than in my connection with the organization of the medical clinic (department) of the Johns Hopkins Hospital and with the introduction of the old-fashioned methods of practical instruction.—I desire no other epitaph—no hurry about it, I may say,—than the statement that I taught medical students in the wards, as I regard this by far as the most useful and important work I have been called upon to do.[16]

At Rochester when I was a student, paraphrasing Osler, we began with the patient, continued with the patient, and pursued our studies with the patient, using books, the library, conferences, the laboratory, and a minimum of lectures as tools, as a means to an end. But this was in an era when the public wards and dispensaries were the back-

---

15. *Journal of the American Medical Association* 36 (June 15, 1901), pp. 1673–1670.
16. *"The Fixed Period": William Osler in Aequanimitas* (Philadelphia: Blakiston and Son, 1932).

bone of the teaching services and private patients were in the minority, an era when Francis W. Peabody could say with accuracy that the
first person in a white coat seeing a new patient on the ward was usually a medical student. Peabody continues, addressing the student:

> Do you see what an opportunity you have? The foundation of
> your whole relation with the patient is laid in those first few min-
> utes of contact, just as happens in private practice. Here is a wor-
> ried, lonely, suffering man, and if you begin by approaching him
> with sympathy, tact, and consideration, you get his confidence
> and he becomes *your* patient. Interns and visiting physicians may
> come and go, and the hierarchy gives them a precedence, but if
> you make the most of your opportunities he will regard you as
> his personal physician and all the rest as mere consultants. Of
> course, you must not drop him after you have taken the history
> and made your physical examination. Once your relationship
> with him has been established you must foster it by every means.
> Watch his condition closely and he will see that you are alert pro-
> fessionally. Make time to have little talks with him and these talks
> need not always be about his symptoms. Remember that you
> want to know him as a man, and this means you must know
> about his family and friends, his work and his play. What kind of
> person is he—cheerful, depressed, introspective, careless, consci-
> entious, mentally keen or dull? Look out for all the little inciden-
> tal things that you can do for his comfort."

These too are a part of the "care of the patient," the phrase that
Peabody immortalized in the same essay that concluded with "One of
the essential qualities of the clinician is humanity, for the secret of the
care of the patient is in caring for the patient."[17]

I am afraid that in the current era of medicine and hospital practice and teaching, Peabody's advice, so appropriate for the twenties,
has a hollow ring in the nineties. Hospital admissions are short and to
the point with the ogres of DRG and the bureaucrats of Utilization
Review and Quality Assurance breathing down our necks. In the
major teaching hospitals most patients have their private attending
surgeons and physicians or are assigned to them. The students have
limited opportunity to spend time with patients assigned to them and
are seldom around at night or on weekends. The sickest patients are
in intensive-care units where specialist teams are in complete control

---

17. Francis Weld Peabody, "The Care of the Patient," *Journal of the American
Medical Association* 88 (March 19, 1928), pp. 877–82.

of treatment and management to the exclusion of the family doctor or generalist to say nothing of the medical student. As for patients who are not acutely ill, they are kept busy with diagnostic testing, CT scanning, ultrasonography, MRI imagery, x-ray, echocardiography, cardiac catheterization, endoscopy or nuclear imaging. If they are not, the Utilization Review people will be asking, "Why is the patient in the hospital?" If they are, the UR people will ask, "Why weren't these done as outpatient procedures?" All in all this is not an ideal environment for conducting a first-rate teaching program and, in fact, many teaching programs are second rate. Teaching at the bedside has become a lost art replaced by "corridor or cafeteria-type" rounds, "chart" rounds, and discussions in conference rooms. The essential missing element is the patient. Grand Rounds are no longer Grand. Neither are they Rounds. Instead we have a plethora of lectures or seminars by outside lecturers funded by pharmaceutical houses. Almost never will a patient be shown at today's so-called Grand Rounds. This means that the students and house staff as well as the attending staff have little or no exposure to much of the teaching material in the hospital. Neither do they participate in the preparation or presentation required in the old style Grand Rounds. Ask a medical student in this day and age to make a formal case presentation on rounds without notes and be prepared to witness a shallow and disappointing performance almost without exception. They simply have not been taught how to do this. Osler said the Master Word in Medicine is WORK. The current system of teaching medicine fails to adequately utilize the students, house staff, and attending staff in the teaching program. They should be put to work. I feel this trend is a giant step backward and an abandonment of the teaching methods pioneered by the greatest physician and teacher of modern times. Clearly, the hospital is no longer the ideal place for training and educating medical students for the practice of medicine. For some ailments the hospital setting is superb while for others it is a disaster. Outpatient clinics too, have changed remarkably. Whereas in the distant past their makeup in the major teaching centers consisted largely of poor people with chronic diseases, the shift has been toward alcoholics, drug addicts, welfare recipients, sometimes second and third generation, single-parent children and the mentally retarded or mentally ill, and patients with AIDS. In the decaying inner cities, emergency rooms are flooded with people with minor complaints who do not have a family doctor or cannot afford one. The low-income, elderly middle-class people who used to frequent the outpatient clinics are now seeing private physicians with the assistance of Medicare. Others are enrolled in HMOs and "managed care" insurance plans. Because of this shift in clinic demography, some major medical schools have resorted to assigning their students to preceptors in private practice. The problem is that the large classes in many medical schools are simply too much for the preceptors to cope with and there are not enough volunteers to supply the demand. Faculty group practice, a rarity in Osler's day, is now a major source of income for all medical schools and serves to attract patients to the medical school that may be used for teaching purposes as well as income. Criticism of the burgeoning Faculty Group Practice is that the full-time men and women who should be devoting most of their time to teaching and research are now tied up with "service" demands and competing with local practitioners. Academic recognition for good teaching has, in the past, been niggardly in many medical schools, the major kudos going for research, much of it of pedestrian quality.

As a seasoned clinical teacher, I have witnessed serious deterioration in the teaching of medicine at the bedside with quasi-abandonment of the "natural method" advocated and practiced so brilliantly by Sir William Osler. In evaluating performance, multiple-choice examinations have displaced the essay type and several generations of medical students, who lack the ability to write acceptable prose, have been graduated without experience in case presentation before audiences or their teachers. Jacques Barzun, in his biting comments on Education in general, says much that can and should be said about Medical Education:

> Forget Education. Education is a result, a slow growth, and hard to judge: Let us talk rather about Teaching and Learning, a joint activity that can be provided for, though as a nation, we have lost the knack of it. The blame falls on the public schools, of course, but they deserve only half the blame. The other half belongs to the people at large, us—our attitudes, our choices, our thought clichés. Teaching is a demanding often back-breaking job; it should not be done with energy left over after meetings and pointless paperwork that have drained hope and faith in the enterprise. Accountability, the latest cure in vogue, is to be looked for only in results. Good Teaching is usually well known to all concerned without questionnaires or approved lesson plans. The number of good teachers who are now shackled by bureaucratic obligations to superiors who know little or nothing about the classroom cannot even be guessed at. They deserve from an Education President an Emancipation "Proclamation."[18]

---

18. Jacques Barzun, *Begin Here — The Forgotten Conditions of Teaching and Learning* (Chicago and London: The University of Chicago Press, 1991), pp. lx, 19.

I perceive that the Teaching of Medicine has drifted steadily away from the patient who should have remained at the center of the entire action. In my day at Rochester our clinical teachers were, almost without exception, Oslerians who focused their efforts on the care of the patient, following the Natural Method of Teaching championed by Sir William Osler.

I believe the time has come to return to the Oslerian methods that revolutionized American medical education at the turn of the century. My plea is to return the medical student and his teachers to the bedside and reinstall the patient as the centerpiece of Grand Rounds.

I spent the summer of 1933 in Dr. Whipple's department working as a paid technical assistant in the plasmapheresis project. Our main experiment was to prove that the dog can be maintained in positive nitrogen balance by giving intravenous plasma protein as the only source of protein. As the senior year approached, I had an important session with Dr. Whipple concerning my plans. I had received the Master of Science degree in 1931 from the University of Rochester for my research work during the physiology fellowship, and the question had arisen whether I should write a thesis for a Ph.D. in addition to my M.D. degree. Dr. Whipple advised me that if I took a Ph.D. degree, which he was sure I could obtain, I would always be identified as a laboratory man, despite the acquisition of the M.D. degree, and clinicians would regard me with suspicion. He said that in place of this, the medical school was instituting an M.D. Degree with Honor, which would recognize the thesis and be the equivalent of a Ph.D. without the actual title. This seemed very good advice to me, and I accepted it and wrote the thesis for which the award was made to me in 1934, the first such award at the University of Rochester's School of Medicine. It read as follows:

> Michael J. Lepore, having completed with distinction the four-year course in the School of Medicine and Dentistry of the University of Rochester, having spent an extra year in 1930–1931 as Fellow in Physiology in teaching and research work, and having demonstrated in this year and in subsequent summers and spare time an unusual ability and inclination for research work, as evidenced by this thesis and the accompanying publications, is hereby recommended by the Advisory Board for the Degree, Doctor of Medicine with Honor.
>
> G. H. Whipple
> Dean
> June 5, 1934

The senior year at Rochester was then an easier one than the junior-year experience. We were more confident, and we knew that no one had ever been failed in his senior year. The assignments were in the outpatient department and the hours of work were different and lighter than in the junior year. The people we saw were not very sick and diagnostic problems became our main concern. We also had opportunities to follow patients who had been treated for years for various chronic diseases, diabetes, anemias, ulcers, heart disease, renal disease, arthritis, etc. The teachers in the outpatient department were, most of them, leaders in medical practice in Rochester who enjoyed telling us about their experiences. Some were extremely effective teachers. The senior year was also our time for quick exposure to the various subspecialty areas. I must confess that most of this experience was quite superficial and mundane—at least at that stage in our careers.

Two types of training assignments brightened up the year. One was the opportunity to substitute for two weeks on one of the inpatient services, working as an intern. I did this in surgery and had a wonderful time, and even enjoyed the drudgery of holding retractors and assisting at various operations. The surgical resident under whom I served was Dr. Louis Goldstein, who was an excellent teacher and, predictably, had a stellar career in surgery at Rochester rising to professor of surgery and chief of orthopedics. I still remember the long hours of standing by while Dr. William P. Van Wagenen did a craniotomy on a patient with multiple meningiomata. He said to me that I would probably never see another such patient, and he proved to be absolutely correct. Another two-week stint was spent riding the ambulance in the days when ambulances always had a doctor when they were sent out on a call. One dramatic experience was being called out to the local airport to a smoke-filled tavern where a tall, obese man was stretched out on the floor, unconscious, the bartender claiming that he had nothing to drink but one Bromoseltzer. The man was an aeroplane pilot who had just landed his plane with passengers, complained of severe headache, and had gone to the tavern for a Bromoseltzer and then passed out. We put him on a stretcher and placed him in the ambulance and headed for Strong Memorial. On the way, I attempted to give artificial respiration and discovered that I could not push on his abdomen because it seemed to contain a mass. His blood pressure was quite high. By the time we reached the hospital, we had decided correctly that the man probably had polycystic kidneys with hypertension and had suffered a stroke secondary to his hypertension. I could never understand why this man was flying an aeroplane without adequate medical clearance.

During the senior year we had to make plans for our internships and it was not easy. First we had to decide what we really wanted to do. Dean Whipple felt that any graduate of his medical school had the equivalent of a rotating internship by the time of his graduation and he advised all of us to take straight internships, i.e., medicine, surgery, obstetrics, pediatrics, etc., rather than to waste our time in a one-year rotating internship with superficial exposure of short duration to a variety of specialties. So it was that most of us applied for straight internships. Nowadays, applying for an internship is much simpler than it used to be, largely because of the so-called matching plan and the agreement upon a uniform acceptance day. For those unfamiliar with the matching plan, each applicant lists his choice of hospitals for internship in the order of his own preference, and the hospitals list their preferences. These applications are then matched by a computer, and on a day in the middle of March, the decisions for all internships in America are made. In my day, hospital internship acceptance days varied from right now to April and there simply was no rhyme or reason except for old established traditions. Many of the major hospitals still adhered to "examinations" to gain appointment. One of these was the Presbyterian Hospital in New York City, which usually held its examinations in March or April, long after other hospitals had made their selections. Dr. McCann had offered me a position in medicine at Strong Memorial, which I declined with thanks, indicating that I had spent five years and several summers in Rochester and thought I should try my wings somewhere else. He appreciated my feelings and offered to hold an opening for me at Rochester pending my receipt of an appointment elsewhere. Elsewhere was the Presbyterian Hospital in New York, where I was attracted by the presence on their staff of Dr. Robert F. Loeb, a brilliant clinician, teacher, and investigator, the son of the renowned Jacques Loeb.

I had made rounds with Dr. Loeb and seen his work with Addison's disease, to which he had made a great contribution in finding that he could prolong lives of those afflicted by supplying large amounts of plain table salt. Loeb had encouraged me to apply to Presbyterian for my internship and indicated that he would support my application. The late acceptance date at Presbyterian meant a real gamble because if I waited, I would be placing all of my eggs in one basket by passing up hospitals whose acceptance dates were earlier in the year. I decided to take my chances, secure in the feeling that with my sound scholastic record, membership in Alpha Omega Alpha, the medical school equivalent of Phi Beta Kappa and Sigma Xi, the Science Honor Society, my M.S. in physiology, my M.D. with Honor, and research publications, there should be no great problem. I came home for the Christmas holidays in December 1933, and telephoned

Dr. Loeb who asked me what had happened to me when the examinations for Presbyterian were advanced to November, and wondered whether I had decided to stay at Rochester. Apparently, through a secretarial error, I had not been notified of the change in the date of examination. Loeb was greatly upset and suggested that I call Dr. Walter Palmer, the Bard Professor, at his farm in Lee, Massachusetts and gave me his telephone number. I did so and, of course, nothing could be done about it, and Dr. Palmer apologized for the error. My next telephone call was to Dr. McCann at Rochester who had held a job open for me until the last minute and had only within the previous twenty-four hours released it to a woman graduate of Johns Hopkins. The telegram had not yet been delivered, but it was too late to call back, and several days later she accepted the internship and I was left high and dry at a bad time of the year. Dr. McCann who had always advised us against going to Boston, now suggested that I try for a position at the Boston City Hospital, where Soma Weiss was the charismatic, brilliant young professor on the Harvard service. Weiss said the competition was keen and the decisions almost made, but thought I should come up and try for it. I took the train to Boston and when I arrived at the Boston City Hospital I found an interesting collection of medical seniors milling around outside the Board Room, where the inquisition called an "examination" would be held. Here I met Gene Scadron from Duke University Medical School who was also applying for an internship. Gene knew everybody and he quickly apprised me of the real situation. He said it was almost a waste of time to have made the trip to Boston because there was really only one medical job open and that was almost certainly going to Charlie Janeway, a Harvard graduate and the son of the great Theodore Janeway of Hopkins and Columbia University College of Physicians and Surgeons' fame. Nevertheless, I went through the charade. When I walked into the large room, it was filled with some of the greatest men in America medicine, among them George Minot, Soma Weiss, Bill Castle, Chester Keefer, Max Finland, and many others. It was a rather frightening experience for a raw recruit and I know I didn't set any track record by my answers to their questions, one of which I remember, "What is the Teleoroentgenogram?" I guessed at it and finally confessed that we had never used it at Rochester. Neither have we any place else where I have been. The job went to Janeway. Later, I talked to Gene Scadron, who told me about the new medical school at Duke and suggested that I apply there. When I returned to Rochester after the holidays, I went to Dr. Whipple with my story and he was very sympathetic. He said he knew Dr. Frederic M. Hanes, the new professor at Duke, from Hopkins days and he would write to him. Almost by return mail, sight unseen, I received a letter of acceptance as an intern in medicine at Duke. Several weeks later, Dr. McCann saw me in the hall and said he had just received a letter from Dr. Longcope telling him that a vacancy had developed at Hopkins when a student selected for internship had become ill, and asking Dr. McCann to recommend someone to him. Dr. McCann said he was recommending me and was quite certain I could have the position. I then told him that I had only recently accepted an internship at Duke with Dean Whipple's intervention and could not go back on my word. He was disappointed because he would have liked to place me at Hopkins. I have told this anecdote in some detail because it illustrates the muddle we were in at that period in medicine, with no real system for filling internships. Many good people failed to get appointments matched to their competence. It was a haphazard, unimpressive way to launch idealistic young people into the most important phase of their careers. Reform was needed but it would be a long time in coming. In retrospect, I must confess that the Duke appointment turned out to be one of the best things that ever happened to me in more ways than one. I have tried to describe what it was like to be a medical student in this exciting new school at Rochester in 1929–34. As I look back, I realize that the educational experience was beyond belief, solid, inspiring, scientific, humane, and incredibly personal.

What a wonderful start for the lifetime of learning and practice that lay ahead. Dean George Whipple, with George Eastman's strong financial and personal support plus that of the Rockefeller General Education Board spearheaded by Abraham Flexner, had succeeded almost overnight in establishing a great medical school with a brilliant future. Even in his wildest dreams Flexner could not have hoped for anything better. True it is that at one point, when the medical-school faculty decided to modify its full-time plan, he tried to browbeat them and threatened all sorts of dire developments and predicted that the compromise could ruin the future of the school. In this prediction, he was of course, terribly wrong. But more on that later.

On 14 March 1932, a little after noon, our medical school was shaken up by a tragic occurrence. Its greatest benefactor, George Eastman, who had been sick and getting weaker each day, had died by his own hand from a pistol shot, leaving this note. "To my friends: My work is finished. Why wait?" The sense of loss hung heavy on the institution, for Eastman was not only the source of financial support, he had become a great and true friend of the medical school, its Dean, and the faculty families. The loss was irreplaceable, but it served to stimulate all who knew him to forge ahead to fulfill the great expectations Eastman had for his medical school.

Tangible evidence of the fulfillment was not long delayed, for in 1934 George Hoyt Whipple, with Minot and Murphy, shared the Nobel Prize in Medicine for the liver treatment of pernicious anemia. Years later Dr. Whipple was to say, "A Nobel Prize announcement comes to any individual with a shock which cannot be defined, disbelief, doubt and self examination, excitement, curiosity as to the official protocol, and so on." The announcement electrified our medical school and each of us seemed to grow a foot in stature as we shared the honor with our less fortunate schools.

The announcement of the award reached us at Duke, where I was interning in the fall of 1934, and caused quite a stir. Duke, like Rochester an offshoot of Hopkins, together with Dean Wilburt C. Davison and Professor of Medicine Frederic M. Hanes (both disciples and students of Osler), celebrated as if Dean Whipple had been one of its own.

Dean Whipple, an Oslerian to the core, had this to say about Osler in his "Autobiographic Sketch":

> Our class (Hopkins 1905) looked forward with great expectations to our contact with Dr. Osler, and we were not disappointed. Many believed him to be the greatest clinical teacher of his generation and I am among that number. His personality was magnetic, and a smile would make a friend for life. Clinical diagnosis came with rare insight. He loved students, both junior and senior types, and enjoyed having a fringe of them at hand for his rounds on the wards. He was very proud that he was largely responsible for first bringing the medical student in the wards for active teaching and diagnosis. His large clinics were never to be forgotten, and he usually added important points because of his knowledge of pathology, often presenting autopsy material. When he decided to accept the regius professorship at Oxford, it might be said that the school and hospital went into mourning. We felt most fortunate that he completed our clinical teaching courses in 1905 before he left Baltimore—we said he graduated with us.[19]

In 1968, Dr. Wallace Fenn, in honor of Dr. Whipple's ninetieth birthday, said of Whipple's medical school:

---

19. G. H. Whipple, "An Autobiographical Sketch," *Perspectives in Biol. & Med 2,* no. 3 (Spring 1959), pp. 253-89.

This is the House that George Built.
These are the students that George allowed
To enter the school so well endowed
To train in the House that George Built.

These are the teachers of wisdom and wit
Thought by George to be worthy and fit,
To teach the students who came to sit
Here in the House that George Built.

So this is the George, New Hampshire-born
Who mastered the art of living long,
And whose ninetieth birthday finds him still
Working away at his desk with a will,
In his brick-lined room, still unadorned
With paint or plaster he so much scorned.

So, courage my friends and be of good cheer
For we can be sure that George is still here
Watching his school grow year by year
Guarding the House that George Built.[20]

To this day, I marvel that one man, Dean Whipple, could plan and build a great medical center from scratch, interview most of the applicants for admission, administer a great and growing organization, personally teach us pathology, engage in productive research, remain an excellent fisherman and hunter, win a Nobel Prize and almost every other conceivable honor, and to the very end of his 97 years recognize his students and continue to be interested in them and to follow their careers with concern and obvious enjoyment. George Whipple said in an interview late in life that he wished to be remembered as a teacher. This he was in the grand tradition. His students will never forget and they will strive to keep forever verdant the memory of this amazing man.

---

20. Dr. Fenn's discourse was published under the title "Nonagenarian Nobelist is on hand at 'his' school's 50th birthday," *JAMA,* 233/8 (August 25, 1975), pp.851-6.

Chapter 6

※◆※

Duke University Hospital and Its Medical School, 1934–1935

For a young man who had never been below the Mason-Dixon Line, my first intimation of what was to come was when I woke up in my Pullman upper berth 30 June 1934 and felt as if I were in a hot shower. But it was only Baltimore in late June with its usual sweltering and oppressive heat in an era before there was any air conditioning. By the time we reached Durham, North Carolina, I began to wonder whether I could take the climate or whether it would take me. I thought back to my Southern Italian ancestry and was comforted by my belief that I must have some genetic protection against the heat. I was mighty glad to get off that train to head for Duke Hospital. That year, I was the only "northerner" or "Yankee" on the medical house staff; in fact I was the only non-Duke graduate. Clearly I was a marked man right from the start. The house staff already on the scene had appropriated the best rooms and I was treated to a hot-box facing an inner courtyard that was virtually without air circulation, resounding, especially in the early morning hours, with bedlam in the kitchens and laundries as well as the roistering of the almost entirely black staff of employees. To top it off, Howland Ward, the appropriately named pediatric unit, abutted the courtyard and was filled to the rafters with howling noisy infants and children whose clatter was enhanced by bouncing off the walls of the courtyard. Clearly, my friends-to-be on the house staff had done a job on the new man from Rochester. It took me a while to adjust to these conditions and it was not easy. Years later, Dean Davison said "our worst error [in the construction of Duke Hospital] was in having interior courtyards, which in Durham summers before air conditioning were a foretaste of Hades." The heavy demands of my new job soon took my mind off the climate. My first assignment was one month on the laboratory service. I believe they thought this was the best way to introduce a stranger, a "Yankee" no less, to a different world. I also learned that the assignment was tough and demanding and one that was not too popular with the house staff—"too much scut work," they said.

My duties involved almost full time in what was then called bacteriology under the aegis of Mary Poston, chief technician, who was meticulous and demanding but, I learned, a topflight bacteriologist and human being. I was responsible for all cultures and smears of blood, urine, sputum, spinal fluid, stools, and autopsy cultures for the medical service.

I was also responsible for cross-matching all donors and recipients on the medical floors and administering whatever transfusions were needed using the citrate anticoagulant technique. This wasn't as bad as it sounds. There were no blood banks and transfusions were few because people could not afford them. Since we had a good deal of brucellosis, tularemia, typhoid, and dysentery there were many agglutination titres to be done in addition to blood cultures and thick and thin smears for malaria. There was a great deal of interest in fungal diseases, including blastomycosis and coccidioidomycosis, histoplasmosis, and others. Dr. David T. Smith was the professor in charge of bacteriology and also was a professor of medicine. He was a charming man, beloved by all of the students, the house staff, and patients. He had the uncanny knack of being able to pluck a suspicious piece of gunk out of a sputum we had already examined to no avail, coming up with a critical demonstration of a fungus or acid-fast organism.

He was a superb teacher who brought out the best in his house staff by his own brilliance and enthusiasm. He had been ill with tuberculosis and spent time at Saranac's Trudeau Sanitorium, where he learned a great deal about his ailment and led research in this field at Duke. He was in a great measure responsible for setting the policy that tuberculosis be treated at Duke within the framework of an active general hospital like any other disease rather than a pariah-like illness to be treated with fear, isolation, and trepidation. As a result, my training in chest disease, mycology, and tuberculosis was far superior to that available in most large teaching medical centers. This would pay several dividends in my future. Another part of the work of the laboratory intern was supervising the "hot box." This was a primitive home-made wooden box resembling a pine coffin filled with large electric light bulbs generating a great deal of heat used to raise the enclosed patient's temperature to high fever levels, 104–105 degrees, a part of the therapy for syphilis or gonorrhea. After watching some of the patients suffer, I could almost believe that the Lord had invented hyperthermia as punishment for transgressions. I had no experience with fever therapy with patients and did my best to understand its hazards and indications. During the first month I had a run-in with an obnoxious attending physician who tried to blame me for the collapse of his patient who had undergone 4–5 hours of fever therapy, denying that he had ever given an order for it.

This shook me up a bit until I checked with Miss Tinsley, the nurse in charge, who fortunately for me, kept a separate order book that contained the required order by that attending physician to administer fever therapy at 104–105 degrees for 4–5 hours. I checked with Everett Pool our chief resident who said to me not to worry— that Dr. H. P. frequently made these threats and claims without reason or justification.

One good thing that came out of this experience was that I used my physiology training to measure sweat volume, urine volume, and chlorides in patients undergoing fever therapy and discovered large losses that demanded aggressive IV replacement to avoid dehydration, hypovolemia, and shock. Certain patients were more apt to do this than others. I was invited to go to Dayton, Ohio, in May 1935 to present a paper on this subject on a program organized by the famous Boss Kettering, the inventor of the self-starter, who was interested in fever therapy for arthritis and had designed an elegant hotbox that was easy to run and humidified so that water and electrolyte losses were kept to a minimum. Boss Kettering was an interesting man and quite likeable. I was disappointed that he did not offer to give or lend us one of his hotboxes for Duke Hospital.

I had a good time at this meeting and met some other interesting people. In passing, Dr. Hanes had provided the funds for this trip and he also offered to send me to nearby Louisville, Kentucky, for the Kentucky Derby. I had already made plans to get back to Durham on Derby Day Saturday to escort my girlfriend (later my wife) to a dance at the Washington Duke Hotel with Johnny Long's band providing the music, and there was no way I was going to miss this part of our courtship. I was reluctant to tell this to Dr. Hanes, who was a strict and dedicated Oslerian who believed in refrigerating the emotions until completion of residency training. I had the gall to tell the professor that I couldn't accept his kind offer because I thought the money would be better spent on research.

Duke Hospital and its medical school were very interesting places in 1934. They were both young, in fact, almost brand new, growing, innovative, and extremely informal. I found southerners to be warm and outgoing and friendly. A word of greeting was always passed when strangers met in the halls or on the street and good manners were the order of the day. The Dean of the medical school, Dr. Wilburt Cornell Davison, son of a Methodist minister from Long Island, was a former Rhodes Scholar, a protégé of Sir William Osler, and a graduate of Princeton University, Oxford University, and the Johns Hopkins University School of Medicine. He was a big man in many ways, over six feet tall and weighing over 200 pounds. He was warm and informal, often working without a necktie and in short-sleeve shirts. His concern for his students and house staff was legendary and set the tone for the entire medical school. In the early years he personally interviewed every applicant for his medical school, mirroring the approach used by founding Dean George Hoyt Whipple at Rochester, one of his former teachers at Hopkins.

A Hopkins graduate and teacher of pediatrics, he was a devotee of that institution and he filled most of the key positions at Duke with Hopkins graduates or faculty. When I arrived at Duke, the chairman of the department of medicine was Dr. Frederic M. Hanes, a Hopkins graduate class of 1908, a student of Osler's, and a student and friend of my mentor, Dean George H. Whipple of Rochester, who had arranged for me to intern at Duke Hospital. Dr. Hanes was on summer vacation when I arrived. The medical service was being administered by Dr. David T. Smith.

Interning at Duke Hospital in 1934 meant that you were really "interned" in the hospital and not living off the premises. Only one of the interns was married. She was a very bright and pleasant woman known to us as "Sis" Easley. We were on the Hopkins plan, on 24-hour call with no nights or weekends off. The only way we could get away from the hospital was to ask one of our peers to take our calls for a few hours. The problem with this, I soon found out, was that you might be suckered into accepting calls for an intern who had already assumed responsibility for the calls of several other interns. Being on call around the clock could be heavy duty but it really was not as difficult as it seemed at first glance. For example, if your ward were full, there simply was no room for an additional patient. If the ward was half empty, you were a sitting duck for new admissions. Turnover and length of stay were much slower than in the present era, and intensive-care units did not exist. Duke Hospital was at the end of a quadrangle terminating in the cathedral-like chapel and on opposite sides flanked by a movie house and a so-called "dope" shop, the dope of that era being Coca Cola made up fresh at a soda fountain pump for a nickel with lots of ice. Movies were shown twice weekly and we could sign out to the on-campus movie where the telephone operator could call us. Of course, there were no beepers. There was no code 99 signal to alert us to an emergency. Meals were served to us by waitresses at tables covered with linen. The food was generally good to excellent. There was plenty of ice water.

The month on laboratory service was a fine experience for me. I was fresh from reviewing my bacteriology for the New York State Board examinations and found that my superb course in bacteriology (now called microbiology) at Rochester, taught by our famous professor, Stanhope Bayne-Jones, was serving me well. Miss Mary Poston, a hard taskmaster from Hopkins, found me to be an excellent student and we were able to turn out some topflight work. In fact, my first intimation that things were going well at Duke was when our chief resident, Everett Pool, announced to our house staff that "we finally have an intern in the lab who can really grow things out of our cultures, a far cry from his predecessor who couldn't grow E. coli out of a barrel of feces." However, he used a four-letter word for the latter.

In those days, we served every afternoon in the outpatient clinic, working up new patients, most of whom had been driven considerable distances to keep their appointments. Gas was cheap and so were the cars, mainly model-T Fords. Every Thursday evening, in the Hopkins tradition, we held "L" Clinic (Luetic Clinic) for the many syphilitics who needed long-term treatment. The clinic would start at six or seven P.M. and continue until we finished with the last patient. Not infrequently this would be midnight.

The clinic clientele was almost entirely black. I had never seen a clinic like it. The women were dressed up for the occasion, wearing castoff evening gowns and slippers probably given to them by their employers. The chatter was active and boisterous and there was much laughter. The atmosphere was that of a social event of some importance for these people and an opportunity to meet old friends and make new ones. The staff encouraged this ambience because it led the patients to keep their weekly appointments and to continue with their treatment protocols.

In those days, 606 (arsphenamine) and Bismuth were the therapeutic agents of choice. The 606 could be toxic and extreme care was needed to be certain it was administered into a vein and did not infiltrate into adjoining tissue where it would be very irritating leading to necrosis and phlebitis. For this reason the 606 injections were given by "Smitty," an expert technician who was better with intravenous therapy than most doctors. The interns were not allowed to give IV 606. The Bismuth injections were given intramuscularly and were safe for the interns to administer. There was a Bismuth room for the women and another for men. Three of them would enter the room, drop their drawers or pants, bend over a table and then were zinged in a buttock with the viscid gooey Bismuth sub-salicylate via a large-caliber steel hypodermic needle. The trick in giving it was to zap the needle into the target area, almost like shooting darts—the quicker the better. After each injection a sterile needle was inserted onto the same loaded syringe for injection into the next patient. The viscosity of the Bismuth sub-salicylate required a strong hand to push in the injection. Fortunately my work in the ice business had given me excellent hand muscles. I soon got to be quite expert at this, treating 40 or 50 patients a night. I knew I was doing well when I could hear my patients in the outside corridor yelling, "Ah wants the little doctor. He don't hurt."

As a "reward" for this work in the injection rooms, the interns were allowed to do the spinal taps required for followup of all patients with syphilis. These were done at the end of the clinic and it might be pretty late at times. This is where I learned to do spinal taps with skill, speed and accuracy, an asset that would come in very handy later when we were faced with a polio epidemic, and various types of meningitis.

The patients making up the teaching material at Duke differed quite a bit from those at Rochester where there were very few black patients and a majority of better-educated individuals who could give accurate histories of illness. It took me a while to learn the nuances of communication with some of the Duke patients. In the syphilis clinic it was useless to ask the patient whether he had ever had a chancre. The code word was to ask him if he had ever had a "haircut," the local term for chancre. The word clap had no geographic boundaries and was universally recognized. When we questioned them about buboes, the term "blue balls" rang a bell. Among some of the white Tarheels, there were curious words derived from old English such as "the boil swaged down," meaning "assuaged." One of the our chief residents, Bob McMillan, a native of North Carolina, claimed that he could tell what town in that state any patient came from by his accent and manner of speaking. I tried him out on this several times and he was indeed accurate.

A number of exotic and unusual diseases found their way to Duke for diagnosis and treatment. One day I was called to the emergency room to see a young black male writhing in severe abdominal pain and crying out in distress. His story was that he and a friend decided to use a two holer on the farm where they were working. They sat on the toilet seats for several minutes and suddenly were bitten in the scrotum and very quickly developed a terrible bellyache. The doctor who was called was a very bright young physician newly arrived in the community. He suspected a black widow spider bite, saw them on the toilet seat, captured a number, placed them in a Mason jar and immediately sent the two young men and the jar to Durham in a funeral hearse, the usual emergency vehicle in those days. One patient was sent to Lincoln Hospital, and the other to Duke. When I saw the patient I recalled having read somewhere that calcium gluconate intravenously was the remedy for a black widow spider bite, so I started an IV infusion and gave the patient calcium gluconate. Fortunately he responded well and recovered. His friend was not so lucky; he was thought to have a perforated ulcer and underwent an unnecessary operation at the other hospital.

For some reason we were seeing a high incidence of patients at Duke with Hodgkin's disease at that time. For several years, the Duke staff thought that Hodgkin's was caused by brucella infection, but the final judgment was that the two diseases were not causally related but commensal. One day I admitted a young man with fever, sweats, and markedly enlarged lymph nodes in the neck and axillae and diagnosed him as having Hodgkin's disease with Pel-Ebstein crises. On rounds the next morning I presented the patient to my attending, thinking I had touched all bases. To my dismay, the attending asked the young man whether he was a hunter and, getting an affirmative reply, elicited a history of rabbit hunting and skinning the rabbit and then cooking and eating it. The attending then asked the patient to extend his fingers and noted an ulcerated area on the tip of an index finger. The actual diagnosis was tularemia, the first case I had ever seen. The attending physician was not one of my favorites and he knew he had shafted me and he gloated and rubbed it in. This was a mistake because he should have known that by the rules of the academic medical game I would be looking to catch him the next time around.

The next time around was when I was making rounds on the private service and learned that a medical student had been admitted during the night with fever thought to be due to a respiratory infection. I looked in on the student and noted that he appeared quite lethargic and had a headache and slight stiffness of his neck. I also learned that he and his partner had been doing a sacrifice experiment on a cat two weeks before. While being anesthetized the cat had managed to scratch both of them. The cat's brain was sent to the State Laboratory in Raleigh, North Carolina, for rabies testing as a routine measure. The cat did have rabies, Negri bodies were found, and the two medical students were started on anti-rabies vaccine. My patient had received his twelfth injection a few days before becoming ill. I quickly got in touch with our professor, Dr. Hanes, who was an excellent neurologist. He dropped everything and came right up to the floor and pretty soon the place was flooded with people, including the chagrined attending who had missed the diagnosis. We did a spinal tap that revealed lymphocytic pleocytosis and elevation of spinal-fluid protein. A quick review of the literature established that this was not an unheard-of complication of rabies vaccine therapy and for some odd reason it usually occurred with the thirteenth injection. The prognosis was serious. We called Dr. Thomas Rivers, world-renowned virologist at the Rockefeller Institute Hospital in New York, and he discussed the case with us at some length. His final words were "in the event of a fatal outcome please send me a specimen of the spinal cord." You may well imagine how we felt when the conversation ended. There was nothing we could do except to wait, using supportive measures and excellent nursing care. The patient just happened to be a bright and charming student, the son of the Dean of the Duke University Law School. We were all very upset and felt so helpless. We had a number of very anxious days but slowly the patient improved and he made a complete recovery without any neurologic sequelae. In fact, he lived to write an excellent paper on rabies vaccine reactions.[1] The other medical student had no adverse reaction to the same vaccine. He went on to become a distinguished pathologist and chairman of the department of pathology at Duke University. I saw him again twenty-five years later when he gave the George Hoyt Whipple Lecture at the University of Rochester School of Medicine. With Dr. Whipple, then in his eighties, in the front row, Dr. Kinney regaled us with the story that years before he had applied for an internship in pathology under Dr. Whipple. He said he was turned down, but his letter of rejection was so warm, complimentary, and kind that he continued to carry it in his pocket until it was worn out.

Duke had more than its share of nutritional disorders filling the wards. This was in the midst of the worst depression this country has ever seen. The share-croppers were relying on the tobacco crop for money and were said to be too lazy to plant gardens and raise crops and vegetables. It was not unusual for them to come to us with scurvy, beriberi, pellagra, and other nutritional ills. Illegal stills abounded in the hills and moonshine liquor called "Cawn" was abundant. They could not afford medical care of any sort and resorted to patent medicine advertised and sold over the counter. One of the most popular was something called B-C. The tablets or powders containing Bromide were used for everything from headaches to rheumatism, "nerves," backache, or flu, and it was not unusual for people to take them three or four times a day. As a result, many patients coming to Duke had chronic bromide intoxication manifested sometimes by severe psychoses and erratic behavior. On occasion, bromide intoxication was lethal. I soon learned that one of the manifestations of bromide intoxication was severe nightmares. When I made night rounds on my ward it was not unusual to spot a patient with unsuspected bromism by witnessing a severe nightmare. A blood bromide

---

1. Harold M. Horack, "Allergy as a Factor in the Development of Reactions to Anti-Rabic Treatment," *Am J Med Sci* 197 (January–June 1939), pp. 672–682.

level would seal the diagnosis and treatment with plain IV normal saline would cure the condition.

The most lethal of the nutritional disorders seen at Duke in those days was pellagra. I quickly learned the acronym for this disease, the four D's—Diarrhea, Dermatitis, Dementia, and Death. Dr. D. T. Smith and Dr. Julian Ruffin were studying this disease intensively and seeking out its etiology. One of the problems was that when patients with pellagra were admitted to our wards, they were placed on the ward diet and this alone seemed to cure the pellagra if they were able to eat. For purposes of clinical investigation, on admission they were served a special control diet similar to what they were eating at home without the corn liquor supplement. Some of the patients would become very ill on this regime and they needed to be watched very closely. On occasion one of the patients might die, probably of cardiac arrest. In those days there were no flame photometers or autoanalyzers and it was impractical to perform serum electrolyte studies that today would be routine for any patient with severe malnutrition, diarrhea, and dehydration. During the course of this study, it was found at Duke that a positively vile-tasting crude-liver extract made by the Valentine Company of Richmond, Virginia, could cure pellagra. The biochemists on Drs. Smith and Ruffin's team were busy trying to isolate the curative factor and seemed hot on the trail but failed to find the Holy Grail before a team of investigators headed by Conrad Elvehjem at Wisconsin discovered that it was nicotinic acid, a member of the B complex, present in considerable quantities in Valentine's Liver Extract. Nicotinic acid tablets were cheap, easy to take, and soon intravenous preparations were made available. A life-threatening disease could now be turned completely around, cured, and prevented by a good diagnostician and a few inexpensive tablets costing less than ten cents a day.

Remember that this was in the pre-antibiotic era, when little or nothing could be done for most infections. Typhoid fever remained a menace, its treatment differing not a whit from that used by Osler before the turn of the century. Observing a patient with typhoid fever with a bellyache could be scary and very worrisome for a young intern fearing perforation, hemorrhage, and general sepsis. Malaria was not uncommon on the wards, its treatment with quinine being one of the few "specific" remedies available. We had nothing for the many cases of brucellosis, tularemia, and tuberculosis. Staphylococcal and streptococcal bacteremia were lethal disorders, our professors saying that of the two, they would rather have streptococcal sepsis with its acute demise or recovery than the staphylococcal with its prolonged and painful course. Subacute bacterial endocarditis was a death warrant when diagnosed. We were pretty clever at spotting it on clinical grounds but helpless to treat it for there was no cure.

Gonococcal endocarditis was usually fatal unless it responded to fever therapy. We learned at Duke that there was a strain of clap in a small town near Durham that was extremely lethal, a killer. I believe the town was Lumberton. If a patient was referred to us from that town with gonococcal disease we knew we and the patient were in for a hard time. Tuberculosis was treated mainly by bed rest on the sun porch at the end of each ward. We were very aggressive with therapeutic pneumothorax, the house staff becoming quite expert at performing it. We had a large outpatient clinic for these patients who returned for periodic treatment and refills to keep the affected lung collapsed. Pneumonia remained the bugbear of our lives and it was a frequent cause of hospital deaths. Antibiotics were not available until the later 1930s when sulfa drugs arrived.

Rapid Neufeld typing of pneumococci made it possible for us to type the pneumonia and if we found Type I pneumococci we could use the Felton antiserum with dramatic effect. A few victories but too many defeats was the story of pneumonia in the hospital in those days. The cause of rheumatic fever was not known but was under study by various groups, rumors reaching us that the streptococcus was involved. Alvin Coburn at Columbia-Presbyterian and Duckett Jones in Boston were hot on the trail of the streptococcal theory. The latter's sister was an assistant resident in medicine at Duke and kept us informed.

We had a polio epidemic in North Carolina while was I was there. Fortunately it proved to be non-paralytic but we did not know this until the epidemic was over. The house staff took care of the patients regardless of the risks. We accepted this as part of the price we paid for being doctors. I know of no house staff who refused to treat patients with polio. Things have changed quite a bit since those days. Thanks to the Sabin and Salk vaccines, polio is gone only to give way to AIDS.

When Dr. Hanes returned from his summer vacation, it was not long before I was asked to come to his office to meet him. He said he wished to discuss my future plans. I told him that I was interested in metabolic diseases and physiological and biochemical aspects of illness. He then told me clearly and unequivocally that I would be a professor of medicine at Duke University. I recall that he also said that he could not promise me that I would be the chairman of the department for this would depend on many other factors, some of them unpredictable at this stage. Here I was a 24-year-old intern being offered a future few might ever achieve. It was pretty heady stuff. He then asked me where I would like to go for the next year. He said that his friend, Mr. Bowman Gray, would provide for a fellowship paying $1,200 a year, so that I could go anywhere in the world for training in the field of my choice. To an intern being paid exactly nothing the stipend seemed generous. I told Dr. Hanes that I would like to go to Yale University medical school and New Haven Hospital to study under Dr. John P. Peters, the great expert in this area, whose textbook, *Quantitative Clinical Chemistry*, written with Dr. Donald Van Slyke, was already my bible. Dr. Hanes said he would arrange it. I emerged from the professor's office walking on air. It seemed to me that I had hit the jackpot.

Let me tell you a little more about Dr. Hanes. He was a tall, handsome man with a regal air and striking presence, always immaculately attired, clean-shaven, a Hapsburg chin, and gray haired, the picture of an outstanding clinician. In 1933, at the age of 50, he was selected by Dean Wilbur C. Davison to replace Dr. Harold L. Amoss as professor and chairman of the department of medicine at Duke University School of Medicine. Dr. Hanes was then and had been for years a practicing consultant in neurology in Winston-Salem, North Carolina, his clientele consisting of many of the most prominent citizens of North Carolina. He was a talented member of a distinguished and wealthy North Carolina family. His father was a tobacco tycoon in Winston-Salem and amassed a large fortune. He had six sons, all successful executives, four of them in *Who's Who in America*, an achievement matched only by the Rockefellers. Dr. Hanes' brother, John, became president of the U.S. Shipping Lines and served as U.S. undersecretary of the treasury. He is credited with having rescued the Hearst empire from financial ruin and became something of a hero in the Wall Street community. Another brother was president of the Wachovia Bank of North Carolina, destined to become one of the most successful in America. The Haneses Knitting Mills are world-renowned. In the recently published *Diary of H. L. Mencken,*[2] I learned that Dr. and Mrs. Fred Hanes were his good friends and that he spent many vacations with the Hanes at their summer retreat at Roaring Gap, North Carolina. This acerbic critic had nothing but warm and kind things to say about his hosts, revealing aspects of Dr. Hanes's life previously unfamiliar to me. In my book, *Death of the Clinician: Requiem or Reveille?*, I said:

---

2. Charles A. Fechner, ed., *The Diary of H.L. Mencken* (New York: Vintage Books, 1991).

The Hanes appointment will go down in the annals of Duke University Medical School as one of the wisest made by Dean Davison, although at first the comment of academicians was adverse—"Hanes, who is he?" Hanes was a graduate of Johns Hopkins, Class of 1908 and a student of Osler who interned in medicine at Hopkins and then had gone on to occupy positions as Assistant Professor of Pathology at Columbia University, P&S, briefly as a staff member of the Rockefeller Institute and also on the teaching staff of Washington University Medical School followed by one year as assistant in neurology at Queen Square Hospital in London. During World War I, he commanded the North Carolina Base Hospital No. 65, and on his return he entered practice in Winston-Salem, North Carolina, concentrating chiefly on neurology. While Hanes was not a research scientist, he was a superb clinical teacher, a perfectionist in the Osler mold. He had a commanding presence and knew how to handle the powerful and the rich as well as the poorest sharecropper. He could make decisions without vacillating and he was one of the most frank and open men I have ever known in his discussions with patients.

His experience in private practice was extensive. From him I learned a great deal about communicating with patients, responding to their needs and demands. More than anything else, he insisted that there was only one class of patient, whether he was on the ward or in the most expensive private room. Davison, a staunch Oslerian, was now joined by an equally ardent disciple of Osler and this was to influence a number of critical decisions that were soon to be made.[3]

Shortly after my meeting with Dr. Hanes, word was received from Dr. Peters at Yale that he would be happy to accept me as a Research Fellow starting 1 July 1935. In the meantime I continued to work hard, learning as much as possible and getting to know my colleagues. One of the best friends I made at Duke was Jay Arena, a Duke graduate and a former intern in pediatrics at Strong Memorial Hospital, Rochester, New York, who became a renowned pediatrician and professor at Duke University Medical School and, among many achievements, was the first to establish and direct a poison-control center, published a fine pediatric text and the now classic *Poisoning: Toxicology—Symptoms—Treatments*. Jay was a close friend and protégé of Dean Wilburt C. Davison and in my judgment is one of the finest physicians every graduated from Duke University School of Medicine.

---

3. Michael J. Lepore, *Death of the Clinician: Requiem or Reveille?* (Springfield, Ill.: Charles C. Thomas, 1982) p. 181.

Another friend was Dr. Donald Martin, a Rochester graduate who had also held a student fellowship there in the department of physiology. Don was second to Dr. D. T. Smith in the bacteriology department at Duke and subsequently left to become Dean of the University of Puerto Rico Medical School. Don told me that Dr. Hanes had spoken to him after receiving Dr. Whipple's letter recommending me for an internship at Duke. He gave me a strong recommendation and added that Dr. Hanes's only reservation was that, "if Lepore is as outstanding as George Whipple says he is, why is he willing to come here to work under me, a quasi-unknown in academic medicine?" A good question, but Dr. Hanes knew nothing of the fiasco at Columbia-Presbyterian and I never told him about it.

From this time on, I was a marked man at Duke. This had some advantages, also some handicaps. My work was being very closely observed by my peers and superiors.

Another contemporary member of the medical house staff, Jasper Lamar Calloway, had been singled out by Dr. Hanes to be the future head of dermatology at Duke and was being sent to the University of Pennsylvania for further training in the specialty. "Cal" was a very bright young man and also lots of fun. He was overweight in those days and on a high-protein, low-calorie diet that entitled him to steak when we might be having chicken. Then he would reach over and appropriate a fried potato or a dessert from anyone seated near him. I had not been at Duke very long before I learned of one of his pet pranks. There were times when the telephone lines between the undergraduate girls' dormitory at Duke (Aycock House) and the interns' quarters at the hospital would be crossed up. When this happened there was a characteristic ring quite different from the usual one. When this ring sounded in the evening, the interns would rush to Cal's room while he prepared to answer. He would then, in a falsetto, feminine tone, answer. The caller, usually male, would ask for Miss so and so, Cal's reply would be that she could not come to the phone. Why not? Well, she is in the toilet. "What! Say, is this Aycock House?" "Young man I'll have you understand this is not a cock house so stop calling." Down would go the receiver and everybody would burst out laughing, putting us in a good mood before going down to dinner.

Another of my friends was the chief surgical resident, Paul Sanger, who was quite talented and later pioneered with Dacron grafts for abdominal aneurysms. Paul had a sideline to supplement his meager income as resident to accommodate the heavy demands of his courtship. The side line was to pick up suits for the cleaners when we left a note on the door. He promised excellent service for less than that charged by his competitors. One day I thought I would give him a little business, and asked him to pick up and return a suit for dry cleaning. The only problem with this was that it was the only suit I had beside my white uniforms and I had a date for that Saturday night.

When the suit had not arrived by 5 o'clock, I became very anxious, contacted Paul who assured me that it would be there very soon. It arrived two hours later and when I got into it, I discovered to my horror that the cleaner had shrunk my suit so that the trouser legs reached up far above my ankles. I tried every means to stretch the trousers and finally by dint of lowering my belt and extending the cuffs by cutting their attachments, if I waddled slowly and carefully I could wear the suit. My date was with the wonderful and beautiful head nurse who would later become my wife. Going anywhere to dance was out of the question. A trip to a movie was clearly the only option I had. As darkness settled, I waddled up the walk to the nurses' residence to pick up my date. Once we were settled in the cab, I told her of my predicament. She giggled and all was well. I knew then she had a good sense of humor.

In December 1934 I spent some vacation time at home in New York with my family. While there I received a call from Dr. Hanes, who wondered whether I could have lunch with him at the Hotel Pierre. The elegance and ambience of the Pierre stunned me. The luncheon was superb. I had onion soup for the first time in my life. Dr. Hanes told me that he had just returned from the Philadelphia meeting of the American College of Physicians, where he had entered my name in competition for the Research Fellowship of the American College of Physicians. There was only one; it paid $1,800 a year, and Dr. Hanes wanted me to win it because of its prestige and the honor it would bring to Duke. He said the competition would be very keen. I thanked him and hoped that we would make it. If I won it, the Bowman Gray Fellowship would be used for another purpose. In May 1935 I received a telegram from the American College of Physicians stating that I was the winner of this prestigious award.

Medical Grand Rounds at Duke in 1934 were in the Hopkins tradition, with two formal case presentations in the conference room. This teaching exercise was traditionally the crème de la crème of the educational experience in most of the major medical schools, its only competitor being the Clinico-Pathologic Conferences, or CPC. The patient, the center of attraction, was wheeled into the room, usually in bed, and the intern, acting and speaking like a doctor and dressed like one, in an immaculate starched white uniform and clean white shoes, clean shaven with a recent haircut, would present a detailed and concise history, the physical findings and the laboratory data from memory without notes or referring to the chart, an art that seems to have gone out the window in the present era of medicine. The professor, and there was only one, would then take over, conducting the remainder of the clinic by actively leading the discussion and eliciting comments from the teaching faculty and questions from the house staff and students.

The essential quality of the Grand Rounds format is that it deals with current medical problems on the medical service of our own hospital, involves the students and house staff in the presentation, meaning that they have to do some work, and allows the faculty ample opportunity for spontaneous discussion and argument. It may on occasion encourage participation of the patient himself in the proceedings, providing the conductor has the communications skill to control the process and direct it into productive channels. When the Grand Round is conducted along these lines, there is simply no better way to teach medicine.

This was the situation at Duke, where some of the most exciting experiences in my medical career occurred. During my first year at Duke I participated in a number of extraordinary Grand Rounds and never missed one. One I shall never forget centered about a 45-year-old woman with a history of diarrhea, weakness, extreme weight loss with emaciation, sore tongue, and a macrocytic hyperchromic anemia, with acid secreted in the gastric juice. She was presented as a patient with probable carcinomatosis, primary site unknown.

As she was being wheeled out of the conference room an intern rose to question the diagnosis, which he felt was undocumented. This was almost unheard of for an intern and led to a rather spirited debate. During the course of the discussion, Dr. Frederic M. Hanes asked whether the intern had an alternative diagnosis. The intern proposed nontropical sprue, a wasting, diarrheal disease often associated with macrocytic anemia. When pressed for tests to substantiate this diagnosis, he suggested a glucose-tolerance test, which had been reported by Danish investigators to be flat in this disease and interpreted as evidence of malabsorption of glucose. The test was done and turned out to be flat, the blood sugar remaining essentially unchanged from its fasting level for three hours despite the ingestion of 100 grams of glucose. The patient was treated with liver extract and responded dramatically with weight gain, remission of anemia, and abatement of diarrhea. This was case number one of sprue at Duke Hospital. I was the intern who broke up the Grand Rounds with this diagnosis. After the conference, Dr. Hanes congratulated me and asked how I had learned about sprue. I answered that before leaving Rochester for Duke, I had prepared myself by reading a good bit about tropical diseases and in the process had noticed a new monograph in our library that had just arrived from Denmark with the title "Non-Tropical Sprue" by Hess-Thaysen. Dr. Hanes checked with the Duke librarian who reported that the monograph was not in the Duke medical library and on Dr. Hanes' order she sent for it post-haste.

In retrospect, we were fortunate that this patient responded so well to liver extract and a high-protein, high-caloric diet. Many years would pass before the real villain in sprue was discovered to be the gluten in the cereal grains of wheat, rye, oats, and barley. Their elimination from the diets of patients with sprue leads to remission and restoration to normal health.

It was not long before another patient with severe diarrhea and weight loss was presented at Grand Rounds. The diagnosis of chronic amebic dysentery had been made by the ward teaching staff based on the presence of cysts of Entamoeba histolytica in the stools. Antiamebic therapy had failed. Once again I had the pleasure of breaking up Grand Rounds, questioning the diagnosis and ending with the statement that the patient's emaciated appearance and clinical features closely resembled that of the first patient with sprue seen earlier that year.

Subsequent studies confirmed my suspicions and this patient became case number two of sprue at Duke. At a later Grand Rounds, she was again presented for follow-up and further discussion. It was clear to me that sprue was not a simple disorder and I felt that it should be studied thoroughly as a systemic disease with serious gastrointestinal, nutritional, and hematological manifestations. I remember the discussion of 59 years ago as if it were today. The teaching staff, led by the chief of hematology, said that "Dusty" Rhoads and "Bill" Castle of the Rockefeller Institute in New York and the Thorndike in Boston were studying a large series of patients with tropical sprue in Puerto Rico, where it was endemic. They felt that they were better equipped to study the disease than we at Duke where there were so few patients with sprue. My audacity and enthusiasm for research came to the fore and I reminded the staff that this was the second case in three months at Duke and both diagnoses were made at Grand Rounds. I predicted that there were many more, perhaps some with milder grades of the disease. Besides, I said, the investigators in Puerto Rico were interested mainly in the hematological aspects of sprue and not in its gastrointestinal and metabolic features. Fortunately Dr. Hanes agreed with me. I had whetted his interest and he decided to pursue the challenge. Dr. Hanes was then 51 years old and had been out of academic medicine for over 20 years. His original appointment at Duke was as professor of neurology. Dean Davison said years later that Hanes was his first choice for the chair in medicine but his (Hanes's) friends told him that "Fred" would not be interested in the administration required of the chairman of the department. "I was never so greatly misinformed," said Davison. "From the day of his acceptance to his untimely death on the 25th of March, 1946, his and Deryl Hart's leadership were responsible for the progress of Duke University Medical Center." In 1934, when I first met him, Dr. Hanes appeared ten years younger than his stated age. His mind was keen and I was quite impressed that he seemed to be reading the literature more than most of his staff. Having accepted the chair of medicine at Duke, he was totally immersed in teaching, administration, and an active consulting practice and in learning something new every day.

I could see that he was really enjoying his new position and giving all of his energy to it. He was independently wealthy and had no financial problems. I learned later that he turned back his salary as chairman to fund departmental activities. Our house staff had a standing invitation to attend his weekly Sunday evening "at home" social sessions in his beautiful on-campus home, where he and his charming wife entertained and extended their hospitality to sometimes boisterous house staff and their friends. Years later, I learned that this was an old Hopkins custom originating with Sir William Osler.

Dr. Hanes attacked the problem of sprue with vigor and provided funds out of pocket for technical and biochemical assistance. As I had predicted, there were many more patients with sprue in the Carolinas and it was not long before Dr. Hanes became a world expert on this disease and the writer of the sprue chapter in the leading medical text of the day, Cecil's *Textbook of Medicine.*

By 1936, only eighteen months after the first patient with sprue was diagnosed at Duke Hospital, Dr. Hanes was able to report that fourteen cases had been studied intensively in that institution. In the 1941 edition of Cecil's *Textbook of Medicine,* Dr. Hanes wrote the chapter on sprue and reported observations on 28 patients with sprue seen at Duke. He continued to write the Cecil chapter on sprue until he died in 1946.

I am happy that Dr. Hanes was introduced to the enigma of sprue by this young intern from Rochester who dared to disrupt his Medical Grand Rounds. Dr. Hanes never forgot this and I have on my office wall the framed letter he wrote to me on 6 April 1940, saying that he would always remember that I diagnosed the first case of sprue at Duke. He wrote "Since you were the man who diagnosed our first case of sprue it is only fitting that you should follow through and study the cases around New York. I can't help but believe that if all diarrheas were carefully considered from the standpoint of sprue a good many would turn up. Snell, at the Mayo Clinic, sees quite a lot of sprue originating in the northwestern states. We have our thirty-seventh instance of the disease in the hospital now."

Dr. Hanes knew, of course, that I had worked in the great departments of physiology and pathology at Rochester on problems of fluid balance and plasmapheresis and had heard me lecture on the Starling hypothesis for fluid exchange as it related to edema formation in patients with nephrosis, a renal disorder I was engaged in studying and treating. This hypothesis was developed by Ernest Starling of London, a famous physiologist, who should have been given a Nobel Prize for at least one of three major discoveries but was cheated out of it by WW I when no awards were made. In essence, the hypothesis is that the net transport of fluid through the capillary wall is dependent on the difference between the effective hydrostatic and the oncotic pressures of the plasma proteins within the capillary. Dr. Hanes told me he was preparing for a Grand Rounds Clinic the next day on a woman with severe trichinosis, wasting, generalized anasarca, and hypoalbuminemia without renal or cardiac disease. He asked me to explain the Starling hypothesis to him. I did this as concisely and clearly as possible, drawing a simple diagram on the blackboard. He took no notes, just listened and observed. The next day, I was at Grand Rounds when he discussed the patient. He gave a masterly, brief description of the Starling hypothesis to explain the patient's edema and then continued on to other aspects of the woman's illness. Some months later the case report was published in *International Clinics of North America*. I tell this story not to stress my erudition but to indicate that Dr. Hanes was studying medicine and staying up to date and not too proud to ask a fellow student for some help. I am sad that Dr. Hanes, who died in 1946 at the age of 63, did not live to witness and participate in the further unraveling of the enigma of sprue with the discovery that gluten in the cereal grains of wheat, rye, oats, and barley was the villain. He would have enjoyed the fun and excitement. He also tried to get me involved in the sprue research, but I felt this was now his project at Duke to develop and expand. At one meeting, when I was pursuing my work on nephrosis and nephrotic edema, he said to me, "Why don't you get away from these nephritics and nephrotics. They all seem to die. Why not try a disease that has a higher cure rate?" It planted a seed in my mind and influenced some later decisions.

Let us return to my internship at Duke. My skills in getting into veins developed during my research work on plasmapheresis were great assets during my internship. In those days there were no IV teams of technicians or nurses; the interns had to do the work and there was plenty of it. Think of all the money that was saved! When I witness how helpless the average current breed of intern is when faced with patients with "difficult" veins I am reminded again that our educational and training programs have failed to teach our medical students the basic skills that a physician needs. There are times in medicine when the physician himself must be the treatment.

During my internship, Mrs. Sarah B. Duke was admitted to the private service for regulation of insulin-dependent diabetes. She had suffered a stroke in the past and it was next to impossible for blood specimens to be obtained from her veins. Fingersticks were not being used in clinical practice in that era except for blood counts. Mrs. Duke complained vigorously about the venipunctures and told Dr. Hanes that no one was able to get blood without sticking her three or more times. The blood sugars were essential for monitoring her diabetes that seemed to vary greatly despite diet and insulin. Later on we found that her chauffeur was sneaking in some snacks without our knowledge. Dr. Hanes said that he would ask one of his residents who was an expert on taking blood to come to take the specimens. The resident was "MJ," the nickname assigned to me by the house staff after they got to know me. Bright and early one morning I arrived at Mrs. Duke's room on Drake floor with my equipment, was ushered in by her private-duty nurse who awakened the patient. She took one look at me and said "Young man, just what do you plan to do to me?" I introduced myself as Dr. Hanes's resident, ordered to take a blood specimen. She adamantly refused and said that the day before they had tried 3–4 times without success. I examined her veins and told her that I was certain I would succeed. She still refused. I then said I might lose my job if she didn't let me try. She mellowed and issued this edict. One attempt and no more. I agreed to this, picked up a sharp narrow steel hypodermic needle and slipped it into her vein without any difficulty and drew the blood for testing. She was so happy at the result that from that point on the nurses would call me whenever they needed blood from Mrs. Duke. One day when the surreptitiously given snack did not arrive, I was called to see her because of insulin shock. I paged the diabetes specialist who was following her and gave her intravenous glucose. When she emerged from the hypoglycemia she was quite angry with the specialist and berated him and demanded to see "Fred" Hanes. Dr. Hanes lived on campus and quickly came to the hospital. His management of Mrs. Duke was firm and in marked contrast to the diabetes specialists who became quite shaky when confronted by Mrs. Duke. Dr. Hanes took her hand in his and said "Sarah, I'm very sorry you have had a reaction to insulin, but you are over it now and we know how to prevent it. You must adhere to your diet. When food is brought in to you without our knowledge, there is no way for us to know how much insulin you need to take," said he, looking her straight in the eye. Mrs. Duke said she was sorry and promised to adhere to her diet and there were no further hypoglycemic episodes. About one week following this episode Dr. Hanes called me and said that Mrs. Duke had asked that her grandchild from Philadelphia, Miss Mary Duke Biddle, sixteen years of age, be admitted as my patient for a thorough checkup. Dr. Hanes said he was arranging all of this and admitted Miss Biddle to the room adjoining her grandmother's. Dr. Hanes's instructions were that I should take my usual thorough history and examine her as I would any other patient on the wards of Duke Hospital.

She was an attractive, pert, slender young lady who gave a good history and presented with no significant medical complaints. When I finished her examination she charmed me by saying it was the most thorough examination she had ever had and expressed her thanks. Even at sixteen, I could see that this was a very exceptional person. Little did I know that she would, in time, become the president of the Duke Endowment. In 1972 my wife and I were privileged to be in the audience in the Duke Chapel at the memorial service for Dean Wilburt C. Davison when that young girl, now Mrs. Mary Duke Biddle Semans, gave a wonderful eulogy in honor of our beloved "Dave." The tears that came to our eyes were not those of sadness but of joy and pride at the accomplishments of our youngsters. Getting old is a joy when we have memories like these. She finished her eulogy with "Thanks be to God for sending him here," and I added "Thanks be to God for sending *her* here."

On another occasion, I was alerted by Dean Davison that Dr. William L. Poteat, the president of Wake Forest College, was coming in for a checkup. The Dean said he was an old friend and he wanted me to do everything possible to make him feel at home and appreciated as a very important person (a V.I.P.) in our midst. Dean Davison had no occasion to worry about Dr. Poteat. He was an alert, keen, rotund, beaming man who was soon surrounded by former students now on our house staff and quickly making new friends. His checkup failed to reveal any serious ailment, and I had occasion to spend a good deal of time with him learning something of his interesting life. He was a Baptist minister and teacher of biology who had participated in the Scopes trial. He described this ordeal as if it had been yesterday, and his tale fascinated me. Dr. Poteat knew he was going to have to testify because he had been subpoenaed. He said to his wife "Mother, I am going to have to tell the truth when I testify tomorrow. I must say that I have been teaching evolution and I believe Darwin is right. We live here and like it but we may have to leave because there are some who disagree with me." His wife replied that he must do what his conscience demanded and if there were repercussions, they would move on together as they always had.

He testified. His testimony was very convincing and the only reason he left the community was to move on to higher and higher office in educational institutions culminating in the presidency of Wake Forest College. He was indeed a scholar and a man of integrity, courage, and high purpose. Years later, when he died, I recall a major editorial about him in the *New York Times* characterizing him as the Great Scholar of the South.

Before leaving Dr. Poteat, I will share with the reader a story about him that I have recently seen in *American Heritage* magazine of November 1993. Laurence Tucker Stallings, destined to become famous in 1924 for *What Price Glory*, had been expelled from Trinity (later Duke University) after being caught drinking and smoking during a poker game. Dr. William Louis Poteat accepted him at Wake Forest, a Baptist institution (although "Doctor Billy" was surprisingly liberal). Within months Stallings was again caught in a poker game, equipped with a cigar and a bottle of moonshine. "Young man," Dr. Poteat asked the culprit in his office, the following morning "can you give me one good reason why I shouldn't expel you?" Stallings thought fast. "Yes sir, I'm engaged to your daughter." On reflection Dr. Poteat decided that did indeed constitute a good reason; Stallings was retained on probation. He then scurried off to find Helen Poteat, whom he hadn't yet actually met, before her father sent for her, and threw himself on her mercy. She thought it hilarious and agreed to play along to save Laurence's academic career. The war (WW I) came and Stallings went overseas as a marine and married Helen Poteat when he returned a wounded hero minus a leg lost in combat. You can understand why "Dr. Billy" was so beloved by his students.

My marvelous year of internship at Duke was drawing to a close. When I look back I realize what that year really meant for me. The loss of the Columbia-Presbyterian appointment, through a secretarial blunder, may have been one of the most fortunate breaks in my life, for it led to my appointment at Duke through Dean Whipple's intercession. It was a very hectic busy year. The long hours of duty under the Hopkins twenty-four-hour on-call system showed me how a doctor should be trained. I was young, dedicated, idealistic, and healthy. Quoting Wordsworth (*The Prelude*, Book XI), "Bliss was it in that dawn to be alive but to be young was very Heaven." I emerged, a veteran of combat, knowing I had endured, performed, and won the battle. On the road, many wonderful things had happened. Years later,

Dean Wilburt Davison of Duke would write Colonel Marshall N. Fulton, a fellow Rhodes Scholar at Oxford and my chief of medicine at Valley Forge General Hospital, that "Mike Lepore was one of the brightest and best interns to ever serve at Duke Hospital." In the midst of a very busy year I had managed to court and win the heart of a charming, idealistic, and beautiful young woman who would soon be my bride. The next stop was Yale, its hospital and medical school and the challenge of the American College of Physicians Research Fellowship under Dr. John P. Peters.

Chapter 7

~ॐ~

Yale Medical School, 1935–1936

I ARRIVED IN NEW HAVEN 30 June 1935, ready to start work the next day. I had already arranged for living quarters in Harkness Hall and they were really quite comfortable and attractive. My sisters went to work decorating the studio, adding drapes and other niceties, so that it looked warm and home-like.

After a hectic year's internship at Duke on twenty-four-hour call, it was a great relief to know that I had no on-call responsibilities for the coming year. Getting through a night without being called out would be a really miraculous change. What I had not figured on was that my studio was on a courtyard adjoining Mory's, the renowned watering hole frequented by sons of old Eli and immortalized in the famous Yale drinking song of the lost sheep saying baa, baa, baa. It would get pretty noisy at times but I slept so soundly that it rarely awakened me. I do recall one night when I was awakened by the rollicking singing in Mory's that was so melodious that I lay awake listening and enjoying it. There was a rendition of "On the Road to Mandalay" that was superior to any I had ever heard and there was one especially good baritone voice. Next morning I inquired at the dormitory office and learned that I was being serenaded by Lawrence Tibbett and the Yale Glee Club who were continuing in Mory's the concert they had started elsewhere on campus earlier that night.

Dr. Peters was extremely gracious, assigned me to a laboratory opposite his office, and introduced me to his staff consisting of Paul Lavietes, Alexander Winkler, and "Chunky Robins." Ann Eisenman and Pauline Hald were the chief technicians, the backbone of the research division. The house staff included Bill Bruckner, Max Miller, and Cal Klinghoffer. It was a small, friendly, and compatible group of very intelligent and idealistic people loyal to their chief and on their way to careers in teaching, research, and academic medicine. I soon learned that there were really two major services in medicine at Yale, one directed by the Sterling Professor, Dr. Francis G. Blake, chairman of the department, and the other by Dr. John P. Peters, the John Slade Ely Professor of Medicine. Dr. Peters's service was devoted to metabolic diseases but not limited to these. Dr. Blake's service was a general medical service with a wide variety of case material. Infectious-disease patients, Dr. Blake's forte, were housed in a separate building adjoining the main hospital. Dr. Peters's interest in disorders of metabolism attracted a wide variety of patients to his service. In addition to my research activities, I made rounds with Dr. Peters regularly and I attended the large diabetic clinic and was assigned patients in the metabolic outpatient clinic.

I was much impressed by the very practical and down-to-earth management of patients with diabetes in vogue at Yale in those days. We did not require that patients carry a scale with them to measure all food intake. Our patients were given instruction by the clinic dietitians on estimating the caloric and carbohydrate content of foods by visual inspection. Fractional specimens of urine were tested by patients before each meal and at bedtime for glucose and acetone and the insulin dose regulated according to the findings. Blood-sugar tests were done infrequently if the urine values were stable and controlled. Most of the patients were on regular or clear insulin. Longer-acting forms were being studied, e.g., protamine zinc insulin and globin insulin. One of the highlights of my stay at Yale was the appearance of Dr. Charles Best, of Banting and Best fame, as visiting professor. One of our residents, presenting a patient at bedside rounds, had the misfortune to say "this patient is on 'ordinary' insulin." "Call it regular or clear but *never* ordinary," well said by the co-discoverer of insulin. I learned in Dr. Peters's diabetic clinic that most diabetics could be treated effectively as ambulatory patients providing they were well instructed, compliant, and cooperative. Hospitalization was needed only for complications and complex problems. The secret to preventing complications was a good working relationship with the patient and access to the staff at all times. When I returned to Duke in 1936 I put into effect, in the newly created diabetic clinic, many of the concepts I learned at Yale.

Dr. Peters's bedside rounds were most informative. His knowledge of biochemistry and metabolic diseases was encyclopedic, but to my amazement he was a thorough and sound clinician with a very practical bedside approach to problem-solving. His method of teaching was Socratic. Oftentimes the answer to our questions would be another question. At all times he kept us on our toes. Like all stellar teachers of medicine he stimulated us to ask why and take nothing for granted. I remember one day when we were discussing a patient's diarrhea and dyspepsia. As Dr. Peters singled out each of us for comment, he reached me and asked whether the patient was achlorhydric and what this had to do with his symptoms. Knowing I was up against a very keen and critical observer, I asked whether the test for acid was done with histamine stimulation and he answered with a grin that it was, so what? I was now cornered because I really knew little or nothing about achlorhydria except that it occurred with pernicious anemia, which the patient did not have. The next question was how would you treat it. I had read somewhere that hydrochloric acid drops could be given with each meal and mentioned it. As I remember his reply, it was that the amounts given were for all practical purposes homeo-pathic and could not influence the patient's condition. You can bet that I went to the library that afternoon to look up the topic and came away with the feeling that Dr. Peters was correct, that treatment with then prevalent doses of hydrochloric acid was ineffectual and proba-bly a form of psychotherapy. Many years later I would learn that dur-ing the Civil War, President Abraham Lincoln was petitioned by a group of homeopathic physicians for their assignment to military duty. In support of their plea they described homeopathy for the president. He was not impressed and terminated the session by saying homeopathy seemed like manuring a field with a fart.

During my year at Yale, I attended as many of the teaching ses-sions in medicine as I could without neglecting my research activities. The CPCs were excellent and well attended, conducted by Dr. Milton Winternitz and Dr. Harry Zimmerman and junior members of the staff including a very bright one, Dr. Averill Liebow, who became an outstanding pathologist. Dr. Winternitz, a Hopkins graduate and fac-ulty member, had been the dean of Yale Medical School and was a runner-up to Dr. George H. Whipple for the position at Rochester. I had heard that Winternitz could be a real terror, but I must say that in 1935 he seemed quite benign and pleasant and I admired him for his having made a second-rate medical school a great one during his tenure as dean. One of my schoolmates at Rochester, Michael Carpinella, was a New Haven resident who had gone to Yale as an undergraduate, commuting to and from his home. His father was a successful barber in the city. Mike applied for admission to Yale Medical School and was interviewed by Dean Winternitz. It was not a pleasant ordeal, the worst of it being the question "What does your father do for a living?" Mike replied "He has a barbershop in New Haven." "Why don't you go cut hair like your father? Do you think you are better than your father?" Mike was devastated by these ques-tions and the way they were expressed. He managed somehow to hold his tongue but emerged from the session swearing he would never go to Yale Medical School. He subsequently took the train to Rochester where his interview with Dean Whipple was far more pleasant than that with Dean Winternitz. He was accepted at Rochester and was a good student who entered general practice in Branford, Connecticut, where for many years he was a beloved physician to many families.

I never doubted the accuracy of Mike's story, but it was really hammered home in print by Sigmund Wilens in his very funny book,

My Friends the Doctors.[1] Wilens, an undergraduate at Yale, applied for admission to Yale Medical School in 1925 and describes what it was like with Milton Winternitz as Dean. The entire pre-medical group from the Sheffield Scientific School at Yale was interviewed by the Dean in person.

> We sat (in alphabetical order) in a row on a bench in the foyer just outside the dean's office. The door was left open and as each candidate went in we could hear semi-audible questions the dean was delivering in a voice that fluctuated rapidly from a low raucous bullfrog-like croak to a high-pitched whine as he rose to the assault. Naturally, I was last in the row, and as each successive interviewee emerged red-faced and in a great sweat, my apprehension increased. As I inched along the bench to the threshold, the questioning became more audible and ominous. The student who was to go in just preceding me was a brassy type who was firmly convinced his success depended on his standing up to the withering interrogation. By the time he went in, I was just outside the door and could hear the questions quite clearly, although I could not catch the response. "Why do you want to be a doctor? What does your father do for a living? Why don't you go into the grocery business with him? Do you think you are better than your father? You mean you want to make a lot of money? Was your name always Stuart? Why did you change it?" and so on, deadlier and deadlier. I wasn't feeling so good when it came to my turn. When I went into the inquisitorial chambers, I met a real Mussolini setup. The five-foot-five Mephistophelean dean was well submerged behind an enormous desk at the end of a large room. Adjoining the dean was a secretary, who sat poised with a stenographic pad, obviously prepared to take down every grunt I made. A spotlight was directed, third-degree fashion, on the seat in which the student was to sit. I did the only thing any sensible person would in such a situation. I promptly swooned. Days later, while I was reading a brochure on how to become a master plumber, a letter arrived informing me that I had been admitted to medical school.

I guess that Mike Carpinella was not exaggerating when he described his 1928 interview at Yale Medical School. Dean Winternitz made some friends at Yale but they were outnumbered by his enemies.

On one occasion, a premedical student being interviewed by the Dean was greeted with a large book thrown at him. The student managed to catch the book before it had inflicted any harm and for this

---

1. Sigmund Wilens, *My Friends the Doctors* (New York : Atheneum Press, 1961).

he was rewarded by being admitted to the Yale School of Medicine.[2] No wonder that Winternitz's mentor, Dean William Henry Welch of Johns Hopkins, expressed the caveat to President Rush Rhees of the University of Rochester who was looking for a founding dean for this new medical school, that Winternitz was "brilliant but needed restraint"—the understatement of the year.[3]

Given these weaknesses and flaws and despite his outstanding performances as an administrator, teacher, and Dean at Yale since 1917, it was almost inevitable that sooner or later his enemies would organize a coup to remove him from office. This was led in 1934 by Dr. Stanhope Bayne-Jones, the first chairman of bacteriology and my teacher at Rochester. Dr. Bayne-Jones left Rochester at the behest of Dean Winternitz (whose medical student he had been at Hopkins) to accept appointment as chairman of bacteriology at Yale and master of Trumbull College. Bayne-Jones was a Yale graduate, member of Skull and Bones, a member of an old southern family, and an excellent diplomat with impeccably good manners. Susan Cheever believes that "Winter" had lost his will to fight in 1934 for a variety of reasons. The faculty voted not to renew his appointment as Dean and President Agnell requested his letter of resignation. Winternitz submitted it without argument and continued as chairman of pathology. Bayne-Jones took his place as Dean.

In 1935 Harvey Cushing was in residence at Yale having been lured from Harvard and the Peter Bent Brigham Hospital by an endowed chair in the history of medicine and excellent housing for his valuable collection of rare medical manuscripts in the Sterling Library. He was suffering with what was believed to be peripheral vascular disease found later to be due to an abdominal aneurysm, but he was mentally clear and was the center of attraction at any of the conferences or receptions that he attended. His friend, John Fulton, was working with him and gathering material for his biography of the great neurosurgeon. At one cocktail reception, I was introduced to Harvey Cushing by my former professor of bacteriology at Rochester, Dr. Stanhope Bayne-Jones who was now the Dean of the Yale Medical School. At the time I was unaware of the events that had led to Dr. Winternitz's dismissal as Dean. I reminded Dr. Cushing that

---

2. Susan Cheever, *Treetops—A Family Memoir* (New York: Bantam Books, 1991), p. 87.

3. Michael J. Lepore, *Death of the Clinician: Requiem or Reveille?* (Springfield, Ill.: Charles C. Thomas, 1982) p. 104.

Dr. George Corner and I had appreciated his letter of 1931 asking why Molière was the Cervantes of French medicine. Dean Bayne-Jones recalled that he had been in the audience at Rochester when I lectured on Molière and enjoyed it.

My research at Yale was focused on the role of the plasma proteins in the dynamics of the Starling Hypothesis of Fluid Exchange, continuing my undergraduate studies. Patients with nephrosis were directed to me for appropriate investigation. Plasma-volume studies were performed on normal medical students as controls and on patients with nephrotic edema. I used the Brilliant Vital Red Dye method I had employed at Rochester in my studies of plasmapheresis in dogs. This dye had been used for most of Dr. Whipple's research on anemia in his dog colony in California and Rochester but it was coming under fire because the red color could be affected by hemolysis of red cells, so that the values for plasma volume might be inaccurate. This could be obviated if the dye content were measured by spectrophotometry rather than colorimetry. This would have complicated a very simple technique and some were claiming that a blue dye, Evans Blue or T 1824, did not have this flaw, making it a more satisfactory dye for plasma-volume measurement. My research studies on medical students and patients at Yale and careful review of the literature suggested that all of the dyes used for measuring plasma volume attached themselves to plasma protein, chiefly albumin, and it was because of this affinity that the dye could be used to measure plasma volume. In other words, we were really tagging serum albumin and using it as the marker for measuring plasma volume. I felt that color did not matter; the common bond was attachment to plasma albumin. I therefore continued to use the Brilliant Vital Red Dye in my experiments. The patients had no complaints, for the red dye gave them a rosy glow whereas the blue dye T 1824 would, in repeated studies, make them look blue. Years later, when radioisotopes became available, the dyes were displaced by I–131 tagged albumin. I also studied colloid osmotic pressure in a wide variety of patients using a newly devised compact osmometer designed by Dr. Carl Wies, a member of Dr. Peters's staff. These studies brought me in touch with a number of people doing research at Yale. One of those was Dr. Marion Howard, a keen internist who was following a large series of patients with lymphogranuloma venereum. These patients, as a result of their disease process, had very enlarged lymph nodes especially in the inguinal and femoral regions. They also had greatly elevated levels of total plasma protein, as high as 10 or 12 grams per dl as opposed to the normal of 6–7 grams, with most of it what we called "globulins" in those days, while the albumin levels would be normal or slightly low. The globulins, being large molecules, have much less osmotic pressure than albumin, so that despite levels of total plasma protein of 10–12 gm or more, there was no significant change of plasma colloid osmotic pressure in affected patients. We did not know the cause of lymphogranuloma venereum in 1935. It was not until 1942 that the cause was found to be chlamydia, curable with appropriate antibiotic therapy. It was also during my stay at Yale that I wrote a paper on Acacia Therapy in Nephrotic Edema, published in the *Annals of Internal Medicine.* This was in an era when we did not have albumin available for intravenous therapy. This would have to await the advent of the plasma separator of Cohn, et al, a product of WW I research. Intravenous acacia, a colloid, relieved nephrotic edema, but I recall that Dr. George Whipple expressed some concern that there might be adverse side effects from that portion of the acacia stored in the liver.

Life at Yale was not all work. We had our share of fun. Alex Winkler and I became good friends. He had a very keen mind, was good in mathematics, and planned experiments very well. He also taught me the wiles of Aschenbrodel's, a perfectly wonderful barn-like restaurant in New Haven with a tremendous open-hearth oven in which wonderful small steaks were burned to our satisfaction while we watched. The beer was also great. It was affordable and within the means of my stipend.

Yale had a fine football team in those days, including the small but quick quarterback, Albie Booth, who became a legend. One of the high points of my year at Yale was a wonderful visit to New York and New Haven by my fiancèe, Ardean Everett. She arrived by train from Durham, North Carolina, at Penn Station in New York where I met her and drove her to my parents' house in the Bronx where she met my family for the first time. They were simply enchanted by her and embraced her as if she were already one of us. My mother, who could be quite critical, was completely won over. That night Ardean and I went to the Rainbow Room in Rockefeller Center where we had dinner in that beautiful setting with all of New York visible from our aerie. We danced to the music of Ray Noble and his orchestra. The service and ambiance were impeccable and all in all it was simply a great night, one that Ardean and I would never forget.

The following day we drove to New Haven and the Yale Bowl to see the Yale-Princeton game. Unfortunately for Yale, Princeton under Fritz Crisler had a championship team that scored touchdown after touchdown out of their huddle formation. One Yale alumnus who arrived carrying a large flask, saying he would have a drink for every Yale touchdown, was so dry and depressed that he finally cried out that he was going to drink for every Princeton score. He was quite loaded before the goal posts were taken down by the victorious Tigers. While at Yale I managed to send flowers to my fiancée, usually red roses, and occasionally a box of Whitman chocolates. We wrote frequently to each other and on occasion had long-distance telephone conversations.

The medical staff at Yale was small and, except for the senior professors, quite young. It was also notoriously underpaid. Full-time instructors were paid in the range of $2,500 a year and assistant professors no more than $3,500. I wondered how they managed to pay their bills. A few were wealthy but most of them survived on their meager pay. I soon learned that most of them would stay in the department for a few years and then they would leave for other positions or enter private practice in or around New Haven. Practices in the depression were not very remunerative anywhere, for paying patients were few and far between. The depression had seriously hurt the New Haven area and I had the impression that there were too many doctors competing for a relatively small population. The affluence of Yale University was not evident in its medical school and one could not escape the impression that the medical school and the hospital were regarded as a burden on the university and accorded second-class citizenship when it came to the budget.

One of the assistant professors was John Lawrence, the brother of the cyclotron wizard and Nobel laureate of California, Ernest Orlando. John had served his residency at Strong Memorial Hospital in Rochester. His stay at Yale was short. He left for California where he joined his brother and had a successful career in oncology and radiotherapy and achieved recognition as the father of nuclear medicine. Another promising young man was Theodore Klumpp in hematology. He was very bright and I knew of him because he had written a good paper on the treatment of sprue with liver extract. With the few full-time chairs filled with vigorous men and with little or no prospect of change or the creation of new medical schools, Dr. Klumpp accepted the offer of the position of FDA commissioner in Washington and did so well that ultimately he was asked to become the head of Sterling Drugs and wrote back to his friends at Yale that he was now being paid $75,000 a year. A friend who received the news said he was sure that the New Deal spending was affecting Ted; he must have misplaced a decimal point. But of course, Ted was telling the truth and in the years that followed he went far above this figure and, I am told, earned every bit of it.

I tell these stories because they concerned me quite a bit, for it would not be long before I would have to face up to the economic facts of life that full-time was no time for one without family wealth and with modest but worrisome debts accumulated during the long educational process in medicine. I saw some of the most promising young people leave academe because they could not meet their financial obligations. The teaching of medicine was being taken over by default by those who had either inherited wealth or married it, by some who eschewed marriage and family life and by others who were willing to subject their families to deprivation in order to further the "breadwinner's" professional career.

I was still old-fashioned enough to believe that it was the obligation of the eldest son to provide adequately for the needs of his dependents and if necessary, those of his parents. I would never forget that my own education was paid for by the sacrifices of my parents and my brother and five sisters. I was the result of a concentrated family effort to produce one well-educated physician despite serious economic handicaps owing to the worst nationwide depression in modern times. This was done without seeking government assistance, welfare, scholarships, or any charitable help. We paid our way and did so without whining or demanding special treatments. I am the product of that system of "free enterprise" and I have never forgotten from whence I came.

One of the major advantages of a Research Fellowship year is relative freedom from routine clinical assignments and ample time for thinking, planning, and discussing future moves with peers and elders. Frankly, even in 1935 I was beginning to question some of the Flexnerian views of a "full-time" career in medicine because I felt that research and laboratory work were being over-emphasized while serving patients was being neglected. In my book *Death of the Clinician: Requiem or Reveille?*,[4] I discussed at length the full-time system advocated by Abraham Flexner and took a strong position against it, siding with Sir William Osler, whose arguments against it are as valid today as they were in 1911 when he expressed them in his now famous-letter to President Ira Remsen of Johns Hopkins.[5]

I was at a point in my career in 1935 when I knew that I liked personal contact with patients and enjoyed helping them. This was more than I could say for some of my rivals and peers in the field of academic medicine, who seemed more interested in diseases than people

---

4. Ibid.

5. Alan M. Chesney, *The Johns Hopkins Hospital and University Medical School*, Vol.. 3 (Johns Hopkins Press, 1963), pp. 176–78.

and were focusing their sights on the oil-immersion lens rather than the low-power objective in the study and care of human beings. I was also troubled by observing academic role models at the bedside who might know a great deal about a single disease and little or nothing about others. I could see that the way the system was evolving, narrow subspecialists were going to take over the teaching of medicine and the direction of departments. I was certain that no matter what happened I did not want to become that type of teacher. I wanted to be just as comfortable at the bedside discussing malaria, diabetes, tuberculosis, brucellosis, nephrosis, ulcerative colitis, sprue, pneumonia, heart failure, or fever of unknown origin. Above all, I was intrigued and challenged by diagnostic problems. I felt that if I could put my finger on what was wrong, I could find someone to fix it.

Many years later, I would realize that my thinking must have been greatly influenced by the teaching and example of my revered, brilliant, and beloved first professor of medicine at Rochester, Dr. William S. McCann. His philosophy was well expressed in his comments on the first twenty-five years of his tenure as the chairman of the department of medicine at Rochester. Dr. McCann had this to say:

> At the outset it was decided that the head of the department of medicine could not afford to be a specialist. A rounded well-balanced program devoted to the best interests of patients and of medical students would preclude such specialization on the part of the professor. As the clinic got underway an effort was made to develop semispecialists within the broad field of internal medicine among the associate and assistant professors; yet care was taken to see that each of these men was given periods of clinical responsibility of the broadest and most varied nature possible, in order to keep him from being overspecialized in practice, even though his researches might follow a narrower field of activity.[6]

What a pity that Dr. McCann's precepts fell by the wayside in many academic departments as the chairs were filled, all too often by individuals with narrow perspectives and minimal qualifications as clinicians, lacking breadth and experience in general medicine, governing by committee or consensus rather than by charismatic leadership. Is it any wonder that long tenure in the chairs has virtually disappeared and half-lives of chairmen seldom exceed ten years? Is it any

---

6. *The Quarter Century, 1925-1950: A Review of the First Twenty-five Years,* (Rochester, N.Y.: The University of Rochester Medical Center, 1950), p. 77.

wonder that our students show little interest in general internal medicine? Where are the brilliant charismatic role models of yesteryear?

Let us now return to New Haven of 1935–36. I shall never understand why Yale University, with its enormous endowment could not, somehow, have established a second Sterling Professorship in Medicine, awarding it to the brilliant and dedicated physician-scientist Dr. John P. Peters, who was world famous, deserving of every bit of recognition and financial support the university and the community at large could give.

Years later I was dismayed that during the Senator McCarthy era, Dr. Peters was being pilloried by that man and accused unfairly, as were many others, of being disloyal, and clearance for government-supported research denied. Dr. Peters was never a communist. He was a sincere and honest man who favored liberal causes. I did not share Dr. Peters's enthusiasm for some of his liberal causes but I respected him for what he was, a loyal and dedicated American. He always gave more to society than he took. He was an unusual individual with independent views. Limited as his financial resources were, he was one veteran of World War I who refused to accept his bonus and turned it back to the government saying he had merely done his duty as a citizen. He had served with distinction in the AEF in France with the famous 2nd General Hospital. I have in my possession a copy of a photograph of that unit with all of the medical officers in service caps and Sam Browne belts with polished brass and shining boots, all except for one individual in the middle row, who was wearing a peaked service hat. By now you must know it was Jack Peters, bucking the rules. Dr. Peters fought McCarthy and his slanders to the point that it impaired his health. While President Eisenhower, who should have known better, failed to attack McCarthy with vigor, Dr. Peters, almost single-handedly beat back McCarthy's accusations and emerged victorious and was given the clearance that should never have been called into question. Not long after, Dr. Peters died, worn out by the bitter fight, vindicated, but at what a cost! At his funeral a devoted friend said that if Dr. Peters had any faults it was that he failed to realize when a good cause had become a lost cause. I differ with that statement. Dr. Peters was fighting for his reputation and his character against a vicious adversary who would stop at nothing to achieve his nefarious ends. Peters was a man of proven integrity, a fighter for the underdog, and a superb human being and loyal citizen of the United Sates. He was to my mind an unfortunate casualty of the McCarthy era of innuendo and character assassination. I mourn Dr. Peters's premature death and pay this delayed tribute to a wonderful man who taught me so much during that splendid year spent on his service at Yale. R.I.P.

Unbeknownst to me, a young man, J. Peter Grace, was a senior at Yale University while I was there, living in nearby Berkeley dormitory on the quadrangle. The scion of a wealthy and prominent family and the son of Italian immigrants from the Bronx, an iceman's son, were each pursuing destiny at a great university under their own head of steam. Our paths would cross again many years later when I was destined to become Mr. Grace's personal physician and consultant. His spectacular accomplishments in the business world as C.E.O. and chairman of W. R. Grace and Company ware paralleled by those in public life as chairman of the Grace Commission, in religion as president of the Knights of Malta, and in philanthropy as president of the Grace Foundation, to name only a few. We shall meet again with "Sir Peter," my favorite nickname for him, later in this chronicle. He illustrates why the personal practice of medicine can be and should be a joy for the physician as well as the patient.

As I look back, the award of the Research Fellowship of the American College of Physicians in 1935 was a milestone in my life. The year with Dr. Peters at Yale was surpassed only by my marvelous year with Dr. Edward F. Adolph at Rochester as his student fellow in physiology. The prize was established by the board of regents of the American College of Physicians in 1934 to promote and advance clinical research by assisting young physicians "in the early states of preparation for a teaching and investigative career in medicine." The fellowships were for one year and only one was granted each year at the time of my tenure. The annual stipend during my year was $1,800. The competition was fierce. It was not an award for which you could apply. The successful recipients were nominated by the ACP Committee on Fellowships and Awards after combing them from a carefully culled list attained through communicating with the professors of medicine and pediatrics in the country, with the officers and regents of the College, and with the National Research Council.[7] The amazing thing was that there was little or no paperwork required of either side, in great contrast to the current procedure with major fellowships. No progress reports were requested. It was as close to a handshake deal as one could ever desire and I was very happy with it. Dr. Reginald Fitz, chairman of the Committee on Fellowships and Awards of the ACP, decided to review the careers and accomplishments of the recipients of these fellowships, with a view to deciding whether the funds had been well spent. He published his findings in

---

7. *Directory, American College of Physicians,* 1955, p. 49.

1947, as an editorial in the *Annals of Internal Medicine* under the title "A Preliminary Note on an Interesting Experiment." Dr. Fitz reported "Up to the Beginning of the War (WW II) 16 Fellows had been appointed in this fashion. While their number is small and the possible years of follow-up on their careers are few, yet it has seemed worthwhile to attempt to evaluate their work. One might argue that if, on the whole, the holders of such fellowships had by now succeeded in accomplishing demonstrably satisfactory results in research the continuance of such appointments was justified; if not, the funds of the College allocated for their maintenance might, perhaps, be used to better advantage for some other purpose." Dr. Fitz chose two criteria to measure the accomplishments of the Research Fellows: bibliographic and academic. He concluded that the publications of the Fellows were serious and impressive. "There has been almost no literary padding," a real compliment especially in the current day and era of bloated C.V.s. Dr. Fitz was impressed by the diversity of interests pursued and the teamwork needed to pursue these goals. "Most of them have approached clinical research through the disciplines of physiology, chemistry, bacteriology or pharmacology rather than the more ancient ones of anatomy or pathology; they have probed almost every corner of medicine with new instruments in an effort to lay bare the fundamentals of disease." On the academic side, Dr. Fitz was much impressed by the track record of the Research Fellows. "The most venerable has scarcely passed his fortieth birthday and yet among the group there are now one professor of medicine, one associate professor, and six assistant professors serving on medical facilities; almost all the rest occupy positions weighted with research or teaching responsibilities; so far the lure of private practice has proved a poor competitor against scientific ambition." Now, forty-four years after Fitz's paper, the record of these first seventeen fellows is most impressive. Almost everyone of the group eventually reached the rank of professor of medicine in a prestigious medical school. Some achieved worldwide fame. Many were heads of departments. By any criteria this was an extraordinary group of men.

I agree with Dr. Fitz's statement that "private practice has proved a poor competitor against scientific ambition" in this group of physicians. In 1947, Dr. Fitz knew that the period of observation was of rather short duration. For reasons I have clearly stated in my book, *Death of the Clinician: Requiem or Reveille?*, many outstanding young men of that era had to enter private practice in order to pay their debts, support dependents, and pay their bills. Full-time salaries were grossly inadequate and after a few years in academe many deserted the ranks for greener pastures. Among these defectors were some of those awarded the Research Fellowships. This was in an era when it was possible to be competent in teaching, research, and clinical medicine, and individuals dubbed Renaissance figures were on the faculty of most of our best medical schools.

Dr. Fitz concluded his sprightly paper in his inimitable style with a caveat. "The College, through its Research Fellowship, has conducted an interesting experiment in medical education which already has yielded interesting results. The continuance of the experiment for a longer period of time seems justified. The Fellows, however, must always be chosen with particular care, and especially so in times when fellowship funds are prevalent. Those selected must appear to offer promise of achieving national prominence in medicine from the impetus they obtain at the beginning of their careers as Research Fellows of the American College of Physicians. If other than young people of rare ability and earnestness of purpose receive it, the Fellowship will degenerate and its maintenance will fail to promote and advance clinical research in any distinctive fashion of which the college can be proud." To this I say AMEN!

I was the youngest of the seventeen recipients, being only 25 at the time of appointment. As the clock inexorably moves ahead and the obituary columns record the passing of most of the original group, I know I express not only my own gratitude but also theirs to the American College of Physicians for its wonderful gift.

We have lived and served in the Golden Era of American Medicine and I do not believe there will ever again be an age so remarkable, exciting, and productive. We did not all travel the same path, but we had a common philosophy and faith, to give to medicine our sincere and devoted commitment in the search for truth. For reasons I have presented here and elsewhere, I chose the less-traveled road, trying to combine the practice of the art of medicine with its science, trying to wear the three hats of teaching, research, and personal care of patients. Recognition was slower than on the full-time track, but with God's help it has arrived in full measure to brighten the closing days of a life devoted to serving my patients as physician and friend striving to live up to the fifteenth century French folk-saying, *Guerir quelquefois, soulager souvent, consoler toujours.*

The first of July 1936 was coming close. The year had passed so quickly and pleasantly. I was ready and eager to return to Durham, North Carolina, and Duke Hospital, where I would be a senior assistant resident in medicine and reunited with the young lady who was destined to be my bride.

Chapter 8

Return to Duke, 1936-1937

O N ONE OF MY RETURN VISITS TO DUKE I made sure that a nice room would be assigned to me in a well-ventilated and quiet area of the residents' quarters. This was quite an improvement over the internship year. I also found that while I was at Yale, the house staff at Duke had rebelled against the twenty-four-hour on-call schedule patterned on the Johns Hopkins model. Instead, the house staff was now on call every other night and every other weekend. This was a lark compared to the old schedule. My duties as a senior assistant resident placed me in charge of one ward each month, supervising the work of the interns; teaching the assigned medical students; making certain that work rounds and attending rounds were well attended, efficient, and stimulating; and responding to my rotation for medical consultations on the other services of the hospital. In addition, afternoons were devoted to ambulatory patients in the outpatient clinics. Since Duke Hospital was in its infancy, the outpatient clinics were being gradually developed and there was considerable room for expansion and innovation. I have already described the "L" Clinic (Luetic Clinic), one of the largest and busiest. With my experience in New Haven I was well prepared to help expand the diabetic clinic, where I soon applied much that I had learned from Dr. Peters. One problem at Duke was that most of our patients had to come from quite a distance. It was not unusual for them to have to travel 100–200 miles for their appointments. As I recall it, the clinic visit was paid for with a fifty-cent piece—this was *frequently* canceled for tenant farmers or share-croppers who seldom saw any cash. Patients often came to Duke without any appointments, arriving late at night, expecting to be admitted to a hospital already filled to the rafters. This took careful triaging by the house staff and around-the-clock attention of the social-service people, plus a great deal of understanding, compassion, and simple patience on the part of the house staff.

Since the Duke Endowment paid one dollar a day for an inpatient, a substantial contribution in those days, and was committed to serve the poor of North Carolina and South Carolina, we had our hands full. Duke Hospital, in keeping with the customs of its community, was a segregated institution, and this led to further problems. Black patients were admitted to the black wards, whites to the white wards, and pure-blooded Indians (native Americans) to the white wards. To one from the North, unaccustomed to these considerations, adjustments were necessary and there were some uncomfortable experiences. The black ward seemed always overflowing. It was not unusual to have no "colored" beds but ample numbers of beds for white patients. When we were dealing with an emergency, it was especially difficult to tell a colored family that they had to take the patient to Lincoln Hospital, the institution serving black patients in Durham. There were no ambulances. The vehicles used to transport emergency patients to Duke were often funeral hearses provided by the local undertakers. Saturday nights in the Duke Hospital Emergency Room were like working in a war zone populated by warring factions and wounded black patients. After sewing up some deep razor-blade or knife-inflicted wounds, the patient would be offered a bed in the hospital, only to reply "No, I'm goin find who cut me and take care of it myself." The perpetrator would soon be brought to Duke Hospital for repairs. To my knowledge, the only drugs involved in those days were moonshine and other alcoholic beverages.

There were no intensive-care units or coronary-care units, so that every ward had its share of very ill patients as well as those with chronic illnesses or diagnostic problems. With good judgemnt and careful management, it was possible to have a balanced service with a good case mix providing excellent teaching material for students house staff, nursing staff, and attending staff.

In those days general internal medicine ruled supreme. There were no subspecialty units and almost everybody was a generalist. Fellowships were few and far between. Board certification was practically non-existent. The Oslerian tradition of long service in the outpatient clinic and experience in the autopsy room and teaching at the bedside and in amphitheater clinics remained in vogue as the ideal preparation for the diagnostician and consultant of the era. In the tradition of Osler, the emphasis was on meticulous observation of the patient, careful history taking, thorough and systematic physical examination, and an attitude of therapeutic nihilism in an era when few if any medications were of any value.

Open-heart surgery did not exist and the technology for bypassing the heart was only a dream. I remember how excited we were at Duke when I admitted a young woman with ascites who had undergone abdominal exploration elsewhere revealing a normal liver and no clear explanation for the ascites. My examination revealed an elevated systemic venous pressure without valvular heart disease or myocardial disease, leading me to the diagnosis of constrictive pericarditis. I presented this patient at Medical Grand Rounds to Dr. Paul White, the eminent cardiologist who was then a visiting professor at Duke. He agreed with the diagnosis, and the next day the patient underwent resection of the pericardium by Dr. Deryl Hart who, as I recall it, had never before operated upon the heart. The operation went smoothly and the patient's ascites disappeared. Today, this is regarded as a fairly simple operation; back then it was a milestone. Another visiting professor at that time was Dr. Claude Beck, the pioneering cardiac surgeon from Western Reserve medical School. I had measured the patient's venous pressure by an indirect method devised by Eyster of Wisconsin. Dr. Beck taught me that the best and simplest technique for measuring venous pressure was to insert into a brachial vein at heart level, a large-bore needle attached to a manometer used for measuring spinal fluid pressure. For years this method was extensively used in many teaching centers, and then was abandoned because of careless technique and sloppy care of the apparatus leading to infections. I still believe it is a simple and very useful technique in good hands. Now that we have sterile disposable equipment, I can see no excuse for failing to measure venous pressure at the bedside or even in the clinic or office.

Another distinguished visitor was Soma Weiss from Boston, newly appointed to succeed Henry Christian at the Brigham. He remembered me from my internship application at Boston City Hospital described in chapter 5. One comment he made to Dr. Hanes after he had completed teaching rounds was to the effect that he wondered how Dr. Hanes had been able to attract so many unmarried residents to Duke. Dr. Hanes smiled in his Oslerian way. Of course, the real reason was that most of us were in poor financial straits, i.e., broke. The internship at Duke, as in most of the major university hospitals, paid exactly zero money and the assistant residency paid $500 per annum. Who could afford to get married?

During the fall of 1936, our chief resident in medicine, Bob McMillan, took his one month vacation and I was made acting chief resident. I enjoyed a very active month, especially the consultations. I answered these promptly and wrote concise and appropriate notes signed M. J. Lepore. By this time my nickname had become "M.J." and this is the way I was addressed by my peers. Among several innovations I introduced at Duke for the medical house staff was "quickie" rounds of the entire medical service at 5 P.M. for sign-off purposes. I had participated in these at Yale and learned that they served a real purpose. You learned something about every patient on the medical service and were informed as to the severity of illness or change in status. The presentations were extremely brief and very much to the point. These rounds were especially helpful for those covering the service that night. When I introduced these rounds at Duke, they became very popular and well attended. They also served another purpose. It had been the custom at Duke for some of the house staff to partake of a cocktail or two prior to going down to the dining room for dinner. I ran the "quickie" rounds in such a way that the last stop would take us right by the dining room, where the smell of good food persuaded most of our house staff to eat rather than drink. I don't know whether this custom still prevails.

While very busy with my house-staff duties, I was doing a lot of thinking about my future plans. I had several conversations with Dr. Hanes and learned that I was to start on 1 July 1937 as an instructor in medicine on a salary of $2,500 per annum. I also learned that living expenses in Durham were not cheap and rent was high. I had never worried about these matters because in the past they had been provided by my hospital.

Since the time was drawing near for a final commitment, I wrote to my mother (in Italian as were all of my letters to her) advising her that I would be staying in Durham and be receiving a salary of $2,500. Her answer was absolutely devastating and unexpected. In brief, she said that I had been away for nearly eight years but they had always expected me to come home to New York City to practice. Substantial sacrifices had been made by my family to provide me with the education and training I had sought and obtained. There were some debts that had been incurred and these had to be taken care of. Mom said she had spared me these problems because there was nothing I could have done about them in the past. Things were getting very precarious in the depth of the depression and there was even some fear that mortgage payments on our house could not be met and we were in danger of losing it. Pop had lost the ice business through no fault of his own but because electric and gas refrigerators had ruined it. He had opened a latticini-and-pork store, but it would take time before a profitable business could be built up. My brother, Frank, who had been contributing to meet family household expenses, was about to be married as were several of my five sisters, all of whom had been putting something into the family purse. My mother, a thrifty and sensible woman who had made every dollar go a long way, told me that the salary promised me would be grossly inadequate for my own needs. She knew I wished to marry and she could not imagine how I would manage on that small salary. But, most important, she said, she was depressed and sad that I was not coming home to fulfill the plans they had all sacrificed to bring to fruition. In fact, she told me it would break her heart if I did not come home, that she was at the end of her rope and without the sustaining hope that I would come home, all of her sacrifices would have been in vain. This letter was a shocker for me and it also made a lot of sense. The dream of full-time medicine was not for me unless I chose to abandon my family and its obligations. I knew I could never do this. The family ties were much too close. I owed them so much. Our general practitioner, family doctor, and friend, despite his good intentions, poured oil on the fire by constantly asking "Why doesn't Mike come home? He can make a good living here and I'll help him." He meant well but he really didn't understand my dilemma. His goals and mine were miles apart. I simply had to discuss this matter once again with Dr. Hanes and I did so as soon as I could. I was very reluctant to raise the question of money with Dr. Hanes and I really could not see the solution to my problem if I stayed at Duke. He was very kind and told me that if I needed more money, he could arrange for me to work part time in the PDC (Private Diagnostic Clinic) at Duke to augment my income. At that time, I was not enthusiastic about this option because it was common knowledge that promising young men at Duke who should have been focusing their energy on research, teaching, and publications were expending it on more remunerative private practice. Dr. Hanes also offered to lend me money to pay off my debts, but I felt that I could not accept his generous offer. My feeling was that after many years of preparation I should be able to earn enough from my professional work to pay my bills. I did not tell Dr. Hanes very much about my mother's depression and heartache expressed in her letter because it was very clear that she simply did not want me to remain in faraway Durham no matter what they offered me. I left Dr. Hanes in a troubled state of mind and sat in my room trying to sort things out. There was no one I could turn to for further advice. Clearly this was a decision I had to make for myself. If I stayed at Duke, I would be abandoning my family that had been sacrificing and planning anxiously for my return for eight years. I could not bear the thought of shirking my family responsibilities as the eldest son of a close-knit Italian family. I could not be guided solely by my own personal desires. My mother's wishes and those of my family had to be considered. I was also beginning to question the "full-time" future laid out for me. During my internship, residency, and fellowship, I had felt the tug of the patient in a way I had not quite anticipated. I liked research and its challenges and had succeeded in doing some excellent things, but I seemed much more attracted to my patients than many of my peers and competitors in the field.

I did not wish to be a one-month-a-year teacher on the wards with little or no close contact and follow-up of the sick. I wanted to be with my patients, responding to their needs, curing some, healing others, alleviating suffering, and above all serving the sick. My happiness would never be satisfied in the laboratory. I was meant to be a real practicing doctor, a healer, and I would settle for nothing less. On ward rounds I did not wish to be a teacher who knew all about diabetes and little or nothing about malaria, pneumonia, meningitis, tuberculosis, syphilis, or sprue. The model that the full-time system seemed to be cranking out was not for me. I wanted to become an outstanding and perhaps famous clinician and diagnostician. Narrow subspecialization might come later but for the first ten or more years I wanted to be a first-rate general clinician with wide interests and perhaps a hobby or two. I wanted to apply the superb education I had received at Rochester, Duke, and Yale to tackling clinical problems that cried out for their solution. I wanted to use the tools of the physiologist and the biochemist to save lives. I dreamed of doing the kinds of things Frederick Banting had done with insulin and Dean Whipple with anemia. I wanted to serve my fellow man at the bedside in the home, in the clinic, in the office, and in the library and laboratory. I wanted to share his suffering, to understand it, to comfort him, to heal if I could, to find new cures, and above all bring hope to the bedside. This was my wish list in 1937, but I knew deep in my heart that to achieve real happiness, I must also accede to the demands of my mother and my devoted family.

Clearly, the full-time arrangement at Duke, attractive as it was, could not resolve my personal problems and desires. After mulling this over I made the decision to leave Duke. I am sorry that I made this abruptly and without seeking further advice. This was perhaps in character because I have always been fiercely independent and proud of being able to support myself, even if it has meant carrying fifty-pound blocks of ice on my back and driving an ice truck. I also knew that I would not be able to marry if I relied on the modest salary then available at Duke. I had met the girl of my dreams, she had met my family and enjoyed their love and admiration, and they looked forward to our marriage. I knew that I must return to new York as soon as possible, roll up my sleeves, set up practice in our house in the Bronx, and begin to pay off the debts and save the family home from foreclosure and earn an honest living.

I knew that my decision would disappoint many people interested in my professional career. As I look back over the years, the basis for the decision was sound but its execution and timing left much to be desired. Years later, I would learn that I was not alone in defecting from full-time medicine, leading the Rockefeller Foundation to establish the Welch Fellowships for young investigators that would pay an annual stipend of $5,000 plus $1,500 for laboratory support. My deep regret is that I was hasty in my actions, and above all, I am sorry that I caused my friend and mentor, Dr. Hanes, any discomfort or embarrassment. I derive some satisfaction from knowing that with the passage of time and further reflection, Dr. Hanes forgave me and was pleased with the "less-traveled" road I had taken. Dean Whipple understood, and since he outlived Dr. Hanes by many years, there was additional time for him to view my career. Several years after I left Duke, Dr. Whipple and I had a meaningful discussion about my future. I said to him that I felt that I could combine a career as a practicing clinician, teacher, and clinical investigator without being on full time. His words were prophetic. "It depends upon how you use your spare time and I believe you can do it, but it will not be easy." Dean Whipple and I became close friends and I knew from him that I had fulfilled the promise he had seen in that teenaged youngster from the Bronx during that fateful admission interview at Rochester in the Spring of 1929.

Discipuli victoria magistri est gloria.

Chapter 9

You Can Go Home Again

M Y MIND MADE UP, I left Duke in 1937 to go home to start a private practice in general internal medicine. Home was a comfortable and well-built three-story brick house in the Wakefield section of the Bronx in what was then a white, middle class, largely Catholic neighborhood. There were three apartments, three rooms on the ground floor and the middle floor of six rooms with the top floor of seven rooms. Our family occupied the middle floor while the other two were rented to reliable tenants, providing income that helped to pay off a first and second mortgage. A few hundred feet away on Bronxwood Avenue the partially completed Our Lady of Grace Roman Catholic Church, presided over by Father Bassi, an Italian priest, enhanced our neighborhood, and our family were communicants. Especially for my mother, the church was a very important part of life. She attended Mass every morning until years later, when her terminal illness incapacitated her. Then one of the priests would come to our home regularly to give his blessing. Pop was a fairly typical Italian Catholic who went to church for funerals, baptisms, confirmations, weddings, and little else, but was staunch in his allegiance. As I look back, we grew up as a family that was quite ecumenical and respected all of the great faiths and did not feel that any one religion was the sole keeper of the keys to Heaven. Our friends included not only Roman Catholics but Protestants of many sects, Jews, and an occasional Seventh Day Adventist. We respected them and they in turn, respected us.

Starting a medical practice in 1937 in the midst of a severe depression that was becoming worse rather than better, was enough to scare off all but the bravest and toughest and those without any other options. In those days, anyone who became a doctor to get rich should have first seen a psychiatrist. Doctors' incomes were at the bottom of the scale of any of the professions except the priesthood or the ministry. Many doctors were relying on sidelines to pay their bills. Some were driving taxicabs. Others were being supported by their families or spouses. In the great cities, especially New York, hordes of displaced Jewish refugee doctors were competing for patients and struggling to make both ends meet. House calls were the mainstay of cash flow and income. Hospitals were used sparingly. There was almost no hospital insurance and few carried health insurance.

City hospitals, Fordham and Morrisania in the Bronx, were available to the indigent, who feared them and avoided them like the plague. The numbers of unemployed beggared description. Many families were on welfare if they could pull enough strings to get on it and not too proud to accept it. The W.P.A. and other projects kept many families from starving and helped to preserve the dignity of those on public assistance. Social Security was unheard of in more ways than one. Responsible people were frightened and uneasy. There were some compensations. A gallon of gasoline cost only ten cents and a good used car could be bought for two or three hundred dollars. A haircut was thirty-five cents. A good Fruit of the Loom cotton shirt could be bought for less than one dollar and an excellent pair of leather shoes for five dollars. Food was cheap and plentiful for those who had some cash. A hot dog with all the trimmings cost a nickel as did a bottle of Coke or an ice cream cone or Eskimo pie. Trolley and subway fares for long rides were only a nickel. It is said by some that a dollar in those days had the purchasing power of fifty dollars of today. What this adds up to is that *at least* the overhead for a doctor could be held down by good management and frugality and no frills. I quickly and at minimal expense turned the three-room apartment in our house into a suitable medical office consisting of a waiting room, a consultation room, and an examining room. One of my sisters, Annette, had worked as a receptionist for a general practitioner and had been trained in practical nursing skills. When I started practice, she took over these duties. There were no telephone-answering services in those days. We covered our telephones as best we could, usually with family help. My initial consultation fee was five dollars and included a comprehensive history, thorough general physical examination and pelvic and rectal examination, weight and height, urine examination including microscopic and a complete blood count, ESR and Kahn test for syphilis. The latter was sent to the Board of Health where it was done without charge. The other laboratory tests were done by me. It was not unusual for me to spend two hours or more on a new patient. At first we were plagued with patients who only wanted their blood pressure taken and nothing else. I refused to do partial and inadequate examinations at the initial visit and, despite the need for creating income, if I could not persuade the patient to have a complete examination, I would recommend that she consult someone else and ushered her out of the office. The news circulated around the neighborhood and it was not long before all of our patients understood the importance of a thorough examination and cooperated fully. As time passed, diabetics, syphilitics, arthritics, and patients with anemia were discovered and treated effectively while the word got around that a good diagnostician was practicing first-rate medicine in the neighborhood. Since I spoke Italian fluently, many of the old timers sought me out and gave my practice a good start. When a new young doctor started practice in a new area in those days there was no ethical way to advertise. Communication had to be chiefly by word of mouth. One satisfied patient would refer others. But it did help if, on occasion, you could do something spectacular.

John Bunyan (1628–1688) said it with eloquence, "Physicians get neither name nor fame by pricking of wheals, or picking out of this-tles or by laying of plaisters to the scratch of a pin; every old woman can do this. But if they would have a name and fame—if they will have it quickly, they must, as I said, do some great and desperate cures. Let them fetch one to life that was dead; let them recover one to his wits that was mad; let them make one that was born blind to see; or let them give ripe wits to a fool; these are notable cures; and he that can do thus first, he shall have the name and fame he desires; he may lie abed till noon."

One of these occurred when a devoted daughter of an elderly woman rang our doorbell and asked me to make a house call on her mother who was seriously ill and delirious. She said her mother had been hospitalized for two months in St. Vincent's Hospital in Greenwich Village where she had remained demented, picking at the bedclothes, incontinent of feces and urine, and unable to take any-thing by mouth, fed only by intravenous glucose. She was advised that her mother was senile, had "little strokes," and would never recover. She brought her home by ambulance to die in familiar surroundings. The daughter had heard of me because of a rather dramatic recovery that I had brought about by medical therapy and begged me to visit her mother.

I feared for the worst but the love and dedication and devotion of the daughter for her mother was so compelling that I simply could not refuse to go. This I did. They lived in a small and very clean and neat-ly kept home nearby. Her mother, white-haired and flushed, was pick-ing at her bedclothes, disoriented, hallucinating, and crying out. I could not detect any focal neurological signs indicative of an organic brain disorder or stroke. She was incontinent and soiling the sheets with loose stools and urine. There was no evidence of a dermatitis but I noted that her tongue was very beefy and red, the picture of chron-ic pellagra. She was obviously demented and had diarrhea fulfilling two requirements for the diagnosis. The other two, dermatitis-absent and explained by lack of exposure to sunlight and the final D, death, was something I hoped to prevent. I told her daughter that my diag-nosis was pellagra, a condition I had seen a great deal of at Duke but seldom diagnosed or recognized by doctors in New York. She clearly needed specific therapy—vitamins and fluid replacement best administered in a hospital. The daughter refused to consider hospitalizing her mother and begged me to try to treat her at home. At that time the cause of pellagra was unknown, but I did know that a vile-tasting crude liver extract made by the Valentine Company of Richmond, Virginia, could cure pellagra. We sent out for several bottles of this and administered it by nasogastric tube into the patient's stomach and added some vitamins then available. I instructed the daughter on how to use the nasogastric tube and left for the night. Within 24 hours, improvement occurred and within 48–72 hours the patient cleared her dementia, the diarrhea stopped, and she went on to a complete recovery and was well for many years. The news of this awakening of the dead by the new young doctor on the block was heralded as a miracle and did much to publicize my work in that neighborhood.

On another occasion I was called to see a teenager, the only son of a widowed mother, a juvenile insulin-dependent diabetic who had developed a chill, fever, and right-chest pleuritic pain followed by a cough productive of rusty sputum. I hastened to make an emergency house call, quickly made the diagnosis of lobar pneumonia, hospitalized the patient in a local private hospital where Neufeld typing revealed a sputum loaded with type-I pneumococcus. He was a good candidate for anti-pneumococcal serum therapy. It was a Saturday evening and Board of Health stations were not open and they did not carry the preferred and more effective Felton serum. I discussed this with the mother who begged me to spare nothing to get her son well. I drove to an all-night pharmacy on the Grand Concourse and obtained the Felton serum and paid for it out of my own pocket. There was no house staff in this private hospital. I personally started the IV and slowly administered the Felton serum and the response was dramatic. Remember, this was in the pre-antibiotic era. The diabetes and ketoacidosis responded well to appropriate therapy. The patient left the hospital in seven days, fully recovered from his pneumonia. The sad part of this story is that I was never paid for my call and never reimbursed for the cost of the serum. Sixty dollars was a lot of money in those days. When I told my family doctor this story, he said "Well you have learned a lesson, don't ever pay money out of your pocket for any patient's medicine. Put it on the hospital bill." Was he right or was I? All I know is that after saving that young boy's life I knew I was doing what was right even if it left me without the rent money. I would do it again under similar circumstances.

I resisted every effort to install expensive and elaborate equipment in my simple office primarily to generate income. The pressures on me to purchase x-ray equipment and a fluoroscopic unit were heavy and clearly income-related for the salesman and myself. I had learned to use fluoroscopy at Duke and felt that it should be used by a well-qualified radiologist. To this day, I have always referred radiologic work to radiologists and limited my own activities to internal medicine in the Oslerian tradition. In the current era of income-motivated, procedure-oriented medicine, I still stand for the old-fashioned virtues of laying on of the hands, communication, verbal and nonverbal, meticulous history taking, thorough physical examination, wisdom, experience, and the selective and discrete use of laboratory, radiologic, and ancillary aids. Early in my career I learned the real secret to cost-containment in medicine. First, keep the patient out of the hospital if possible. Second, train the gatekeepers extremely well in internal medicine and diagnosis, reward them appropriately for cognitive work, and trust them to make sound decisions without second-guessing on the need for further studies and procedures.

On another occasion, I was consulted by a North Italian, an intelligent artisan who was ill with chills and fever and left-flank pain. He had been hospitalized several times in what was then the Italian Hospital in lower Manhattan where he had been treated by a urologist and told he had an infected left kidney. A variety of medications had been administered to no avail. Here again the era of antibiotics was yet to come. I examined the patient very carefully and checked his urine, found it full of clumps of white blood cells and some red cells. In addition to a gram stain of the urine sediment I did a Ziehl-Nielsen stain for tuberculosis. The latter was strongly positive, a Gafkey IV. Certain of the diagnosis of renal tuberculosis, I referred the patient to the Squier Urological Clinic at Columbia-Presbyterian Medical Center and I gave him a note on my prescription pad stating the diagnosis and enclosed in the envelope the slide that was positive for acid-fast bacilli. This created quite a stir at Columbia-Presbyterian, where he was seen by the chief resident in urology, Dr. Thomas Killip. Dr. Killip called me and congratulated me on making the diagnosis. He also told me that he was from Rochester and had practiced internal medicine in Rochester, New York, for several years before deciding to become a urologist. Dr. Killip removed the patient's left kidney and cured him of the disease that had plagued him and incapacitated him for several years.

One night I was called by telephone to make a house call in a slum section of the Bronx to see a man with chills, fever, chest pain, and cough. I arrived there and could not believe what I was seeing. The house was a small bungalow with a gas-burning stove and five or six little children running around crying, some of them coughing and

sneezing and all of them with colds. The mother seemed ill and mentally disturbed, the father was acutely ill and in respiratory distress
with a temperature of 104°F, chills and cough. It was winter and an
epidemic of flu was raging. I knew the man belonged in a hospital. He
said he would rather be dead than to go to Fordham Hospital. That
day I had received a notice from the Hospital of the Rockefeller
Institute that they were interested in treating and studying patients
with pneumonia and would do this free of charge. I called the
Rockefeller, where a nice chap named Paul Beeson was the resident
on call. I described the patient to him and he seemed reluctant to
accept him because I had not detected any clear signs of pneumonia
on physical examination.

When I explained how difficult the situation was in this home, he
agreed to accept the patient. I then persuaded him to send an ambulance. At first reluctant, he finally agreed. The patient did not develop
pneumonia and responded well to good nursing care. This was my
first contact with Dr. Paul Beeson, whose career in full-time medicine
is legendary. You know, of course, that I was never paid for my efforts
nor did I expect to be. A follow-up on this case report is that six
months later the mother of the brood of children committed suicide
by gas, taking all of the children with her. The father was at work and
was spared.

On yet another occasion, I was prevailed upon to make a house
call on an impoverished family living in the Bronx in a rambling old
house with a wood stove for heat. The patient was a woman in her
forties, the second wife of an elderly widower who had raised one
family and started another with his new wife. There were several
young children in the house. The patient had some form of cirrhosis
of the liver with marked ascites. She had been in Fordham Hospital
on several occasions for belly taps but she was now refusing to go
there because there was no one to take care of her children. I knew
she had to be tapped and I boiled water and sterilized the equipment
on the wood stove and proceeded with the paracentesis. It went very
well and she was much relieved. When it recurred some weeks later, I
repeated the procedure. The following morning I was awakened by
severe itching and found I had brought bedbugs home to my bed and
wife. I knew where I had caught them and they had caught me. After
this I simply had to insist that the patient go to a hospital for treatment.

I was holding office hours one day when the doorbell rang and a
highly excited neighbor asked me to hurry with him to a house across
the street where he said one of his relatives had turned on the gas and
was unconscious, seeking to cash in on a $25,000 insurance policy that

he had purchased with the aim of using it to pay off some debts. I grabbed my bag and hurried down the street. The front door of the apartment was ajar but the place reeked with gas from the oven. Someone had turned it off. On the floor was a stocky, swarthy man in his forties, unconscious and not breathing. I could not get a pulse or hear any heart sounds. He clearly needed intracardiac adrenalin that I had in my bag. However, my syringe and long needle were not sterile and would have to be boiled but there was no time for this. Besides I did not dare strike a match in that kitchen filled with gas. It took me a one second to make up my mind. I used the unsterile syringe and needle to zap one cc of 1:1000 adrenalin into the patient's heart. The response was dramatic, his heart resumed beating, and I continued artificial respiration and he emerged from his coma. By the time the ambulance from Fordham Hospital had arrived the patient was out of immediate danger. The resident riding the ambulance congratulated me and I was glad to turn the patient over to him for transportation to Fordham Hospital. This man recovered and was alive and well and quite prosperous thirty years later when I last inquired about him. Had he died, the policy would not have been valid because it did not cover a suicide.

By this time you must be aware that many of my patients, when I started private practice in 1937, were poor. Many had been abandoned by their doctors because they were unable to pay and almost all refused to go to available city hospitals. I responded at all hours of the day or night and tried to do what I could in a very difficult period for both patients and doctors. The response time of city ambulances in that era in the Bronx was an abomination. In essence, neighborhood doctors functioned as the 911 of that day. Not infrequently I would be called out during the night, travel over icy and slippery roads looking for a house number in a strange neighborhood, and on arrival be met at the door by someone saying "Sorry Doc, we already got our own doctor." Getting back to sleep after one of these adventures was not easy. In my day it was not unusual to be called out to a seedy neighborhood to see a patient and family completely unknown to me, my name having been plucked from the classified phone book at random. Their own doctor had either refused to come or was otherwise "unavailable." Diagnoses had to be made firmly and quickly and appropriate action taken. I still vividly recall one dimly lit hovel of a home, the patient sitting up and wheezing away in considerable respiratory distress, his bed surrounded by many anxious relatives eyeing the strange and very young doctor with anxiety and suspicion. Just a few months before, a doctor who had finished injecting diphtheria antitoxin into a seriously ill child was blamed for causing her sudden death, and her father, carried away by his grief, stabbed the doctor to death.

Also there came to mind the passage in A. J. Cronin's best-selling novel, *The Citadel*, where the new young doctor (played in the movie by Robert Donat) in a Welsh mining village answering an emergency call from the family of one of the coal miners, had to face the hostility and suspicion of the many relatives who missed their old doctor and feared what would happen with the new doctor. For the patient I myself was seeing in 1937 his apparent cardiac "asthma," due to acute left-ventricular failure, called for an injection of morphine for its relief, and he would have gotten it if he had been in a hospital. Fear of an adverse reaction to morphine or respiratory depression caused me to first try an injection of phenobarbital and calm reassurance. The last thing I wanted to risk in a shaky situation was sudden death. I elected to go with the phenobarbital and fortunately it calmed the patient down and he soon became comfortable and I was able to leave the house with all of us in a good mood. We learned very little about these aspects of the practice of medicine in medical school, but we had good basic rules to guide us and time and experience as solo practitioners out on the firing line would soon make veterans of all of us.

The house call by a doctor has virtually disappeared in modern-day medicine. It has been deemed wasteful, impractical and anachronistic and not cost effective in the present era of medical practice. 911 is called and management of the serious emergencies is turned over to paramedics or medical technicians. I have never understood why, in New York City and similar areas, an intern is not assigned to ambulance duty to accompany the paramedics as part of the rotation as it was in the old days. This is not intended to displace the paramedics, who may be much better at resuscitation and handling emergencies than a doctor. It is to give the intern an opportunity to witness crises at the site of origin and in a two-week rotation appreciate what it is really like out there in the streets when the 911 calls come in. At Rochester as a senior medical student I rode the Strong Memorial Hospital ambulance for two weeks, accompanying a surgical intern. I have never forgotten that experience and I strongly recommend that every medical student should be required to ride the ambulance as an observer for two weeks. It might inspire some. It might also serve to improve the image of doctors if the public could see them, as they did in the old days, as dedicated young people responding to the call of people in distress.

Let's do something about bringing the doctor back to the streets and out of the ivory tower, and let's do this while the young men and women are still young and idealistic. Beyond this, let us reinstall the house call at the central core of primary care medicine. It brings us closer to our patients and serves to cement the bond between physician and patient that is at the basis of all good medical practice. I have seldom made a house call at night that failed to send me home tired but happy with my lot as a physician serving my patients to the best of my abilities. That's what doctoring is all about.

In my early days of practice in New York City over fifty years ago, I made house calls in some very rough and rundown neighborhoods but I never once had a hand laid on me in anger or with bad intent. The people were poor but they respected the doctor, they would carry his bag without stealing it, kept neat and surprisingly clean homes and apartments, were not on drugs, and were all for law and order. Family life was the key to survival. People tried to help each other. Property was not defiled or destroyed. There was no graffiti. The police would almost never give a doctor a ticket, and the doctor's insignia was a permit for parking almost anywhere except on top of a hydrant. Compare this with the present era when doctors in New York City no longer carry the black bag for fear of attracting muggers. The attaché case has taken its place. In at least one major hospital in New York City, the attendings coming in for a nighttime emergency put a ten-dollar bill in the upper jacket pocket so that the would-be mugger may quickly remove it without harming the doctor. The streets of New York in these rundown areas are dominated and populated by muggers, panhandlers, hookers, and hustlers, most of them on drugs, who are a menace not only to outsiders but also to the poor people who are forced to live there, innocent victims and sitting ducks for many brutal assaults and random violence and shootings. When our politicians rail against doctors for avoiding practice in these run-down communities, why doesn't someone take steps to stop the crime, clean up the mess, and revitalize the slums created? During the years of the Great Depression, poverty was rampant in our city but law and order and civic responsibility did prevail and things were never as bad as they are today.

Why don't we have a Marshall Plan to rebuild America's inner cities? A nation that put a man on the moon should have the commitment and capacity to restore our inner cities and their residents to the world of peace, order, and productivity. All Americans must participate and share in this. A crusade must be organized to accomplish this. We simply cannot abandon our future to the status quo.

I close this chapter by contradicting Thomas Wolfe, for I did go home again and served my people at a very trying period of their lives and mine. I knew I was succeeding against great odds in giving my patients and my people the best of medical care. When feedback reached me that I was becoming known as the second Dr. Antonio Stella, I appreciated that my people were awarding me a very special commendation.

Dr. Antonio Stella (1868–1927) was a distinguished physician from the small mountain town in southern Italy, Genzano, in La Basilicata, that was the birthplace of my father and home of the Lepore family. Dr. Stella was educated in Italy and came to New York City, where he practiced and developed a great reputation as a diagnostician and consultant in internal medicine. Overcoming great odds and bias, he rose to eminence as a physician, educator, and influential citizen. He was the first Italian appointed to the staff of the original New York Hospital as a professor and a Fellow of the New York Academy of Medicine.

In 1924 he published a small gem of a book entitled *Some Aspects of Italian Immigration to the United States*,[1] which clearly expressed his pride in the contributions made by Italian immigrants to America and dispelled some of the myths and anti-Italian bigotry that was rampant at that time. Dr. Stella was obviously well informed about the adverse conditions that Italian immigrants faced and did not hesitate to expose them in public print at a time when the Italian immigrants had few defenders. Witness this excerpt from his book.

> The Italian immigrant may be maimed and killed in his industrial occupation without a cry and without indemnity. He may die from the "bends" working in the caissons under the river, without protest; he can be slowly asphyxiated in crowded tenements, smothered in dangerous trades and occupations (which only the ignorant immigrant pursues, not the native American); he can contract tuberculosis in unsanitary factories and sweatshops, without a murmur, and then to do this country an additional favor, when he is disabled and sick, he goes back to his mother country to die, thus giving the American cities the credit of a low death rate. (p. 94)

In the preface to his monograph, Dr. Stella made this eloquent comment:

---

1. Antonio Stella, M.D., *Some Aspects of Italian Immigration to the United States* (New York and London : P. G. Putnam's Sons, The Knickerbocker Press, 1924). Reprinted by Arno Press, 1975.

As an enthusiastic American of Italian descent and very proud of my ancestry, I can honestly say that, while my sympathies may have somewhat colored the style of my exposition, I have not, to the best of my knowledge, allowed it to color its contents. In fact, I have not failed to point out the negative features of the Italian character, whenever present. Many of the Italian faults are the results of adverse factors in their historical backgrounds. But a race, which, after centuries of oppression, exploitation, and repeated foreign invasions, has not only not surrendered its identity, but has managed to preserve its physical, mental and spiritual vigor and can boast of an intellectual eminence for a period of two thousand years (a record without parallel in the history of mankind) can well be relied upon to give in the future a full measure of contribution to this country and to the progress of civilization.

How prescient a statement! Is it any wonder that I treasure the appellation of my *paesani* that I was "il secondo Stella"?

Chapter 10

My One and Only Wife

THE MOST IMPORTANT DECISION the young doctor must make is to court, pick, and win the hand of a good woman. This decision should not be made too early in life for many reasons. Medicine is a jealous mistress and calls for all of one's energy, passion, and dedication. Osler's admonition to "keep the emotions on ice" during these early years, still makes sense but is seldom heeded. Early marriage is the trend as is the premature raising of a family when study, reading, working with patients at the bedside, in their homes and the clinics and pursuit of experience should be the order of the day. No matter how much I hear in defense of early marriage, I remain convinced that the young doctor or medical student cannot serve two loves and do justice to both. I also know that this advice will fall upon deaf ears and youth will insist on pursuing its own priorities, disdaining the admonitions of senior advisers. I am reminded of the comment of an actor friend and patient who moved heaven and earth to secure a minor role in *Hamlet* with Richard Burton when the latter was at the height of his success. My friend called me to let me know that he had won his bit part and would let me know how it worked out. At his next visit I asked him what sort of Hamlet Richard Burton had been. He replied "Very good. But you know, no one can drink all night, make love to Elizabeth Taylor, and still play an extraordinary Hamlet, but he came pretty close to doing it." The Richard Burtons among medical students are, in my experience, nonexistent. Osler's warnings were issued in a day when internships and residency and fellowship programs were rare, and when Board certification did not exist. However, when I was a medical student at Rochester in the 1930s, I remember very well an epidemic of medical-student marriages, usually involving a secretary or nurse at Strong Memorial Hospital. Dean Whipple, an Oslerian to the core, posted a typewritten notice on the student bulletin board to the effect that we should keep our emotions on ice as advised by Osler. Furthermore, the next medical student who married an employee could find that her job had been terminated. I really don't know how many were deterred by this warning but I suspect there were several secret "arrangements." Marriages consummated by medical students or even premedical students too early in life may be an explanation for the high divorce rates in this group, although I have no statistics to support this belief. One solution I can think of is to accelerate the preparatory course leading to medical school by encouraging the skipping of grades by gifted students so that they may reach medical school in their teens. What is the track record of "gifted children" in medical school? In a recently published monograph entitled "The Academic Acceleration of Gifted Children,"[1] this subject is discussed by a number of scholars who present the pros and cons. On the whole, I believe the evidence for accelerating the progress of such children in the elementary and high school phase of their education is most persuasive. The numbers of students studied and followed are small but almost all who went on to professional and graduate school performed exceptionally well. It would be interesting to pursue this matter further with the medical school deans.

At the time I was graduated from medical school (1934) most of us were single and felt that we should complete our residencies before getting married. In those days, an intern or a resident lived up to this designation by living on the premises. In fact, married interns were not accepted at many prestigious hospitals.

It was my good fortune to meet a most attractive, in fact, a beautiful young woman at Duke who was the efficient and very capable head nurse on Nott Ward. This was the "colored" ward where almost every patient was acutely or severely ill. It was the most popular ward on the medical service because of the superb teaching material. It also called for hard work and long hours. Miss Ardean Clough Everett, the head nurse, attracted me not only by virtue of her beautiful face with high cheekbones, a fair complexion capped by lustrous marvelous jet black hair, sparkling brown eyes, and a charming low-pitched throaty voice. Her double-frilled, pleated Philadelphia General Hospital (Old Blockley) nurse's cap was most attractive, as was the Buster Brown collar she wore. In addition to all of this, she was extremely intelligent, quick, and resourceful, never getting rattled no matter how serious problems were. We hit it off right away. She told me later that she especially appreciated me because I wasn't always hollering for the nurses' help and seemed to be able to get things done by myself.

She also thought my patient case presentations on rounds with the professor were always on target. Well, one thing led to another, and we began dating. I remember returning late from a meeting in Dayton,

---

1. W. Thomas Southern and Eric D. Jones, eds., *The Academic Acceleration of Gifted Children* (New York and London: Teachers College Press, Teachers College, Columbia University, 1991).

Ohio, to escort her to a dance hosted by Dr. Hanes in the ballroom of the Washington Duke Hotel with Johnny Long and his orchestra supplying the music. My guest was this young lady, beautiful and radiant in a striking dress, her attractive black hair seen without the Blockley cap. She was really the "belle of the ball." It was the first time I had gone to a dance in Southern territory and I had a lot to learn. After a few turns on the dance floor, I would receive a tap on my shoulder as one of the other doctors would break in and take her away. She was, of course, charming and having the time of her life. I recall that I spent most of my time off the dance floor or with another partner. But, *c'est la vie.* She was clearly happy and that was all that mattered. We would go, in the very little spare time allotted to us, to nearby Chapel Hill where there was a small restaurant where we would have ice cream or a dessert or watermelon and we would talk about our lives. Money for this was hard to come by but I could sell my blood for transfusion for $25 making this possible. In those days interns at Duke were paid nothing. We were given merely room and board. Stipends were not given by any of the major university hospitals. Hospitals that paid salaries for interns were considered to be second class. I learned that Ardean was helping to support her widowed mother. Her father had died in his thirty-second year of typhoid fever, which was rampant on the Eastern Shore of Maryland as it was in North Carolina and other Southern States. In those days, a head nurse at Duke was paid in the range of $70 a month plus room and board. Within a few months, I knew that I had found the woman of my dreams and I courted her in earnest, somehow scrounging the time to get away for an occasional date. When I was awarded the American College of Physicians Research Fellowship for 1935 at Yale University Medical School and New Haven Hospital, she celebrated with me, even though it meant we would be apart for that year. As I recorded in a previous chapter, when I was at Yale I kept in touch with my fiancée by letter, telephone, Whitman chocolates, and occasional flowers—usually red roses. When I returned to Duke as senior assistant resident in medicine in July 1936, we continued our courtship whenever our work permitted.

For reasons discussed in the preceding chapter, I left Duke and set up practice in the three-room apartment on the first floor of our home in the Bronx in February 1937 with my sister Annette serving as my receptionist. By dint of being on call around the clock, the 911 of that neighborhood, some good luck with my patients and my Italian heritage, despite a severe economic depression, I built a steadily growing practice in general internal medicine, and in September 1937, Ardean and I traveled to her home in Sudlersville, on

Maryland's lovely Eastern Shore, where we were married. After spending a week's honeymoon at Atlantic City at the Claridge Hotel, we came home to temporary housing in my parents' home, pending arrival of our newly purchased furniture at our new apartment on Bronx Boulevard.

No doctor husband and wife could ever have had a happier life than Ardean and I. In the nearly fifty years of our marriage, I do not recall a single serious argument. It was a joy for me to see her beautiful face and listen to her low voice at breakfast. Our love grew stronger with each year and was increased with the birth of our wonderful son, Frederick, who is now a professor of neurology and neuro-ophthalmologist at the Robert Wood Johnson School of Medicine. Ardean was everything a doctor's wife should be. She was tactful, kind, the soul of discretion, never revealed a confidence, and was in every respect very much a lady. I saw to it that she wanted for nothing. My greatest joy was to bring home to her some major triumph or the story of an interesting patient. As a marvelous nurse, she understood what I was saying and trying to do. She put up with delayed meals, my being paged from a social occasion, my intensity of commitment to the care of my sick people, and my love and concern for our families. She never had to worry about a budget or bills. I took care of all of that. She had experienced enough of financial hardship when she was growing up on the Eastern Shore. I knew I had found a gem, a really great lady, loyal wife and companion, beloved mother and daughter. This is what made the life of this doctor possible and attractive.

Ardean taught me to love the Eastern Shore of Maryland, where her forbears came from London on the ship *James* under Captain William Cooper, arriving in America in 1635. "The original family is listed in colonial records. There was no limit to choice of homesite—land was free and no lord was to take his money for rents. He was a free man in a free land."[2] The Everett family prospered on the Eastern Shore and Ardean's mother, a school teacher in a one-room schoolhouse, owned two farms and was known as an excellent teacher, called by all "Miss Annie." When she married, her husband owned a farm and a sawmill. Ardean was the first born of five children whose lives seemed secure and well provided for until the sudden death of their father at age thirty-two of typhoid fever. Ardean's mother returned to teaching, but the expenses of raising and educating five children soon

---

2. The Everett Family Genealogy.

ate up the heritage of the farms and the sawmill. Ardean, as the eldest child, early on was the leader of the family, caring for her younger siblings while her mother was busy teaching school. It was not an easy life but it molded character and a spirit of independence. A family doctor noticed that Ardean handled herself and the other children well in emergencies and suggested that she become a nurse. He thought she should go to Easton, Maryland, for her education. One of Ardean's cousins had graduated from the Philadelphia General Hospital's excellent school of nursing and urged her to apply there for her training. At this time Ardean was only sixteen years of age and had not completed high school. She was interviewed by Miss S. Lillian Clayton, one of the major figures in American nursing education and the head of the nursing school at Philadelphia General Hospital. Miss Clayton, herself an Eastern Shore woman, made an exception for this thin, black-haired, bright, and well-mannered girl and accepted her, perhaps influenced by the fact that she herself had entered nursing at the tender age of sixteen. Her judgment proved sound. Ardean was one of her stars, despite several illnesses she suffered while in nursing school. The most serious of these was diphtheria with myocarditis, which she caught from a patient and barely survived. Her first position after graduating in 1928 was as head nurse of the pediatric ward of the Graduate Hospital of the University of Pennsylvania. There she made an excellent reputation and worked with a number of outstanding and famous doctors. One of these was Chevalier Jackson, who was then the foremost bronchoscopist in the country, with children being sent to him from all over the world for removal of aspirated or swallowed foreign bodies. One Christmas, Dr. Jackson presented Ardean with one of his famous water colors entitled "October." It hangs on our living room wall, a reminder of the past. Other distinguished physicians she assisted were Henry C. Bockus, the great gastroenterologist, and George Morris Piersol, the eminent internist.

It did not take her long to realize that she could not advance in her career as a nursing educator without a high school diploma. In those days, there were no equivalency diplomas. The demands of her daily work were so great that going to night school to complete her high school was too much. Finally, she decided to stop working as a head nurse and returned to Chestertown, Maryland, where she enrolled in the high school and in two years completed her high school education with high grades and was awarded her diploma. She then returned to nursing and in 1933 accepted an assignment as head nurse at Duke University Hospital, where it was my good fortune to meet her in 1934.

I had never known what a summer vacation was like. As a boy, when the rest of the family went to the Rockaways for the summer, I stayed home with my father, working with him in the ice business and traveling with him to the Rockaways on the Pennsylvania Railroad on Saturday afternoon to spend the rest of that day and Sunday with my brother and sisters at the beach. In medical school I worked in the research laboratories during each summer. When I started in practice, vacations meant nothing to me. It was of primary importance that I be able to pay my bills and be available to the patients who needed me. As my practice developed, Ardean and I were able to take one or two weeks off in the summer, usually going to the Jersey Shore, Toms River being a favorite. After the war, several new developments occurred. Having leased a house in West Englewood, New Jersey, and adapted myself to sleeping in New Jersey and practicing in New York, we decided to purchase an old house in Englewood. It was quite modest and we benefitted from a Veterans' Home Administration low-interest loan. My mother-in-law, who had been hospitalized with Alzheimer's disease for the duration of WW II, kept asking to come home. With the purchase of the house at 87 Knickerbocker Road, in Englewood, we had a nice bedroom for "Miss Annie" and arranged for her to come home. Soon she would be joined by Frederick, our son, born in November 1949 amidst great rejoicing. Each summer we would now spend one month, usually July, at Rehoboth Beach, Delaware, close to Ardean's beloved Eastern Shore. Some of the happiest days of our lives were spent at Rehoboth where we entertained family and friends and relaxed. Years later, after Fred had gone to college at Princeton, we purchased farm land on the Eastern Shore near Sudlersville, outside of Chestertown and Church Hill. My brother-in-law, Leroy, who was in charge of the Sudlersville Bank, gave me sound advice about purchasing farm land and he also managed the farm. Ardean's face would always light up when we decided to go down to the farm. The first farm was named Jamaica Farm and it gradually became the nucleus of a sizable piece of land, totalling 353 acres. Leroy saw to it that crops of wheat, corn, soy beans, and the like were grown. He also had a herd of steers. Ardean now had her own automobile and could drive down to the farm whenever she so wished. We derived much enjoyment from Jamaica Farm. Ardean was proud that once again she was in possession of farmland. A favorite down-home saying whenever a blow-hard native was boasting, was "Talk's cheap but it takes money to buy land." I did some of my best medical writing and research planning at Jamaica Farm. I had bought the land for the love of my wife who was always so happy when she was on her beloved Eastern Shore. I had never thought much of it as an investment but it turned out remarkably well. When Ardean became ill and incapacitated, we had no real reason to return to Jamaica and I began to think of how and when to dispose of it.

One day the telephone rang and when I answered it, Miss Janet Nile of the University of Rochester School of Medicine and Dentistry's development staff was on the line. She called to notify me that the school had decided to name the chair in gastroenterology for me and would appreciate my helping them with it. I was rather staggered and greatly honored by this unexpected proposal. Dr. Arthur Localio, who had been approached regarding fund raising for the medical school, said he was getting tired of raising money at NYU for doctors who had died. "Why don't you honor people who are living instead of waiting until they die?" said Arthur in his inimitable way. What could I say? There was no way I could say no to this proposal to help my alma mater and to advance my specialty of gastroenterology.

In a way, it reminded me of Abraham Flexner's comment of 1920 that he would start a new medical school in Rochester that would be the Johns Hopkins of New York and shake up the existing medical schools in New York City. Gastroenterology in New York needed a burr under the saddle. What better place to start than Rochester? I began to warm up to the project. I doubted very much that we could raise one million dollars but I was promised that the school would also do its share. I discussed this with Ardean and she was pleased with the honor and eager to see it come to pass. We raised a substantial amount of money from my patients and family but there was a limit to this and the goal represented a lot of money. Finally, since Ardean and I were not spending any time at Jamaica Farm, we decided to deed the farm to the University of Rochester School of Medicine and Dentistry for the Lepore Professorship in Gastroenterology. A charitable trust was set up and a gift of $350,000 was made to help support the Lepore Chair.

Ardean died in 1987 after a prolonged and agonizing struggle with a severe form of Parkinson's disease. Our fifty years together will never be forgotten. She made it possible for me to be the kind of doctor I have become. As an old-fashioned first-generation Italian-American, in the tradition of my forebears I wear the black necktie in memory of my one and only wife and the mother of our son. I thank the Lord for having sent this angelic woman to be my companion for a lifetime.

Why have I told this story? To pay tribute to a remarkable human being who will never be forgotten by me, my family, my son and grandchildren, and to some degree by posterity. She had a great deal to do with the development of the doctor I have become and perhaps her memory will serve as an inspiration for the wives of other doctors.

In writing this chapter, even though it is more than six years since Ardean's death, this writing, to use a word I learned in the hills of North Carolina, where middle English still exists, has served to *assuage* my grief for a great lady.

Chapter 11

~ɔᴊɕ~

The Bronx Is the Graveyard for Specialists, 1937

MY PRACTICE IN THE BRONX was keeping me very busy and I was learning lots of things they had never taught in medical school. The first unpleasant experience was to find that virtually all of the doctors I encountered were splitting fees and accepting kickbacks. A specialist would charge the patient a fee and then split it with the referring doctor. A surgeon would operate and split the fee with the family doctor. If you called a private ambulance for a patient, the ambulance company would kickback a portion of their fee. If you ordered a back brace or a truss for a patient, the surgical supply firm would kickback part of the fee. I knew this was wrong and I didn't have to take a course in medical ethics to be certain this was unacceptable. I remember how embarrassed I was when I accompanied one of my early patients for an ENT consultation on the Grand Concourse. The specialist tried to slip a few dollars in cash into my pocket as I left his office. I returned these on the spot like a hot potato and told the doctor that I did not split fees. I never sent him another patient. On another occasion, a check for ten dollars arrived in the mail from an ambulance company. It was promptly sent back. A similar check from a surgical supply house for a back brace was returned by the next mail. Both checks were accompanied by a short letter saying that I did not accept these "referral" fees and suggested that they charge my patient less.

To my chagrin, I soon found out these practices were rampant in the Bronx and presumably elsewhere. When I discussed this with some of my colleagues, various explanations were offered. Times were tough and they needed every dollar they could get to meet their expenses. They said everybody was doing it. Some would later, when they were financially better off, deny that they had ever split fees. Others would claim it was merely another legitimate business expense that served to steer patients to them. One of the scandals making the rounds was that a noted ENT specialist, under the auspices of his medical society, was lecturing in Brooklyn on the evils of fee-splitting when a physician in the audience rose up, waved a piece of paper, a copy of a canceled check, made out by the specialist and shouted, "Doctor, this is a check you made out to me when you split a fee." It is said the specialist made a hasty exit via a back door.

Given the existence of this evil and my adamant decision never to participate in it, there was a practical point I had to face. Where to send my patients for consultation or surgery? It became crystal clear to me that I could never be content with a Bronx practice using second-class hospitals and fee-splitting consultants for my patients. I needed a hospital that took care of the poor and medically indigent as well as the well-to-do under the same roof and with the same staff. There was no medical school in the Bronx (1937) and very little prospect of there being one in the foreseeable future. Many colleagues told me that the Bronx was the graveyard for specialists. Beyond this, despite a successful and growing practice, I could not be happy or fulfill my destiny without medical students and house staff to teach. I also had to have day-to-day contacts with my peers and my betters. I proceeded to plan my career in private practice to achieve these goals. I knew it would not be easy but I have never chosen the easy way.

The practice, by dint of hard work and some good fortune, was prospering and I was able to save our house in the Bronx from foreclosure. The Home Owners Loan Corporation (HOLC), set up during the Roosevelt Administration, rearranged our mortgage so that one monthly payment spread out over twenty or more years would not only pay off the debt but also interest and taxes. I remember the agent who worked out the details. He was a very pleasant man who told me that I had no legal obligation to assume my parents' debt. I knew he meant well but my reply was that I had a moral obligation to do this and insisted on doing it. This saved our house and served as a partial payment for the sacrifices my parents and my family had made to provide the superb education I received.

I kept in close touch with my fiancée, who was now a head nurse in medicine at the Billings Hospital of the University of Chicago. We were planning to marry soon and I was saving up for this great moment in my life. The knowledge that I would soon be joined by my beloved Ardean inspired me to work harder and harder with my practice and to willingly accept the vicissitudes and heavy demands of being on twenty-four-hour call. We were married on 18 September 1937 in Ardean's hometown near Church Hill on Maryland's Eastern Shore. All we could afford was a short vacation spent in Atlantic City at the Claridge Hotel and very soon I was back at work. We rented a nice apartment on the Bronx River Parkway where we set up housekeeping.

By this time, I had made up my mind to swallow my pride and approach the Columbia-Presbyterian Medical Center Department of Medicine, seeking an appointment on the staff of the Vanderbilt

Clinic. This decision was not an easy one for me. As I explained in an earlier chapter, I was very upset and disappointed that I had not been notified of the change of date of the internship examination at P&S in 1933. In fact there had been a rather heated exchange on this matter between Dr. Nathaniel Faxon, the director of Strong Memorial Hospital and then president of the American Hospital Association, and Dr. Walter W. Palmer, the Bard professor and chairman of the department of medicine at P&S. I was willing to forget about the past and let bygones be bygones.

Fortunately, Dr. Ashley Weech, professor of pediatrics at P&S and Babies Hospital, remained a good friend since my having worked in his department in the summer of 1931. I had a nice visit with Dr. Weech and explained that I was in practice in the Bronx and hoped to do part-time volunteer teaching. Unknown to me, Dr. Weech had been in private practice for a brief spell before coming to the Babies Hospital and he clearly understood why I was seeking some sort of affiliation with a major teaching center. It would be good for me and for my patients. He subsequently discussed my situation with Dr. Robert F. Loeb, who was in charge of the department in Dr. Palmer's absence due to illness. His reaction was warmly supportive. In fact, Dr. Weech told me that Dr. Loeb said, in the light of the fiasco of 1933–34, the "very least we can do for Lepore is to give him an appointment to the department of medicine starting with the Vanderbilt Clinic." I accepted with alacrity and gratitude.

The chief of the Vanderbilt Clinic in Medicine at that time was Dr. Samuel Waldron Lambert, Jr., son of the former Dean of P&S. We became good friends and he helped me a great deal. I gave two afternoons a week to the Vanderbilt Clinic, where I taught one medical student at each session, reviewing the history and physical findings on a new patient the student had spent the morning examining and interviewing. We would work out a plan of study and management and the patient would be added to my list. The student and I would then proceed to examine and treat the "return cases." Working the Vanderbilt Clinic was very stimulating. In fact, in retrospect, after all these years I feel it was the best-administered outpatient clinic in the country, and, I suspect, the world. Patients came by appointment and were assigned to a specific attending physician whose name was known to the patient and appeared on the yellow appointment card as a permanent assignment. If my name appeared on the yellow card, I was forever that patient's doctor. Conditions in the clinic were excellent. The clerks were alert, well mannered, and well educated. The social workers under Miss Janet Thornton were superior, as was the nutrition staff under Miss Nelda Ross. The nursing staff was of the highest calibre and dedicated to its work. One of the best in the medical clinic was Miss Margaret Reid, whose name will be mentioned again in another context. The spirit of the Vanderbilt Clinic was a joy to behold and it was indeed a privilege to work there. All of us seemed to have a common purpose, to give our patients optimum care. In those days, attendance in the clinic was required of all the doctors, including the senior professors. It was very stimulating to see Dr. Robert F. Loeb, Dr. Walter W. Palmer, Dr. Dana Atchley, Dr. Franklin Hanger, Dr. Dickinson W. Richards, Jr., Dr. Robert L. Levy, and other senior professors working side by side with the junior members of the staff in the Vanderbilt Clinic. It made each of us feel that ambulatory care was important and an essential part of the training program. Privacy was respected in the clinic. Each doctor had a private room for his patients and addressed them as Mr. or Mrs., no first names being used.

On any given day there would be at least twenty doctors in the general medical division of the Vanderbilt Clinic, each one teaching one student and many of them capable of being a chairman of medicine in a major medical school.

Most of the staff served without pay and many of the best specialists in New York were part of the team. Patients were referred from far and wide with all sorts of unusual and serious medical problems. For myself, the Vanderbilt Clinic had a very special meaning, especially after my experience in the Bronx. I knew the tablet on the wall near the Vanderbilt Clinic entrance to the Medical Center meant what it said:

PRESBYTERIAN HOSPITAL FOR THE POOR
OF NEW YORK

WITHOUT REGARD TO RACE, CREED OR COLOR
Supported by
VOLUNTARY CONTRIBUTIONS

High on the list of voluntary contributions were the attending physicians and surgeons who served without pay, year after year, with dedication and enthusiasm, making it possible for the poor to have excellent medical care without bureaucratic government intervention or interference. I became the first new member of the department of medicine of the Columbia-Presbyterian Medical Center who had received all of his training at other centers, in my case, Rochester, Duke, and Yale. For some reason most people referred to me as the new attending from Duke.

With my appointment to the staff at Columbia-Presbyterian, I decided upon another important move. This was to open a second office in Washington Heights near the Medical Center. This I did in 1938, renting a two-room office in a modest private house on 175th Street between Audubon Avenue and Broadway. The house was owned by one of our Italian *paesani*, Mrs. Cardillo, who rented the space to me for thirty-five dollars a month. This was a good decision for me and made a great deal of sense because my earlier roots were in Washington Heights. I already had developed a small clientele in that area and the proximity to the hospital would be a great advantage. My only competition in the neighborhood at that time was a very active and successful general practitioner who was overworked and could not qualify for appointment to the Columbia-Presbyterian staff. It was not long before my practice in Washington Heights boomed to the extent that I did less and less in the Bronx. I was the first staff member of Columbia-Presbyterian to have an office and home in the Washington Heights community.

Most of the staff had offices on the Gold Coast, Manhattan's fashionable East Side and Park Avenue. A small minority had offices in Harkness Pavilion. By dint of hard work and success with my students in the clinic, I earned the respect of my chief, Dr. Sam Lambert, who conveyed his approval to Dr. Walter Palmer, the Bard professor and chairman who had returned to his duties. I referred many interesting patients to the Vanderbilt Clinic and I became known to the staff and was able to select appropriate consultants for my patients. I began doing research on non-tropical sprue and small-bowel disorders, work that I had started at Duke. It was the era of vitaminology, and new vitamins were being discovered at a dizzying pace. With the discovery that nicotinic acid, a member of the B complex, could cure pellagra for a few pennies a day, the search was on for other miracle vitamins, and the B complex was full of these. I had started a sprue clinic and was studying small-bowel function in that disorder using barium and radiologic techniques. I quickly found that x-ray studies of the small intestine were in their infancy and the interpretation of the same set of films could vary quite widely from one radiologist to another. At the time, I was trying out a variety of B complex factors in the treatment of sprue and sought to study the responses not only on clinical grounds but by using the small-bowel x-ray study. Dr. Ross Golden was the chairman of radiology at P&S and renowned for his knowledge and publications on the gastrointestinal tract. Puzzled by the conflicting reports I was receiving from Dr. Golden's staff, I requested an interview with him that he graciously granted, starting a friendship that would last for the rest of his life and most of my own.

Dr. Golden confessed that he knew relatively little about the radiology of the small intestine but indicated that he would be very interested in pursuing it with my collaboration. He then agreed to review all of the small bowel studies that I was requesting. To accomplish this, he set aside a definite time once a week to go over my cases. This proved to be a milestone in my career. It was very instructive for me to see how a superior mind, the best in modern radiology, would approach the problem. The first thing he did was to standardize the procedure. He specified that the patient be examined after an overnight fast. He was given six ounces of barium sulfate by mouth in the morning and then followed with serial films of the stomach and small intestine with fluoroscopy at appropriate intervals.

Dr. Golden then coined the term "transit time," which he defined as the time it took for the barium to travel from the stomach to the cecum. He used the term "segmentation" to describe breaking up of the barium meal. "Flocculation" was coined to describe the appearance of speckling of the barium, like a positive Kahn test. Dilatation or narrowing of the small intestine were meticulously described and other new words were added to the vocabulary of the small-bowel radiologist. Dr. Golden preached and practiced detailed and precise word descriptions of the radiologic findings and felt that the word picture should be so accurate that if the films were ever lost, the written report would serve as a permanent record. What a difference between Dr. Golden's reports and the current one-liners, "the small bowel appears entirely normal."

While Dr. Golden pioneered in the pursuit of the radiologic examination of the small intestine, he encouraged me to pursue my clinical and investigational studies in patients with small-bowel disorders, including sprue and other conditions, among them regional enteritis. In 1945 he published his classic monograph "Radiologic Examination of the Small Intestine,"[1] which included the findings on a number of my patients. By this time he was the foremost radiologist in the field. The second edition (1959) of his monograph[2] still remains the definitive work on this subject. At the Medical Center, during the late thirties and early forties, before going into military service, I became the clinical expert on small-bowel disease and was asked to

---

1. Ross Golden, *Radiologic Examination of the Small Intestine*, 1st ed. (Philadelphia: J. P. Lippincott Company, 1945).

2. Ross Golden, *Radiologic Examination of the Small Intestine* (Springfield, Ill.: Charles C. Thomas, 1959).

see most of the patients in this category or their films. What was it that fascinated me about the small bowel and its diseases? First of all, the ailments were supposed to be rare and very little was really known in clinical medicine about this twenty-foot segment of the intestinal tract, in part because of its relative inaccessibility. I soon became aware of its major importance in human nutrition and general health. Here it is that absorption, digestion, and assimilation of nutrients, fluids, and electrolytes takes place. The human being can live without the esophagus or stomach, without the pancreas or gallbladder, and without the colon, but cannot survive without the small intestine. This should place the small bowel at the head of any list of essential organs, but in the thirties it was the most neglected area in the gastrointestinal tract and the least studied. This was, for me, a very real challenge and an opportunity. Additional stimulus to study the small intestine came with the publication in 1932 by Crohn, Ginzburg, and Oppenheimer of the Mt. Sinai Hospital of their first paper on "Regional Ileitis."

Dr. Ginzburg, a surgeon, thought the disease should have been named after him and he was probably right. Dr. Burill Crohn loved to tell the story that when he was a medical student at P&S in 1905, the professor of medicine, Evan Evans, would advise them to skip the section on the small intestine in their textbook of medicine because there were no known diseases of that organ. In 1937, I diagnosed my first case of regional enteritis and studied her ailment with the best tools I had then at my disposal. I was privileged to follow this patient in my clinics for over fifty years and I learned a great deal from her. I also followed a large series of patients at Columbia-Presbyterian with this disease and had, next to the Mt. Sinai group, the largest series of patients in New York with this disease. This led to my interest in other inflammatory bowel diseases, especially ulcerative colitis, which I shall discuss in a later chapter. While I was in military service at Valley Forge General Hospital, I continued to study regional enteritis and allied disorders on a limited scale. In 1944, I was invited to lecture on small-bowel disorders at the New York Academy of Medicine, where I presented some of the case studies from Valley Forge.

When Dr. Golden first came to P&S in 1922, there was no department of radiology. His first appointment was in the department of medicine as an assistant professor in charge of radiology. He was a 1916 graduate of Harvard Medical School, interned in medicine 1916–17 at the Peter Bent Brigham Hospital, served as a Major in World War I, followed by an assistant residency in radiology at the Massachusetts General Hospital. In 1935, radiology was designated as a separate department at P&S and as the years went by the department grew in stature and fame with Dr. Golden leading the way. Greatly sought after for residency training, many of his trainees rose to positions of eminence in radiology and its subspecialties. The move from the old Presbyterian Hospital at 71st Street in Manhattan to spacious quarters in the newly built Columbia-Presbyterian Medical Center at 168th Street and Broadway in 1928 gave Dr. Golden the opportunity to develop the radiology division along academic and university lines while expanding its teaching, research, and service activities. He was more than equal to this task. This was in the days when continuing medical education of the attending staff was in its infancy. Since all of the departments relied upon the radiology division for assistance in diagnosis, it became a headquarters for exchanges of views and continuing education. Dr. Golden was a superb teacher and the attending staff flocked to him with their problem cases. Dr. Golden not only knew radiology, he was well informed and knowledgeable in the area of gastrointestinal physiology and pharmacology, a worthy disciple of his renowned teacher at Harvard, Dr. Walter B. Cannon. Many of the prominent clinicians at P&S owed their reputations as diagnosticians to Ross Golden, who frequently solved their problems. He worked effectively and energetically with his clinician associates who sought his advice. In effect, he was the main teacher of gastroenterology at P&S, for there was no formal program in this field. The general internist was king of the hill and ruled the roost. Almost by default, Dr. Golden took over the teaching of this important subspecialty working effectively with surgeons and internists in an institution where its leading teacher of internal medicine, Dr. Robert F. Loeb, had as one of his five famous aphorisms, "Keep the patient out of the surgeon's hands." Despite heavy administrative demands, Dr. Golden continued to take his turn in the fluoroscopy rotation and he never lost touch with patients. Throughout his life he maintained his zest for new knowledge and continued to explore new frontiers in gastrointestinal physiology. He was the first at P&S to explore the nuances of cholinergic and anti-cholinergic influences on small-bowel motor function in keeping with his early training in physiology at Harvard.

As I look back, I was blessed to have Dr. Golden as a friend and mentor who taught me many things. A parting pearl from Dr. Golden was expressed one day when I walked into his x-ray department, where he was reviewing a series of chest films that he invited me to examine. I was astonished to see that a right-upper-lobe mass was present on all of the films going over a period of many months. My reaction was one of dismay that the mass had not been excised. Dr. Golden said to me these are the films of Senator Vandenberg, a prominent politician from the mid-West. "I called this a carcinoma and recommended surgery but others disagreed. It is now inoperable and he is dying of cancer. Don't ever be a VIP when you get sick."

Chapter 12

~oiu~

The Columbia-Presbyterian Medical Center, 1937 — The First of Its Kind

A S MY PRACTICE FLOURISHED with my beloved wife helping to run the office and assisting me, my ties to the Medical Center became closer and closer. We finally decided to move our home from Bronx River Parkway to Washington Heights and combined the office and home in a first-floor apartment in a nice building, first on 173rd Street and then in a new building at 200 Haven Avenue. During this period Ardean's mother, a very sweet and charming woman, moved in with us and became a full-time member of our family. We gradually phased out the Bronx office because there was more than enough to do in Manhattan.

As the months went by, my steady and exceptional work in the Vanderbilt Clinic did not go unnoticed. Dr. Samuel W. Lambert, Jr., son of Dean Lambert, who was my chief of clinic, was very supportive and I shall never forget him. Late in 1938 Dr. Palmer asked me to come in to see him. He indicated how pleased he was with my performance and then surprised me by asking me to become director of the personnel medical department of Columbia-Presbyterian Medical Center on a part-time salaried basis with a stipend of $3,000 per annum, some fringe benefits, and a modest budget. The opening had developed with the retirement of the elderly physician who had been in charge. Dr. Palmer indicated that he would like me to take over and update the department's program for the ambulatory care of several thousand non-professional employees, including 500 food handlers and a large number of orderlies. A major activity was the pre-employment examination of all applicants for work and the setting of standards for a multitude of positions. I had never done anything like this before but I quickly grasped that this could be a major challenge in what was then the largest medical center in the world. There was no book or blueprint on how this could be done. This was to be left to my judgment. Dr. Palmer offered his help and support and that was all I needed to know.

The department was housed in the basement of the Presbyterian Hospital, where some space had been allocated for the purpose. An administrative manager and secretary, Miss Martha Swensson, was in charge and the chief nurse was Miss Marie Gaffney, a St. Vincent's

Hospital R.N. who was energetic, good at triage, and had the bright and cheerful personality needed to reassure our clientele. I found Miss Swensson to be an excellent administrator with a valuable background in medicine and sound judgment and tact. These two young ladies were the backbone of the department, and with their dedicated and loyal help I quickly built up the confidence of the personnel of the medical center in the new medical department. The budget permitted me to pay a modest stipend to young physicians on our staff who would assist me with our program. The times were very difficult and many of the young attendings vied for assignments in our clinic. They could work in a nice environment, meet decent people, and practice good medicine without concern, for the costs that were assumed by the hospital and contribute to the welfare of the Medical Center. The doctor's paycheck could pay their rent and could be relied upon as a steady income in an era when few doctors knew where the next dollar would come from. When the caseload was very heavy, we paid selected residents to help out by moonlighting with us.

If an employee became ill, he or she was sent to the personnel clinic to see one of our doctors. If hospital admission were needed, this was arranged and provided at no cost to the employee. This proved to be a great inducement for people to seek jobs at the Medical Center and I made a point of emphasizing this in my discussions on policy with Mr. Luther, the director of personnel. If the employee needed consultation and care in the Vanderbilt Clinic by specialists, this too was given without charge. I soon found out that all too often our employees were kept waiting in the clinic by a resident or intern, losing much time from work. This was especially true in the ENT, dermatology, and orthopedic clinics. I resolved this by arranging to move our employees ahead of the queue by frequent telephone calls to the clinic aide. When the clinic demands were heavy, I made special arrangements for the employees to be seen by a competent attending physician or surgeon rather than house staff. When I took over the service, employee clinical charts were numbered according to a system that differed from that used in the record room for all other patients. This was initially designed to preserve confidentiality, but after some effort we were able to arrange to number the charts for employees in the same manner used for all other patients. This made access to charts uniform and avoided the inability to obtain employee charts when the personnel medical department was closed. Most of the doctors working in the personnel clinic were very capable internists, but to assure uniformity, all problem cases were unobtrusively reviewed by me. Miss Swensson and Miss Gaffney were very adept in selecting cases for my review.

Early on, I discovered that some prospective employees were being started on jobs without undergoing a physical examination. Their supervisors defended this by saying that there was no use wasting time and money examining people who simply could not function acceptably in their assignments. This was an especially dangerous lapse in the case of food handlers who might, if ill, or carriers, expose a hospital full of patients. I insisted that all persons hired by the hospital had to be cleared and examined by the personnel medical department before they started to work no matter what it cost. Dr. Palmer backed me and the policy was enforced. I also required stool cultures on all food handlers before giving them clearance. At the time I took over, this was being done only for typhoid. When the Medical Center was downtown, the notorious carrier "Typhoid Mary" had spread the disease far and wide. This was a raw nerve and I did not have to argue for the stool typhoid tests, even though they had turned up only one carrier in ten years. Since we were hiring many Puerto Ricans, I insisted on having a stool for ova and protozoa on all food handlers and we turned up quite a number of positives. This cost us some money but it was good medical practice. I remember that someone complained that I was running a Mayo Clinic in the cellar at Columbia-Presbyterian and questioned the need for stool examinations for parasites. Mr. Dean Sage, president of the Presbyterian Hospital and Mr. Harkness' personal representative, came by one morning and questioned me about the stool examinations. I answered that if I had to stop anything I would stop the routine typhoid cultures and continue the parasite examinations because of their greater positive yield, but I would prefer to keep both. He agreed. My battle to keep our medical standards for employment at a practical and sound level paid off major dividends in 1940, when an outbreak of bacillary dysentery occurred among the student nurses at Columbia-Presbyterian. Some blamed it on the food they were eating in the hospital but I was skeptical because everyone knew the girls were often eating at the greasy-spoon restaurant on the corner of Broadway and 168th Street when they were bored with the hospital food.

However, the news of the outbreak had reached the Department of Health and I received a call that the associate commissioner of health was coming up to review our methods of checking the food handlers. I remember spending a Thanksgiving Day processing several hundred food handlers, including a proctoscopic examination for those who could not spontaneously pass a stool specimen. Dr. Greenberg of the Health Department was present when this was done. I later learned that he had shut down the private pavilion at Mt. Sinai Hospital for one month because a food handler had transmitted his dysentery bacteria to a number of hospitalized patients. He found that they were putting food handlers to work without examining them. Dr. Greenberg was so impressed by the way we were checking our food handlers that he complimented me at the end and said the next time this happened, he would take my word over the telephone.

Word quickly got around that the personnel medical department had saved Harkness Pavilion from being closed down for a month. That could have paid for quite a few stool examinations.

The personnel medical department was flourishing and had gained the respect and confidence of our employees. We tried whenever possible to have the same doctor follow the same employee. I saw that the blue-collar-type employees were very happy with our care. Another group was quietly coming to us. They were mid-level and at times high-level white-collar workers and supervisors who had in the past been seen and treated by senior professors at the Medical Center. I found that Dr. Robert F. Loeb, the brilliant clinician and teacher, had been taking care of quite a number of our valued personnel. He was becoming more and more busy with his many other obligations and I made every effort to help out when I could, trying to spare him as much as possible. This was not easy for a junior physician but I tried. With the passage of time, more and more employees were being referred to the personnel medical department for their medical needs.

Through my work as the director of personnel medicine, I was now better known to the employees than almost any other doctor at the Medical Center. I also was working closely with the various consultants and learning a great deal from them. I became quite expert in what we now call primary-care medicine. In addition, I introduced a program of preventive medicine for employees, including vaccinations and annual checkups. It was not unusual for me to see and examine fifteen to twenty patients in a morning. During a flu epidemic I actually checked out sixty patients in a four-hour session. I was fast, well organized, and had a superb team working with me. I know that I was not missing much, because the patients were closely followed and not lost in follow-up. One day I tied up the operating rooms in Presbyterian Hospital with three patients with right-lower-quadrant pain. One had an acute appendix, another had a perforated appendix secondary to a carcinoma of the cecum, and the third transposition of the viscera, situs inversus, that led to a prolonged search for what proved to be a perforated acute diverticulitis. That day I had a semi-facetious telephone call from one of the surgical residents to take pity on them.

Many years later, I would learn that my first professor of medicine, Dr. William S. McCann, had told his cousin, Olive Miller, who was an employee of Presbyterian Hospital and one of my patients, that "Mike Lepore took on the tough job of personnel medical director to show the Medical Center staff what a topflight internist could do to improve employee care. His track record will stand for years to come."

My private practice was also going full blast. Dr. Golden thought very highly of me and brought me to the attention of Dr. Fordyce Barker St. John, the charismatic and great abdominal surgeon who filled many of the beds in Harkness Pavilion with patients who were referred to him from far and near. Through Dr. Golden, Dr. St. John asked me to see one of his patients, Mr. J.C.E. who had been experiencing repeated episodes of upper GI tract bleeding with melena and had been referred to Dr. St. John for surgery for a duodenal ulcer. The only problem was that Dr. Golden, a superb radiologist, disagreed with the diagnosis and said he could find no evidence of a duodenal ulcer. In those days, that was the ultimate gold standard. Gastroscopy with the semi-rigid Schindler instrument was inadequate for viewing the duodenum.

I recommended that we do a small-bowel x-ray study to rule out a small-bowel cause of bleeding. None was found. Then we passed a long double-lumen Miller-Abbott tube into the duodenum and aspirated as it moved down the small bowel, looking for a site of bleeding. The findings were negative and he had stopped bleeding. Dr. St. John also had our professor of hematology, Dr. Randolph West, consulting on this puzzling case. Hematological studies were all within the normal range except for mild anemia. One day the patient saw me because of a urinary tract infection for which he was studied by Dr. John Robinson of our urology staff, who found that the patient had a horseshoe kidney. Since congenital anomalies are often multiple, I suspected that the cause of bleeding might be a Meckel's diverticulum of the ileum. It just happened that Dr. Golden in his many years of GI radiology had never been able to demonstrate Meckel's by x-ray. We tried again with a small-bowel enema and series to no avail. The patient continued to bleed intermittently, usually when faced with some crisis at work and often when up for a promotion at Western Electric. In 1942 I saw him again for melena and had a long talk with him. He said he was thinking of going to the Lahey Clinic and might have Dr. Lahey operate to settle the diagnosis. I called Dr. St. John and told him what the patient had said. I also said I thought he should be explored for a Meckel's diverticulum. Dr. Randolph West voted against exploration and advised the patient to take iron tablets. Dr. St. John then said to me "Well I have a dilemma here. My two consultants disagree. What shall we do?" I suggested getting another opinion from Dr. Walter W. Palmer. This was done and Dr. Palmer agreed with me that the patient be explored. I have neglected to mention that the patient's wife was a third-year medical student at Long Island College. I have always made it a practice to be present in the operating room whenever one of my patients is having a major operation. I have learned a great deal by being a spectator. There is no better way to understand what the patient is going through than by being there. The anesthesiologist can be observed, the assistants and nurses are visible, and the surgeon himself is seen in action. There is no better way to monitor a surgeon than by watching him at work.

I don't think there is a substitute for this kind of experience. In the old days at Columbia-Presbyterian, the operating rooms had galleries from which one could communicate with the surgical staff and see what was going on, using binoculars if necessary. This kind of voyeurism has virtually disappeared, the reasons propounded being fear of infection, lack of interest, and waste of operating-room space. This subject has been reviewed in great detail by Dr. Owen Wangensteen.[1] Most of the new hospitals no longer have balconies or facilities for viewing operations that were standard in the old days. I am certain that precautions can be taken with modern construction techniques and laminar-flow devices to avoid infection and contamination in operating rooms. My vote is to reinstall viewing facilities to the operating room. Don't blame the non-surgeons for not visiting the operating room when their patients are there. Don't blame them for their lack of interest in surgical techniques. My teaching has always been that the medical man or woman who has recommended or agreed that a major operation is indicated should be there when it is being done.

At any rate you can be very certain I was in the operating room that morning when Mr. E. was being explored. Dr. St. John, in addition to being a master surgeon, was a dramatic teacher. His hand was the first to enter the abdomen. He palpated and explored the right lower quadrant for a brief interval and then pulled a loop of small bowel out of the incision. He looked up at the balcony and asked "Is Dr. Lepore there?" "Yes Sir!" "Please go down and tell Mrs. E. that you were right. He has a Meckel's diverticulum and I am going to cure him by removing it."

---

1. Owen H. Wangensteen and Sarah D. Wangensteen, *The Rise of Surgery* (Minneapolis: University of Minnesota Press, 1978).

I went out of that operating room at full speed, found Mrs. E., and rejoiced with her over the good news. The Meckel's diverticulum contained ectopic gastric mucosa with a small peptic ulcer in its center, the source of intermittent bleeding. Mr. E. stopped bleeding, was promoted at Western Electric, and lived to a ripe old age.

In a great teaching medical center, news of an outstanding diagnosis spreads like wildfire. This is how reputations are made. These are the home runs that the long-ball hitter produces that create much of the excitement in our profession and separate the men from the boys.

On another occasion, Dr. St. John asked me to see Mr. M., an elderly man who had been referred to him because of weight loss, anemia, and a mass in his right lower quadrant. This proved to be a carcinoma of the cecum that was resectable, without any regional or hepatic spread. Dr. St. John said "Mr. M. was operated upon one week ago and I am certain I cured his cancer, but he is steadily failing, wasting away, has diarrhea, dementia, picking at the bedclothes, and will take nothing by mouth." I entered the room and quickly realized that the patient had pellagra, a disease I had seen frequently at Duke. His tongue was beefy red and slick, plus angular cheilosis as well as lesions in the nasolabial folds consistent with pellagra. I recommended Valentine's Crude Liver Extract via nasogastric tube. The response was dramatic and in two weeks Mr. M. left the hospital in good condition. My training at Duke had once again prepared me well for this small miracle.

One night I made a house call in a walk-up tenement on 164th Street, east of Broadway, to see an elderly man who had fainted. He resided on the sixth floor, a pretty good jaunt but I was a lot younger then. Mr. F. was alert, white-haired and rosy-jawed and comfortable. He described his blackout and denied previous episodes, loss of vision, headache, tinnitus, or vertigo. His blood pressure was normal as was the remainder of his examination. At that time Soma Weiss in Boston had written several papers on something he called carotid sinus syncope. I pressed on Mr. F.'s carotid artery at the angle of the jaw. The response was dramatic, his heart stopped and he began to faint. I immediately stopped pressing on his neck and prayed that his heart would start up again and it did. I thought I had made a diagnosis of carotid sinus syncope and sent Mr. F. to the Medical Center with a note on my prescription pad to the effect that he should be admitted for further investigation and consultation for this entity.

He was admitted to the ward medical service where he remained for several days and then was sent home with the diagnosis of syncope of undetermined origin. I talked to the resident who had admitted him and he said they had been unable to reproduce the syncope during his stay despite multiple attempts to provoke it. This left me in a quandary in my relationship to the patient. I rechecked Mr. F. and had no difficulty in provoking the attack by pressure on his carotid.

I was annoyed by this and decided to telephone the attending physician in charge of that ward. He just happened to be a wonderful man, Dr. Dickinson W. Richards, destined years later to share in the Nobel Prize for Physiology and Medicine for his work on cardiac catheterization. Dr. Richards listened to my complaint and asked whether I could find time to come to his office in Harkness Pavilion with my patient so that he and I could examine him together. It was arranged and we proceeded with the examination. Dr. Richards failed to elicit a positive response and I thought I could see why. He was not pressing on the carotid sinus. I then proceeded with my examination and without any difficulty caused Mr. F.'s, heart to stop and induced beginning syncope. Dr. Richards apologized for the missed diagnosis and re-admitted the patient. A carotid sinus denervation was performed by our senior head and neck surgeon, Dr. John Hanford, and Mr. F. was relieved of his syncopal episodes. In retrospect my admiration for Dr. Richards's honesty and humility never wavered over the many years I was privileged to know him. He was truly a great physician.

On another night I was called out to a small apartment on 175th Street near Audubon Avenue to see a young deaf-mute married woman who had suddenly developed severe abdominal pain localized to the left lower quadrant. I had never learned in medical school or residency how to examine a deaf mute but, at the bedside that night, I learned quickly. Her husband used sign language and transmitted my questions to her while I watched her facial expression and her movements. On physical examination, there were signs suggestive of peritoneal irritation on the left. They had been married for one year. Her menstrual periods were usually regular every 28 days but she was two weeks overdue. I made a diagnosis of a probable ruptured ectopic pregnancy and sent her down to the emergency room at Columbia-Presbyterian with my note on my prescription pad to that effect. The ob-gyn resident who examined her disagreed but he had the good sense to put her in what we called the overnight ward for further observation. Early the next morning, the senior attending in ob-gyn, Dr. Anthony D'Esopo, examined the patient and agreed with me that it was a ruptured ectopic pregnancy and operated upon her, saving her life. Dr. D'Esopo and I became good friends after this experience and he did most of the gyn surgery for my patients over the years. He remarked on a number of occasions that my pelvic examinations and diagnoses were very accurate. "If Mike Lepore says that ovarian mass was not present one year ago, I will operate on his say so."

One day I was asked to make a house call to see one of the "little people" who was having abdominal pain. This young man was one of the famous Rose midgets appearing at the Audubon Theater. They were housed in a large nearby apartment. I think there were about fifteen of the midgets occupying the various rooms. They were well spoken and well mannered and very concerned about the patient. He was very intelligent and gave a good history. I examined him, found no focal signs, and decided that he had some form of acute gastroenteritis. I prescribed an antacid and light diet and suggested they call me again the next day. He recovered. I had been contacted because Mr. Rose's daughter, Dr. Antoinette Rose Parry, was a classmate of mine at Rochester.

My next call was on an adjacent street where a teenage girl was complaining of sore throat, fever, and choking feeling. She had a clear case of rheumatic heart disease with mitral stenosis. The throat difficulty was a swelling in the region of the right tonsil. I thought it was a peritonsillar abscess but I had never seen one before. Her mother was a friend and devotee of Dr. Charles Imperatori, a famous ENT specialist with his office downtown in the thirties. I called him and described my findings. He asked me to imitate the patient's speech over the telephone and to the best of my ability I imitated her nasal tone. Dr. Imperatori said "That has to be a peritonsillar abscess. Bring her down to my office and I will take care of it." He nicked the abscess under local anesthesia and aspirated a large amount of pus, curing the girl of her ailment.

The practice was booming and I was happy helping some wonderful people and earning my way without being obligated to anyone. I was also getting referrals from the hospital as well as from some of my colleagues. Most important were several referrals from my professor, Dr. Walter Palmer. One of these was a lovely Colombian family from Baranquilla, Colombia, the Santo Domingos. The professor asked me to take over the care of Mrs. Santo Domingos' mother, who had been operated upon in Harkness Pavilion and found to have an inoperable cancer of the stomach. I visited this nice woman at home and made her comfortable with symptomatic measures. I also encouraged better nutrition with a special diet and vitamin supplements. To my pleasant surprise, the tumor must have been slow-growing. She improved, had no pain, and was able to make a trip to Colombia and lived for nearly three years after the initial diagnosis. The family moved to America and became my patients until I went off to war in 1942. Dr. Palmer also referred a young man to me in 1940, the nephew of Dr. Dean Lewis, chairman of surgery at Johns Hopkins. He and his family have been patients and friends of mine ever since.

I have watched him with pride rise to a senior partnership with a prestigious Wall Street law firm.

In 1941, my sister Lucille, the eighth and last-born of our flock, sought my advice about entering nurses' training. At the time she was a young and well-paid designer for a novelty company and turned her paycheck over to our mother. Lucille was very bright and was the only one in our family except for me who had graduated from high school. The other sisters left high school for private business schools and to positions in private industry, a common practice in New York City in that era.

Lucille's fiancé had been called to military service with an Anti-Aircraft (ACK ACK) unit in January 1942. Ardean and I were delighted that Lu wanted to be an R.N. as her part in the war effort and I agreed to sponsor her and to pay the bills. She was accepted by the excellent and vigorous school at Bellevue Hospital and entered their program in February 1942. Ardean relived her own career as a student nurse, enjoying selecting her outfits and advising and encouraging her. Eventually Lucille entered the Cadet Nurses Program and in February 1945 she received her R.N. diploma, the Bellevue cap, and pin. By that time her fiancé had been returned from the North African and Italian theater of war because of battle-incurred injuries and ailments. While on temporary duty they were married in February 1945. Lucille was asked to remain at Bellevue as Ward Instructor on Floor A7B, the busiest medical wards there. She performed these duties with dedication and great skill for three years, serving also as head nurse. In the meantime her husband, in the classic Army tradition that those who had already served with distinction should continue to serve, was rotated back to combat in the Italian campaign in early April 1945. Lucille remained at Bellevue until 1948, when I opened my Park Avenue office and persuaded her to take charge of my private practice. This was one of the smartest moves I have ever made. Through her efforts many of my accomplishments were made possible in successfully combining private practice, extensive free clinical work, teaching, research, and administration. She left Bellevue with her colors flying and, in our family tradition, left a fine reputation as a superb and dedicated nurse. This spirit has continued for the remainder of her professional life as the superb nurse administrator of my personal practice unit. God has blessed me with the wonderful women who have been associated with me in my life and work. High on the list, headed by my mother, Filomena, and my late beloved wife, Ardean, is my baby sister, Lucille.

My activities in the Columbia-Presbyterian setting were becoming more and more demanding of time and energy, but I was enjoying every minute. The inpatient medical service of the Presbyterian Hospital was divided into three geographical areas: East, Center, and West, the eighth floor for men and the ninth for women. Each unit was called a team and had a permanent chief, usually a senior attending. Assigned to him were the junior attendings, a mixture of full-time salaried men and women and volunteer faculty in private practice. The overall head of the department was Dr. Walter W. Palmer, the Bard professor of medicine. There was a healthy spirit of rivalry among the three teams that enhanced the quality of teaching and practice. Medical Grand Rounds were held once weekly in the main amphitheater and were called Team Rounds, with each of the services presenting cases. The presentations were first rate and the discussions usually quite informative. It was said, somewhat in jest, that if you attended Team Rounds, you could keep up-to-date on recent trends in medicine without having to spend much time in the library. I tried to do both and continued to be a voracious reader of the medical literature. I also got into the habit of purchasing and reading medical monographs, usually on some topic that had turned up in my daily practice.

Each Saturday during the medical school year at 12 noon the major teaching clinic of the medical service was held in the main amphitheater. If you were not early for these sessions, you would have to stand in the back for an hour and one half. These clinics were superb presentations featuring some of our best teachers and focusing on a major topic of current interest. In later years the best ones were published in the *American Journal of Medicine*. Holding these clinics on a Saturday served several purposes. It was a day convenient for many attending physicians because the Vanderbilt Clinic was closed except for emergencies. It also ensured that the students, house staff, and attending staff did not start the weekend on Friday afternoon. It was one way to preserve Saturday as a workday at the Medical Center. I regret that for various reasons, Saturday clinics have become almost non-existent in many great medical centers. Long weekends, sometimes with a holiday on Monday, have taken over. I know we have lost something in the process.

Whenever I could, I attended out-of-city medical meetings, especially those in Atlantic City in the spring. I recall being in the audience when Dr. Warfield T. Longcope of Johns Hopkins presented his now-classical paper on sarcoidosis. I sat riveted to the edge of my seat when he described some of his patients. One case description fit that of a Mexican patient (Marie Custin) in the Vanderbilt Clinic who had puzzled our entire staff for many months. She had extensive bilateral pulmonary infiltrates that were frightening to see on her chest films, but she did not seem sick, had no cough, and was able to go up and down two to three flights of stairs without dyspnea. She had been seen by many consultants, including a formidable array of chest and tuberculosis experts, and her tuberculin tests were negative. On one occasion she had been admitted for parotitis, and her most recent admission had been to the Harkness Eye Institute for iritis and uveitis. As I listened to Dr. Longcope, a light bulb lit up in my head and I felt certain that this lady had sarcoidosis. The first thing I did when I came home was to requisition her chart from the record room, reviewing every detail in it. I found she hand undergone a partial iridectomy for uveitis and glaucoma in the Eye Institute the year before and I knew that a cell block with iris tissue was somewhere in the pathology laboratory. I located this and asked that additional sections be made and, lo and behold, giant cells and granulomata of sarcoidosis were present, settling the diagnosis. I believe this was one of the first cases of this condition diagnosed at Columbia-Presbyterian Medical Center.

I followed the patient in the Vanderbilt Clinic for some years. The pulmonary lesions slowly faded; she never had to go to a tuberculosis sanatorium and, except for mild GI symptoms, she remained well. The trip to Atlantic City had paid off a major dividend.

During the 1930s, the head of the Vanderbilt Clinic was Dr. Frederick MacCurdy, an outstanding administrator who was highly respected and ran a tight ship. As with the best administrators, he had excellent people working with him, the star being Miss Haseltine, who was the soul of efficiency and diplomacy. It was Dr. MacCurdy who seemed more sensitive to the needs of the Washington Heights community than the Flexnerian full-time professors led by Dr. Robert F. Loeb. It was Dr. MacCurdy who realized that the junior members of the staff were taking care of people of limited means who could not afford the fees of senior staff and the usual charges for x-ray work and laboratory tests. These patients wished to maintain their relationship with their personal physicians who were seeing them at reduced fees, sometimes without a fee, in their private offices. To help with the care of this group of individuals, Dr. MacCurdy set up a classification labeled "Limited Diagnostic," which markedly reduced charges made to them for x-ray examinations and laboratory tests done at the Medical Center. This made it possible for us to do an excellent workup on our low-income patients without swamping them with the costs of the necessary tests. The mechanism for doing this was very simple. The requisitions for the tests had to be labeled "Limited Diagnostic" by the referring doctor. This might have lent itself to abuse by patients who could afford the regular fees, but our doctors cooperated and helped it to succeed. In the Harkness x-ray department, the private side of the medical center, if the referring doctor wrote "Semi-Private" on the requisition, the fees were reduced to half the usual rate. This was so easy to do that the courtesy was abused and eventually had to be rescinded. With the passage of time and the advent of insurance coverage for outpatient studies, the need for these special arrangements disappeared, but they did serve a real purpose during the depression years.

As the director of the personnel medical department, I was obliged to attend budget meetings with the department heads of all of the units constituting the Columbia-Presbyterian Medical Center. I attended but I kept my mouth shut and merely listened. It did not take me long to realize that geographic proximity of the various units making up the center did not of itself create a body with common goals and purpose. In fact, each unit remained semi-autonomous and it would be some years before the dreams of those who started the great medical center could be realized. The greatest unifying force during the severe depression was the need to economize and to reduce waste, reduplication, and inefficiency. When the Medical Center was first established, it brought together the Presbyterian Hospital, Babies' Hospital, the Vanderbilt Clinic, the Squier Urological Clinic, Sloan Maternity Hospital, the Eye Institute, Harkness Pavilion for private patients, and the Neurological Institute. Each of these units had its own administrative staff, trustees, and endowment. Each one treasured its freedom and autonomy and their administrators were dedicated people, most of them highly respected nurse-administrators who felt it was their obligation to represent the interest of their specific institutions. It would be some time before the concept of a unified center would emerge, and much of this had to await the loss by attrition and retirement of the old guard. I was amazed and pleased to see that in those early days Mr. Edward S. Harkness would write a check to cover the annual deficit for the Columbia-Presbyterian Medical Center. This was a Godsend in those days of economic recession.

Despite the heavy pressures of my many activities, I did manage to do come clinical investigation, the first of these culminating in a paper published in the *Annals of Internal Medicine* entitled "The Clinical Significance of a Flat Oral Glucose Tolerance Test." This tied in with my interest in sprue, a condition of malabsorption associated with the flattening of the absorption curve of orally ingested glucose. I know that Dr. Palmer was very pleased with this report and commented to an associate that in addition to my clinical duties, I was doing more teaching and research than some of his salaried people. Miss Margaret Reid, then a head nurse in the Vanderbilt Clinic, helped me greatly in the performance of the absorption tests for glucose and in comparing capillary with venous blood-sugar levels in selected patients. Years later I was able to attract Miss Reid to become the nursing supervisor of the innovative and endowed Upjohn Gastrointestinal Service at Roosevelt Hospital. This is yet another story.

It was during this period that, stimulated by Verzar's superb monograph on absorption from the intestinal tract, I hit upon the idea of using D-xylose, a non-metabolized pentose, as a test for malabsorption in the small intestine. For these research efforts, I had no funds but managed to scrounge around for the wherewithal to get things done. I was able to persuade a cooperative biochemist at P&S to do two tests for D-xylose absorption on my patients with sprue. Unfortunately, the two cases we studied were quite mild and the tests were borderline. Since the D-xylose was expensive and we lacked funds to purchase it, I lost out on being the first to use this test for diagnosing sprue. Others, better funded, established this many years later.

In the fall of 1942 I was asked to make what proved to be the most hazardous "house call" I have ever made. The patient was referred to me by Dr. Bill Stevenson, a pioneering plastic surgeon on our staff. Little knowing what lay in store, I agreed to take him on. The next call was from a shipping line. The patient was a forty-year-old Merchant Mariner on an oil tanker anchored in midstream in the Hudson River west of the 79th Street Yacht Basin. It was wartime and the Port of New York was under strict military control. I was advised to drive down to the 79th Street Yacht Basin and to contact the Coast Guard, who would be responsible for conveying me to the oil tanker. After they had made sure I was not an enemy agent, transportation in a yacht assigned to the Coast Guard was arranged. By the time the boat reached the Yacht Basin, it had become pitch dark and a blackout was mandatory. When we arrived alongside the empty tanker riding high in the Hudson, the cutter made two unsuccessful attempts to reach a rope ladder dropped over the side of the tanker. These failures were greeted with Bronx cheers and some rather choice four-letter words from the tanker's crew. By the third attempt, I was getting a little nervous about going up the rope ladder on a pitch-black night under the guidance of what was clearly an inexperienced crew. To top it off, I had never learned how to swim. The third attempt succeeded and I somehow managed to climb up the ladder onto the deck. I proceeded to the seaman's quarters where I found an acutely and seriously ill man breathing rapidly, coughing rusty sputum and febrile. On rapid physical examination he had classical signs of pneumonic consolidation of his right lower lobe. I felt certain he had lobar pneumonia and had to be moved to Harkness Pavilion. The real problem was how to get him from his bunk to the Coast Guard cutter. After witnessing the problem we had getting aboard the tanker, I was not very happy at the prospect to trying to debark our patient without getting all of us drowned. The patient weighed at least 170 pounds and was too ill to cooperate. Nevertheless, with the help of several crewmen, we approached the rope ladder and started to move the patient down the side. Suddenly, the Coast Guard cutter veered off, leaving me holding the patient by the armpits with a black void between us and the cutter. Somehow, with God's help, calling upon all of the strength I had developed by years of carrying 100-pound blocks of ice on my back, I managed to hang on to the patient until the cutter maneuvered alongside so that I could drop the patient into the arms of their crew. We hurried ashore and I drove the patient in my car, a four-door Pontiac sedan, to the emergency entrance of Harkness Pavilion. Within short order he was in a Harkness room with an oxygen tent and on sulfapyridine. Fortunately he responded well and was able to leave the hospital in two weeks. I had risked my life to help this patient but almost no one knew the full details of this incident. There was no family; he was a traveling merchant seaman making good money during wartime. I submitted a modest bill for my service but it took the assistance of Hayt & Hayt, the hospital attorneys to assure that his bills were paid.

Chapter 13

Pearl Harbor and World War II

December 7, 1941. "A Date which will
live in Infamy."

— F.D.R.

T HE WAR IN EUROPE SEEMED FAR AWAY and many Americans, if
not most, hoped that we would not become involved in it. The
depression was lifting, unemployment was diminishing, and,
once again, America seemed to be on the move. The Japanese attack
on Pearl Harbor on 7 December 1941, "the day of infamy" described
by President Franklin D. Roosevelt, shook us out of our complacen-
cy and self-insulation and isolation from the problems faced by our
friends in Europe. Very soon the impact of entering the war was felt
at Columbia-Presbyterian Medical Center. The first major move was
the organization and mobilization of the 2nd General Hospital, the
Presbyterian Hospital Unit that had served with distinction in World
War I. It was soon apparent that most of our medical staff would be
leaving in a few months. This included not only junior staff but most
of our key attending staff. Very soon the halls of the medical center
were flooded with doctors in military uniform who were making plans
to leave. Practices were turned over to associates or abandoned. Clinic
assignments were canceled and leaves of absence for the "duration"
were granted by the Medical Center and the Columbia University
College of Physicians and Surgeons. In addition to those with the 2nd
General Army Hospital, others left for duty with the Navy and unaf-
filiated units in the various branches of military service. We had a few
artful and agile draft dodgers who sought every means of avoiding
military service, but they were clearly a minority.

As the director of the personnel medical department, I was
informed that I was on the Essential list of the medical center. A
statement to this effect was sent to the Draft Board and higher
authority and I was told I would never be drafted while I held this
post:

THE PRESBYTERIAN HOSPITAL IN THE
CITY OF NEW YORK
THE INSTITUTE OF OPHTHALMOLOGY
THE SLOANE HOSPITAL FOR WOMEN
22 WEST 168TH STREET
NEW YORK, NY

MICHAEL J. LEPORE, M.D.
DIRECTOR, PERSONNEL MEDICAL DEPARTMENT
July 20, 1942

To Members of the Professional Staff certified
as essential for the care of Patients in all of the hospitals at the
Medical Center:

On the recommendation of the Director of Your Service you
have been certified by this office to the Procurement and
Assignment Service as essential for the care of patients. It is the
intention of the state chairman of the Procurement and
Assignment Service to respect that certification. However,
should you receive from your Draft Board or the Procurement
and Assignment Service, or on its stationery, a statement that you
are now regarded as available for military duty and are requested
to fill out the forms and report to the medical Officers
Recruiting Board for physical examination, will you please turn
that request over to this office immediately? At the request of the
Procurement and Assignment Service we have been instructed to
return such papers on the assumption that they have been sent to
you in error.

John F. McCormack
Acting Executive Vice President

    As I bade farewell to my friends and colleagues, who were enter-
ing military service, I felt uneasy, especially since the news from
Europe was more upsetting each day and the war in the Pacific was
going poorly for us. The flood of European refugees, including many
doctors from Nazi Germany, had engulfed Washington Heights and
the community around the Medical Center. Their tales of mistreatment and abuse were almost incredible but well documented. I came
to the conclusion that this was going to be a long and terrible war and
I knew that I simply could not stand by and avoid participation while
so many of my friends were leaving. I asked permission to see Dr.
Palmer in August 1942. I told Dr. Palmer that I felt very strongly that

I could not stay out of the war. As a son of Italian immigrants who had found opportunity and recognition in America I felt I wanted to volunteer for military service. I asked to be released from my assignment as director of the personnel medical department. To replace me I had already started to indoctrinate a competent woman physician, Dr. Gwendolen S. Jones. Dr. Palmer said some very warm and fine things to me and I expressed my appreciation for all he had done for me. His reply was that he never had to worry about anything I did; a high accolade from a New Englander who exuded integrity, decency, and fairness.

In preparation for military service, it occurred to me that Board certification in internal medicine would add strength to my application and assure my assignment in internal medicine. At that time the American Board of Internal Medicine was in its infancy and no one in authority at Columbia-Presbyterian was promoting it. I guess that the feeling was that being a member of the staff of this prestigious hospital spoke for itself and needed no additional sponsorship or credentialling. Nevertheless, I proceeded to study for my American Board examination, somehow finding time for this despite heavy demands of my practice, the personnel medical department, teaching responsibilities, and some clinical research.

I took the whole-day written examination, essay-type then in vogue, in the fall of 1942 and passed without difficulty and was certified to take the oral examination in May 1943, which I did at the Philadelphia General Hospital and passed.

Having received my chief's approval, I volunteered for service in the Army of the United States. The paperwork and processing took several months. The writer of one of my letters of recommendation proposed that I be appointed to the rank of Major. My chief, Dr. Walter W. Palmer, the Bard professor and director of the medical service, Presbyterian Hospital, a renowned clinician and medical educator, wrote a strong letter of recommendation to the Surgeon General on my behalf that carried considerable weight. It was answered on October 27, 1942, by Lt. Colonel Durward G. Hall for the Surgeon General who said, in part, "This office appreciates your excellent letter—It is extremely unlikely that this commission (as a Major) can be granted since our present procurement objective is nearly exhausted, and furthermore, since it is believed that Dr. Lepore is under 37 years of age [I was 32]. However, your letter will be placed in his file and we will certainly tender him the highest possible grade commensurate with his age and training according to our present rules. Furthermore, it will be certainly determined on the basis of your letter that he will be assigned to duty in internal medicine."

On 22 October 1942, I was ordered to appear before the Medical Officer Recruiting Board, 39 Whitehall Street, New York City, for my physical examination and did not anticipate that there would be any problem because I had never been ill or hospitalized except for a tonsillectomy in 1923. While I was stark naked in a cubicle awaiting my examination, the air-raid siren went off and I was bundled up in a sheet and ushered into a makeshift bomb shelter where we sat until the practice drill ended. I was then examined and a chest x-ray was done. On 3 November 1942, much to my surprise, I was notified that I was physically disqualified for military service because of myopia and x-ray evidence of arrested tuberculosis. This was completely unexpected and I appealed the decision. I remembered that I had had a chest x-ray at Rochester in 1933 while I was a medical student. I called Rochester and was pleased to learn that the film was in their inactive file. They quickly retrieved it and sent it to the Army Recruiting Board where it was reviewed and compared with the current films. The decision was that I had arrested reinfective type, pulmonary tuberculosis with no essential change since the film of 17 February 1933. I signed an affidavit stating "I, Michael J. Lepore, being desirous of entering upon active military service during the current emergency, and being aware of the fact that I have the following physical defects:

> 1. Defective vision right 20/400, left 20/300 correctable to 20/20 bilateral.
>
> 2. Arrested reinfective type pulmonary tuberculosis do hereby acknowledge the existence of the above mentioned physical defects, and request that I be placed upon extended active duty.

On 3 November 1942, waiver was recommended for "Limited Service only" and I awaited formal notification of my appointment and orders to active duty. In preparation for Army service, we had to give up our nice office and home at 200 Haven Avenue adjacent to the Columbia-Presbyterian Medical Center, place our furniture in storage, and arrange to transfer my patients to the care of others. We made arrangements to lodge my dear mother-in-law with relatives on the Eastern Shore. My first notification that I had been assigned a commission in the Army of the United States arrived on 28 November 1942 in the form of a telegram. That same day, a popular band leader, Captain Glenn Miller, received his commission.

When I deciphered my telegram and the official orders, I learned that my temporary assignment was in a medical replacement pool at

Army & Navy General Hospital in Hot Springs, Arkansas. I decided to drive down with my wife, stopping overnight in private houses that accepted guests at moderate rates, there being no motels in those days. As we motored south, the friendliness of the people matched the warmth of the climate. In small towns strangers would say good morning with a smile. It was amazing how many salutes I returned with my lovely bride on my arm. I am certain they were meant for Ardean rather than my Captain's bars. We stopped off for a while in Virginia where Miss Wofford, a former head nurse at Duke and a good friend of Ardean's, was stationed near the Blue Ridge mountains. When we arrived at the Army and Navy General Hospital on 12 December 1942 I discovered that I had misinterpreted the orders by arriving four days earlier than expected. I had not figured on being allowed four days travel time to the hospital before reporting in. Housing in Hot Springs was easily arranged. We were able to rent a clean and nice room with a bath in a private house a short distance from the hospital for eight dollars a week. The town was full of people who were coming for the therapeutic baths for which the area was noted. There were also people who were there to gamble at the racetrack and casino, activities we avoided like the plague. Gas rationing prevented us from traveling about, so most of the time was spent in Hot Springs. The people we rented from, a couple named Seitz, could not have been nicer, made us feel at home and treated us to some local delicacies, including quail, which was plentiful.

The hospital was an imposing and handsome edifice on a hilltop. My next visit to it was in compliance with my orders and I was registered in the medical pool, where I joined a large number of doctors who were waiting for their assignments and spending most of their time shooting the bull and griping about the boring existence they were leading. The hospital was full of patients and understaffed, but no one was volunteering to help out. I struck up an acquaintance with Dr. Neil Stone, a pediatrician from Poughkeepsie, New York, who was assigned to the medical service at Army and Navy since there was no pediatric service. We became friends and I asked whether it might be possible for me to help him out with his patient load. It turned out that Colonel Irving S. Wright from Columbia and Cornell was the chief of medical service and he was delighted to have me pitch in. He assigned me to one of the wards where the ward officer really needed help. I saw some very interesting cases and in the process learned quite a bit about Army and Navy General Hospital. There were many patients there who were veterans of World War I, some of whom made a practice of coming to Hot Springs ostensibly for the therapeutic baths for arthritis and peripheral vascular disorders. It cost them nothing, and for some, hopping from one V.A. Hospital or Army General Hospital to another according to the season of the year, had become a way of life. They spent a good deal of time out of the hospital on pass, taking in the sights and activities of the region. One of the first patients I looked after was a World War I veteran with Buerger's disease who spent much of his life in government hospitals. He knew he was not supposed to smoke and always denied that he did. On rounds one morning Colonel Wright questioned him about his smoking, which he denied. Colonel Wright reached under his pillow and pulled out a large supply of cigarettes the patient had stashed away. He then proceeded to order the patient to stop smoking or leave the hospital. The patient left the hospital. He almost certainly went to another V.A. hospital where he could continue to get away with smoking and eventually end up an amputee. On another occasion, the ward officer asked me to check out a young Arkansas native who made his living by fishing from a boat. He had been drafted but when he started basic training, he complained of severe pain in his knees and legs and said he was unable to walk more than a few feet. Since he had made his living as a fisherman, and nothing could be found on physical examination, he was thought to be malingering, and after more study it was decided to get him out of the army with a CDD (Certificate of Disability Discharge). He was going to appear before a Board with this in mind when the ward officer asked me to check him out. He did not strike me as a malingerer. He was quasi-illiterate but convinced me that there might be something going on that had been missed. I examined him from head to toes.

When I palpated the back of his knees, he almost jumped off the bed, saying I had touched a sore spot. The "sore spot" proved to be a glomus tumor, a painful neurovascular growth. Instead of bringing him before the CDD Board, we presented him to Col. Wright, who was fascinated by the case and was indeed a renowned expert in this disorder. The result was a superb Grand Rounds conducted by Colonel Wright with illustrations of many cases he had collected over the years. The lesion was excised, the patient's condition was relieved and he was returned to duty.

The season of the year was a great time to be in Hot Springs. Christmas and the New Year were occasions for merriment, goodwill, and socializing. There were dinners and dances, and we made many new friends. In fact we were getting along so well that Colonel Wright tried to have me permanently assigned to his service. This triggered off some action in the Surgeon General's office in Washington, where apparently I had already been picked by Colonel Marshall N. Fulton of Harvard Medical School to be assigned as chief of the Officers and Women's Medical section of the new Army General Hospital nearing completion at Valley Forge, Pennsylvania. The next thing I received was a New Year's present, ordering me to proceed to Valley Forge General Hospital, dated 1 January 1943 from General George C. Marshall.

Chapter 14

✧

Valley Forge General Hospital, 1942–1945

THE RETURN TRIP NORTH BY AUTOMOBILE was a little hairy, especially in the mountains where we encountered a good deal of snow and ice. There were no snow tires in those days and chains could quickly wear out and were almost impossible to purchase. I breathed a sigh of relief when we finally reached Philadelphia and proceeded to drive to Phoenixville, Pennsylvania, where Valley Forge General Hospital was under construction. We searched Phoenixville for private housing and found to our dismay that almost nothing was available and that rents were simply out of sight. When I applied for extra gasoline to travel to Philadelphia I was told rather bluntly by the commanding officer, Colonel Henry Beeuwkes, that I was asking for more gas than he used and he refused to approve my application. I found out later that the commanding officer obtained his gas on the post at minimal or no cost. This did not make me happy, but perhaps it served a purpose because Ardean and I decided that we would have to set up housekeeping in Philadelphia and I would live on the post in the officers' barracks and commute by train to Philadelphia when I could. We were also quite concerned about Ardean's elderly mother who was boarding with relatives in Maryland. We had friends in Philadelphia and with their help we finally located an apartment at a rental we could afford. Soon Ardean and "Miss Annie" were living together, and Ardean obtained a position at the Graduate Hospital of the University of Pennsylvania as assistant directress of nursing under her good friend, Miss Helen Hawthorne, directress of nursing. Ardean's first position after graduation from the Philadelphia General Hospital School of Nursing in 1928 was as head nurse of the Children's Service at the Graduate Hospital of the University of Pennsylvania; so it was like coming home again. Helen and Ardean, both graduates of that marvelous nursing school at Old Blockley, were almost like sisters, a friendship that endured for the remainder of their lives. Ardean's stipend helped augment my Captain's allotment. Fortunately, she was a good manager and she made a dollar go a long way. Life in the Army in wartime is always unpredictable. There was no guarantee how long we would remain in one assignment or another. We were advised to travel light and be ready to move on short notice.

We simply lived from day to day, doing our best to adapt to a new way of life, expecting no favors and making the best of a difficult situation. Valley Forge General Hospital was a sprawling two-story brick structure designed for 2,000 inpatients, located on what had been a farm of 180 acres on the outskirts of Phoenixville, Pennsylvania, and a short march from Washington's original encampment of December 1777. When I arrived on 14 January 1943 the hospital was in its final stages of construction and the dirt roads of the compound were muddy from the steady rains that had plagued the area for many months. Since there were no patients, there was no professional work for the doctors, but we were soon put to work making up lists of supplies thought to be needed when the hospital opened. This was very boring work, unfamiliar to most of us and customarily performed by nursing and administrative staff in civilian hospitals. In the Army, we were told, the doctor is in charge of his service and is ultimately and personally responsible for every aspect of his assignment, including inventory and supplies. As chief of the Officer's and Women's Section of 100 beds, I had to decide how many bedpans, thermometers, pencils, flashlights, rubber gloves, tubes of lubricant, tongue blades, urinals, sheets, and blankets we needed as well as the medical equipment, instruments, and medical supplies needed to care for 100 patients. It occurred to many of us that some sort of blueprint must have existed for supplying the thousands of Army hospitals being built during wartime. We were told there was nothing of the sort and advised to get our lists in on time. The supply major was an old Regular Army non-commissioned officer, who with the advent of war, had been rapidly moved up to a majority. He seemed to delight in hoarding the supplies and never seemed happy about our requests. The ploy was clearly to keep the doctors busy with paperwork and to let them know who was really in charge. For most of us, it was our first contact with a well-organized and powerful organization, the MAC (Medical Administrative Corps). At Valley Forge, there were forty-nine doctors, several of whom were chiefly administrators, and *twenty-eight* lay administrators belonging to the MAC. Shades of things to come! We soon learned to play hardball within the established ground rules in order to protect our patients, ourselves, and the quality of care.

The commanding officer at Valley Forge was Colonel Henry W. Beeuwkes, age 62, whose chief claim to fame, we were told, was that he had been General John J. Pershing's aide and personal physician in World War I and had been his friend ever since. We did not know much more about Col. Beeuwkes in 1943, but in later years, after I became President Herbert C. Hoover's personal physician, I was privileged to have access to further information about him. Col. Beeuwkes was a graduate of the Johns Hopkins School of Medicine,

Class of 1906, one year after Osler left for the regius professorship at Oxford. Dr. Beeuwkes joined the Regular Army Medical Corps in 1909 and served with distinction in World War I in France, reaching the grade of full Colonel and earning many decorations. He was, for a time, the commanding officer of the hospital to which Harvey Cushing was assigned and was mentioned with approval on several occasions in *From a Surgeon's Journal* by Harvey Cushing.[1]

In 1921, while secretary of commerce in Washington and chairman of the American Relief Administration (ARA), Herbert C. Hoover was asked to reorganize and direct relief efforts in Russia where "one of the most terrible famines in history" was raging:

> We were in fact, confronted with famine in 750,000 square miles of the Volga Valley and 85,000 square miles in the Ukraine. About 25,000,000 people in these regions were in the midst of absolute famine, with death for the whole population of these areas only a few months away. Typhus, cholera, typhoid, smallpox and relapsing fever were sweeping over the area because of lack of physical resistance and medical and sanitary services. Millions of panic-stricken people were attempting to flee the famine on foot and by rail and every other sort of conveyance. They were moving into other parts of Russia which were already short of food, and they were carrying infections with them."[2]

At a meeting in August 1921 with Dr. Livingston Farrand, chairman of the American Red Cross, who was directing Red Cross aid to the ARA, Mr. Hoover met Colonel Henry Beeuwkes of the U.S. Army Medical Corps and was so favorably impressed by him that he arranged for his assignment by the Army to direct the medical staff of the ARA. Hoover said:

> Colonel Beeuwkes selected a group of skilled and devoted men for his assistants, mostly from the Army Medical Corps, and the Army generously assigned them to our service and continued their Army pay. Colonel Beeuwkes and his assistants arrived in Moscow on September 21, 1921. They soon began to send back word of a scourge of infectious disease on a scale unknown in

---

1. Harvey Cushing, *From a Surgeon's Journal, 1915–1918* (Boston: Little Brown and Company, 1936), pp. 433, 459, 462, 464, 465.

2. Herbert Hoover, *An American Epic*, vol. 3 (Chicago: Henry Company, 1961), p. 436.

modern history. Their reports showed that not only the famine area but the whole of Russia was being infected by refugees from the famine-stricken provinces with typhus, relapsing fever, small-pox, cholera, typhoid, malaria, bubonic plague, tuberculosis, trichinosis and pellagra. These infections were running unchecked except by the variation of the seasons. If anyone wishes to read a story of unspeakable horrors and at the same time a record of American men of highest courage, ability and devotion, I recommend Colonel Beeuwkes' reports. And at this point I may mention that the quotations and information in this chapter come from these truly great American medical men.[3]

Hoover continued:

Colonel Beeuwkes rapidly increased his medical staff to an organization of 40 American physicians and specialists, 21 other American staff workers, and supervisory staff of some 800 competent Russians. He established central warehouses in Moscow into which our immense medical imports were received and thence dispatched to the areas in need. He established stations in each of the famine districts and also at points where the refugees could be treated. He put two medically equipped trains on the road to deal with refugees from the famine district. He inaugurated in each famine district sanitary measures in which he employed thousands of Russians who were paid with a food ration. His major methods of attacking the scourge was to equip existing institutions with food, medicines and medical instruments in order to bring life and tools to Russia's own doctors and technicians.

Colonel Beeuwkes' efforts succeeded almost beyond belief. Mr. Hoover concluded that "This, the greatest foreign peacetime medical crusade ever undertaken, stands as a monument to the whole medical profession—and to Colonel Beeuwkes."[4]

This was lavish praise from Mr. Hoover, who was not given to overstatement. I report this now, many years after my sojourn at Valley Forge, because those of us who served under Colonel Beeuwkes during World War II had no knowledge of his World War I experience or post-war involvement in famine and pestilence relief in Russia. In World War II, as the commanding officer of a modern

---

3. Ibid., pp. 467–8.
4. Ibid., pp. 473–477.

2,000-bed Army General Hospital, we felt he left much to be desired. The explanation for this lies in great part with the fact that Colonel Beeuwkes left the Army in 1925 and worked for the Rockefeller Foundation, spending nine years on yellow-fever epidemiology and field research, part of it as physician in charge of the Rockefeller Foundation headquarters in Lagos. It was there in 1927 that Hideyo Noguchi, the famous bacteriologist and member of the Rockefeller Institute, arrived to pursue the etiology of yellow fever. Noguchi had persuaded Simon Flexner, director of the Rockefeller Institute, to send him to Lagos in the hope that somehow he could recover the reputation he had lost when he had erroneously identified Leptospira as the cause of yellow fever. Flexner had been reluctant to let him go but was pressed so vigorously that he finally yielded and prepared the way for the assignment by writing Dr. Beeuwkes to extend every courtesy to Noguchi and to provide him with anything and everything he might need to accomplish his mission. The needed funds would be furnished by the Rockefeller Foundation over and above Beeuwkes' budget. In 1943, when Colonel Beeuwkes was commanding officer at Valley Forge, he would regale our staff with tales about Noguchi that invariably cast him in a bad light. Most of us knew very little about Noguchi but were rather dismayed by the bitter criticism of the eminent scientist. Some of us concluded that there had been some sort of personality clash between the two men. This was amply confirmed recently when I happened to locate the Noguchi biography by Isabel Plesset, *Noguchi and His Patrons*.[5] On page 258 I picked up this revealing remark. "For the entire six months of his stay in West Africa, Noguchi kept up a feud with the people at Lagos and with Beeuwkes in particular—Beeuwkes was a retired Army Officer who was so meticulous, according to one of the junior staff men, he required all personnel to turn in pencil stubs before they could be issued new pencils." Noguchi accused Beeuwkes of failing to supply him with enough monkeys for his yellow-fever research. Obsessed with his desire to repair his tarnished reputation, after the Leptospira debacle, Noguchi risked his life by leaving Lagos, where yellow fever was of a low order of frequency, for nearby Accra on the West Coast of Africa where it was more prevalent. While in Accra for five months, he was convinced that he had succeeded in transmitting yellow fever by inoculating monkeys with "material derived from old preserved specimens

---

5. Isabel Plesset, *Noguchi and His Patrons* (Fairleigh Dickinson University Press, 1980).

of yellow fever blood."[6] Before he could complete his research, he himself caught yellow fever and within ten days, he died, a martyr to his research, on 21 May 1928. The diagnosis of yellow fever as the cause of death was documented at autopsy by an experienced pathologist, Dr. William A. Young. An incidental and unexpected finding was the presence of syphilitic heart disease. Dr. Beeuwkes, who also attended the autopsy, said "Dr. Young had preserved the one interesting part of the organ (the heart) and he promised to run this over to me for shipment to New York."[7] Eight days after Noguchi's death, Dr Young died of yellow fever, another martyr to the cause.

In 1941 Colonel Beeuwkes retired from the Rockefeller Foundation and settled down on his farm in Berlin, Maryland, on the Eastern Shore. With the advent of World War II he emerged from retirement and rejoined the Army. With General Pershing's help he managed to be assigned a real plum as commanding officer of Valley Forge General Hospital in 1942, even though he had been out of touch with Army medicine and hospital administration since 1925.

Fortunately, the medical staff for Valley Forge was carefully screened in the Surgeon General's office in Washington, D.C., starting with Lt. Colonel Marshall N. Fulton of the Peter Bent Brigham Hospital and Harvard University Medical School, who was designated chief of medical service. Fulton was a scholarly clinician and superb cardiologist, a medical graduate of Johns Hopkins and a Rhodes scholar who had been one of the "latch-key" young men allowed free access to the "Open Arms," the Osler homestead in Oxford. Many physicians thought Fulton would succeed Henry Christian at the Brigham, but on the crest of a wave seeking new blood and new directions, the position went to Dr. Soma Weiss, a brilliant young Hungarian refugee.

Colonel Fulton selected as his assistant chief of medicine Major Maurice Schnitker, a top-flight internist and cardiologist who had been Dr. Henry Christian's longtime chief resident at the Brigham. He picked me to be chief of the Officer's and Women's Section on the basis of strong letters to the Surgeon General from my former chiefs, Dr. Walter W. Palmer of Columbia, Dr. Frederic M. Hanes of Duke, and Dr. John P. Peters of Yale. Each of the other sections of our 600-bed medical service was headed by similarly highly qualified internists. In fact, the staff in medicine at Valley Forge was the equal of that in

---

6. Ibid., p. 264.

7 Ibid., p. 268.

any major medical school. As we felt each other out in the subtle and sometimes not so subtle ways professionals do, we quickly realized that we had the makings of an excellent professional team well equipped to provide superior professional care. Assignment to Valley Forge was a real coup, providing us with a wonderful opportunity to serve and also to learn by serving. In point of fact, the high calibre of medical practice in the Army General Hospitals during World War II has received scant attention in the press, books, movies, television, and the like. Most lay people think of Army medicine as the "MASH" type consisting mainly of emergency trauma surgery, first aid, and a fair bit of womanizing and carousing. Without question the medical and surgical activities of these frontline units saved many lives and earned the admiration and respect of all of us in military service. I was never in the frontlines during my nearly four years in the Army. My work was almost exclusively in Army General Hospitals in the zone of the interior and later overseas in the Western Pacific Base Command on Tinian and Saipan, and finally as the professional consultant in medicine in Tripler General Hospital in Oahu.

As I look back, the nearly three years I spent at Valley Forge were the equivalent and more of an additional major residency or fellowship in medicine undertaken ten years after graduation from medical school. By having to live on post, we were really "residents"; there were few distractions and we were in truth on a "full-time" assignment. Grand Rounds were held weekly and daily teaching and treatment rounds were of a high order.

Journal Club meetings were held regularly and Colonel Fulton remained in touch with Dr. Merrill Sosman, the acerbic and brilliant chief of radiology at the Peter Bent Brigham Hospital, who sent him case reports for use in our teaching program. One week the case was most unusual, a patient with pneumatosis cystoides intestinalis presenting with painless pneumo-peritoneum. I had never heard of this disease and said so in my discussion. Colonel Fulton wrote to Dr. Sosman saying that Mike Lepore had not heard of this disease. Sosman's reply was "Tell Mike Lepore to spend less time in the Officers' Club and more in the Library" and sent along a reference. This cutting remark, even though untrue, was stamped indelibly on my memory center and would serve me well in the future when I really did diagnose a similar case some years later.

The named Army General Hospitals in the zone of the interior of the United States were the pride of the medical corps, and assignments to them were avidly sought. To name a few of the most prestigious at the start of World War II there were Walter Reed in Washington, D.C., Letterman General in San Francisco, Fitzsimmons

General in Denver, Colorado, and Army and Navy General Hospital in Hot Springs, Arkansas. In preparation for the advent of World War II casualties, many other named General Hospitals were speedily constructed across the country, raising the total in 1944 to 59 in the zone of the interior, scattered over the nine service commands created by Army planners. Staffing these hospitals was a very important function of the Surgeon General's office and great care was exercised to place the medical officers in assignments appropriate to their experience, ability, and civilian background. This was not an easy task because Board certification was in its infancy and relatively few doctors were certified. Letters of recommendations from leaders in medicine carried a good deal of weight, as did hospital appointments, residency and fellowships served, and academic appointments in leading medical schools. The appointment of Colonel Hugh J. Morgan (later Brigadier General) in January 1942 as chief consultant in medicine to the Surgeon General proved to be one of the best ever made. An impressive and pleasant leader with superb civilian experience as a teacher, clinician, and chairman of a major department of medicine at Vanderbilt University, he was able to reorganize the assignment of internists and to attract outstanding men as consultants and chiefs of service. Under his guidance a method of classification of internists was developed and implemented. It was quite simple, dividing the men into one of four categories—A, B, C, D, in descending order of ability and competence. Internists were assigned the MOS (Military Occupational Specialty) 3139. Mine was B-3139.

As chief consultant in medicine to the Surgeon General, Brigadier General Morgan brought order to a process that needed reorganization and objectivity. He knew most of the leaders in American medicine on a personal basis and had the respect of the men being processed. One of his most important innovations was the assignment of very-high-calibre internists as consultants to the nine Service Commands in the Continental United States. This innovation was at first resisted by some of the Command Surgeons, most of whom were products of the Regular Army, who were not very happy to have doctors from civilian backgrounds taking over some of their power. General Morgan's selections proved to be so outstanding that it was not long before all of the Service Commands accepted them.

Of considerable interest to doctors stationed at Valley Forge General Hospital was the fact that the Third Service Command was the last of the nine to go along with the concept of a command consultant, a delay that cost many of us substantial losses in income and promotions to Field Grade.

Traditionally, the medical department of the Army during wartime stresses the care of the wounded rendered by surgeons while the role of the internists is neglected and regarded by the line as a secondary function. The truth of the matter is that in modern warfare, medical ailments causing disability and ineffectiveness outnumber by far those of the wounded. "In the Italian campaigns of World War II, 80 percent of noneffective soldiers returned to duty by the Medical Department were medical patients; only 20 percent were surgical. The internist, thanks to the developments in medical therapeutics since the early 1920s, has become the most effective therapist extant, and this in fact is reflected in Army records."[8]

The battle of the Solomon Islands was almost lost to the inroads of malaria rather than enemy action. With the introduction and implementation of Atabrine prophylaxis the malaria incidence was markedly reduced, a minor miracle of preventive medicine. Similarly, the British defeat of Rommel at El Almein was in part due to the fact that American research on man in the desert conducted by my former teacher, the distinguished Dr. Edward F. Adolph of Rochester, had demonstrated the critical importance of an adequate supply of water for tank troops in combat in the desert heat, information used by the British in battle to great advantage. Water for the men was as important as gasoline for the engines in tank warfare in the desert.

I admitted the first acutely ill patient to the medical service of Valley Forge General Hospital in February 1943. We had received a call from the nearby Wayne Military Academy that one of its cadets was acutely ill with a severe respiratory-tract infection and fever. The cadets were entitled to Army medical care and instructions were given to bring the patient to us by ambulance. He was to be admitted to the Officers and Women's Section where I was the chief. I waited for his arrival even though I was supposed to be off duty and the officer of the day (O.D.) was covering the service. When he arrived at my building I quickly examined him and knew immediately that he was gravely ill. He was febrile, disoriented, complaining of headache, had a stiff neck and purple spots all over his body. I said this man has acute meningitis and must be taken to the isolation ward and I accompanied him there. Dr. Victor Kugel, an experienced internist from New York, was the officer of the day. We examined the patient together and agreed with the diagnosis of acute meningitis, probably meningococcal, and we called for a sterile lumbar puncture tray. To our dismay, we were told that all sterile supplies were under lock and key in the operating

---

8. *Medical Department United States Army Internal Medicine in World War II*, vol. 1, *Activities of Medical Consultants Office of the Surgeon General Department of the Army* (Washington, D.C., 1961), pp. 2–7.

rooms, which were closed. We looked for the chief nurse who was the only one who had the keys, but she was nowhere to be found. We had no beepers in those days and the overhead loudspeakers were not installed. We called the M.P.s and asked them to find the chief nurse. We were told she was wandering about somewhere in the 180-acre post. Finally, after what seemed a dreadful waiting period, she was located and we obtained a spinal-tap tray. We were all wearing masks and gowns and using rubber gloves. I instructed our corpsmen, my sergeant and a corporal, to hold the patient on his right side in a flexed position. The O.D. had a little difficulty in gaining access to the spinal canal but soon succeeded only to have the fluid spurt out of the needle, spraying his glasses and his eyes. The fluid was turbid and cloudy, consistent with meningeal infection. At this juncture my sergeant, Jack Lerner, who had never witnessed a spinal tap, fainted. Corporal George Meckler restrained the patient and we succeeded in getting spinal fluid specimens for smear, culture, and chemical analysis. We also hastened to get sulfadiazine eye drops for the officer of the day and a supply of sulfadiazine tablets for his use. Sulfadiazine therapy, which was the only therapy available to us in those days, was started on the patient and he was given intravenous fluids and medication for pain. The following morning we had a rather tense meeting with the commanding officer complaining about the delay in getting sterile supplies and the problem locating the chief nurse. We demanded twenty-four-hour coverage on the premises by assigned operating room personnel. Clearly the commanding officer and the chief nurse had not coped with a hospital emergency for many years. Fortunately the officer of the day had no sequelae from this misadventure. The patient recovered from his meningococcal meningitis but was rendered permanently deaf and ultimately had to be discharged for disability. As often happens under wartime conditions, this was the first of a series of young patients with meningococcal meningitis from the Philadelphia area, all of whom responded well to sulfadiazine therapy, later to penicillin when it became available.

It was then that I learned that by pricking the purpuric spots in the patient's skin and smearing and staining the aspirate we could establish a diagnosis of meningococcemia in a few minutes. The C.O. had learned a lesson, so had the chief nurse and so had all of those involved in their first admission of a medical emergency to Valley Forge General Hospital. We had started off with a bang and knew that we had our work cut out for us before Valley Forge could become an outstanding hospital. We also found out that we could buck the system and change it for the better. For instance, the first patient who lost his hearing as a result of his meningitis was a telephone linesman who could never work again at this civilian occupation. Since he could no longer be able to function as a soldier, the administration wanted to get rid of him as soon as possible. We, fresh from civilian life, wanted something done to rehabilitate the man. There was no provision for this in the Third Service Command but we kept pushing for it and hid the patient whenever the C.O. would come in on an inspection tour. Finally we arranged to transfer the patient to Deshong General Hospital near Pittsburgh, where a new rehabilitation service for service-connected hearing disabilities had been started.

My Officers' and Women's Section was the only section where women could be admitted. This included nurses and WACs and officers' wives. This was excellent experience for the doctors assigned, ensuring their continuing experience with female as well as male patients. It also could and did lead to some problems. We had a group of German POWs assigned to us to perform housekeeping duties in each section. Most were quiet and well disciplined. Some were not. One day my sergeant reported that one of the Nazi POWs was actively pursuing and harassing one of the WACs who was on duty as an aide on the second floor of my section. This was not the first time that the WAC had reported this to him. My decision was to order the POW transferred to another unit where there were no WACs. Within twenty-four hours, the Nazi POW Captain asked to see me and demanded that I explain why I had transferred one of his men without his approval. I said I owed him no explanation. "I am in charge." He clicked his heels and left my office but he never bothered me again. It was about this time that our commanding officer called us into his office to tell us that he had received complaints from the Nazi POWs that we were not returning their salutes when they saw us outdoors. Colonel Beeuwkes said he thought it was bad manners for us not to do so. We then asked the C.O. whether he had ever seen their salute. His answer was no. Well, we said they give us an upheld hand and Heil Hitler. Colonel Beeuwkes flushed and said no more.

On another occasion, a problem arose with one of the Nazi POWs who had cavitary tuberculosis and was receiving collapse therapy of his right lung that had been started at a Station Hospital. He was scheduled to be sent to Fitzsimmons General Hospital, TB Center for the U.S. Army, but was waiting for a bed. In the meantime he needed a pneumothorax refill. Colonel Beeuwkes could not understand why his refill could not be done at Valley Forge. Colonel Fulton, our chief of medicine, said there was no one on his staff who could give pneumothorax. This led to some critical remarks by the C.O. about our large medical staff with all of their renowned specialists who couldn't perform a pneumothorax. The C.O. had a point. We had on the medical service highly qualified internists, graduates of Harvard, Yale, Johns Hopkins, and other prestigious institutions, none of whom had been trained in giving pneumothorax. I had received superb chest training and experience at Duke and had performed many pneumothorax treatments in my internship and residency, so I volunteered to do the refill. Dr. Reid Heffner of Johns Hopkins was assigned to the Prison Ward and I said I would teach him how to do it. We located the Davidson pneumothorax equipment, which had never been used, and we put it together. Reid and I then went to the prison ward to see our patient. He was a strapping blond young man surrounded by the rest of his POW friends. I placed the patient in a sitting position on a chair with a medication table in front and proceeded to inject a local anesthetic, and then without fanfare hooked him up to the pneumothorax machine by inserting a needle attached to the machine into the right chest at an appropriate level. I injected the prescribed amount of air and the procedure was over with. I removed the needle, packed up the equipment and went out the door of the prison ward. When we were outside, Reid said to me "That was very slick. You were cool as a cucumber and acted like you had done hundreds of these. Weren't you afraid of a reaction with those tough Nazis looking on?" I said, "No. When I checked his chart I saw that for the first pneumothorax he was given at the Station Hospital, they injected 1500 cc which was too much. I figured that if they couldn't kill him with that, there was no danger of a bad reaction to half that much that I was giving him." Almost all of the section chiefs in medicine were captains although their positions in the Table of Organization called for a majority. They were doing a major's work for a captain's pay. It would not take long before dissatisfaction was being expressed. As the months went by with no upward movement, even the most docile people began to complain. Colonel Beeuwkes's comment to one captain doing a major's job was to the effect that "Captain is a pretty good rank." Then on another occasion, "If I move my captains up to major, they will be taken away from Valley Forge for overseas duty," a thinly veiled threat that silenced some but not all of the rebels.

The final blow was a comment made by the C.O. that no officer at Valley Forge General Hospital would be promoted until he himself was awarded the star of a brigadier general. The inside information was that the Third Service Command in Baltimore would never approve a star for Colonel Beeuwkes. I received dozens of letters of commendation for services rendered by me to grateful patients. Morale began to slip and men sought opportunities elsewhere, and some succeeded in getting transferred. Colonel Fulton constantly pressed the matter of promotion to no avail. The C.O. seemed to be living in his own dream world.

Heaven knows when the logjam would have broken if it hadn't been for the first medical consultant to be appointed to the Third Service Command in the person of Colonel Thomas Fitz-Hugh, Jr., a renowned clinician and professor at the University of Pennsylvania School of Medicine. "Colonel Tom," as we got to call him with respect and affection, came into the Command like a breath of fresh air. He had gone overseas with the 20th General Hospital of the University of Pennsylvania and served with distinction in the China-Burma-India (CBI) theater until he was rotated back to the United States. He was a close friend of General Hugh Morgan, had excellent relationships with his colleagues, and had the knack of getting along well with the Army brass. My first encounter with him was when he visited Valley Forge and made rounds accompanied by Colonel Frank Strome, who was the Regular Army Third Service Command Surgeon. Colonel Strome had apparently been told that I had been conned by a malingering doctor, a captain, with disabling polyarthritis. I had carefully examined that doctor and observed him as a patient on my section at Valley Forge. We had decided that the man was disabled and arranged for him to be sent to Army and Navy General Hospital, Hot Springs, Arkansas, where a special arthritis unit had been set up headed by Dr. Philip Hench, the well-known arthritis specialist from the Mayo Clinic, who would in 1950 become a Nobel Laureate for his work with cortisone in arthritis. Colonel Strome, a stranger to me, bellowed out his defamation of the doctor-patient and thought I had been fooled by the man. I had great difficulty in restraining myself and, had it not been for Colonel Tom, I might have gotten into real trouble. He was positioned behind Colonel Strome and was signaling me to cool down and not let the man upset me. I managed to say that I did not know where Colonel Strome got his information. I was certain of the diagnosis and did not believe the doctor was a malingerer and I suggested that he call Dr. Philip Hench and discuss the case with him. Colonel Strome glared at me and said that he would certainly get in touch with Dr. Hench and Heaven help me if I had made a mistake.

Colonel Strome had been misinformed and the one who caught hell for this was the informant. Colonel Strome admitted, later on, to Colonel Tom that he was impressed by my guts and composure but he did not say that to me. Colonel Tom called me later to reassure me, felt I had handled the dispute well, and he knew that Colonel Strome and I would get along well. His prediction was accurate. By dint of doing a topflight job at Valley Forge General Hospital and bringing substantial credit to the Third Service Command, Colonel Strome and I became good friends and he referred many important officers to me as patients. One day Colonel Strome called me from Command Headquarters in Baltimore saying that he had a general staff colonel serving with General George Patton who had a gastrointestinal problem that was disabling and undiagnosed despite many consultations and tests at numerous Army Hospitals, including Walter Reed, Letterman General, and, of all things, Johns Hopkins. General Patton and his tanks had arrived at Indiantown Gap preparatory to going overseas and he was very concerned over the condition of his colonel and chief of staff. Colonel Strome told him that he had the best diagnostician in the Army at Valley Forge and he would come up with the answers. I agreed to take care of the patient and he arrived at Valley Forge General Hospital several hours later by ambulance. He was a keen young man in his forties who was in a cast for a fractured femur incurred during tank maneuvers some time before. I dropped everything to examine him as thoroughly as possible. His chief complaint was of recurrent abdominal pain and cramps with episodes of diarrhea alternating with constipation. I could find nothing suspicious on physical examination. The patient had brought with him a large bundle of x-ray films that included several barium enemas, one of them done at Johns Hopkins. I saw something suspicious in the splenic flexure of his colon and ordered an emergency barium enema, which was done within two hours of his arrival. As I suspected, the colonel had a tumor of the splenic flexure of his colon, a lesion that had been missed on multiple examinations. I quickly called Colonel Strome in Baltimore and gave him the news. He let out a few choice cuss words about the previous examiners, congratulated me, and contacted General Patton who had paid out of his own pocket for the patient's examination at Johns Hopkins. Patton expressed his thanks and commendation to me in his own inimitable fashion and departed for what was to be the Normandy Invasion. Colonel John Owen, chief of surgery, operated upon the Colonel, resected the tumor, and before long we sent the patient back to full duty and also lost track of him. The tumor was a low-grade carcinoma without visible metastases.

Three or four months later I was advised that General Norman Kirk, the surgeon general, was visiting Valley Forge and was coming to see me. The surgeon general was a man of few words. He had a weather-beaten face with wrinkles at the edges of his blue eyes that stared through you. He said, "Tell me about the colonel." I signaled to my sergeant to get the slides from the pathology laboratory and I recited the history of the colonel's illness for the surgeon general. He listened without saying a word. When I had finished he fixed me with gimlet blue eyes and said, "You certainly wiped somebody's nose this time," and he strode from my office. I am told this was one of the highest compliments he had ever paid any officer. He was from the small town of Rising Sun on the Eastern shore of Maryland near the home of my beloved late wife. The shoremen and their women do not overdo the compliments or commendations.

When I was promoted to Major, 11 August 1944, I was excused from serving as officer of the day, but I chose to continue to take my turn in the rotation for several reasons. The more doctors who participated, the less frequent were the tours of duty. It meant going twenty-four hours without sleep once every two weeks. On this tour, you could see for yourself how the entire medical service functioned in the eerie night hours. You find out whether the corpsmen are asleep at the post, goofing off, or occupying themselves constructively. One night I became worried about a young infantry lieutenant with a severe bilateral pneumonia being treated with sulfadiazine and in an oxygen tent. I had assigned a corpsman to do nothing else but watch this patient and to see that the oxygen tent was functioning properly. In those days, oxygen was fed into the tent through a bedside portable tank because there was no central supply. When I looked into the patient's room, to my horror, I found the oxygen tank nearly empty and no one else in the room. I got another tank in place and then started to look for the corpsman. There he was, asleep on the examining table in my office that adjoined the patient's room. I chewed him out quite thoroughly. The next day we expedited that corpsman's transfer to a unit shipping out for the European Theater of War and combat duty.

I never court-martialed anyone during my tour of duty. I know that some who served under me would rather have been court-martialed than subject to the tongue-lashing they had earned. I have always tried to be fair and to abide by the Golden Rule, but patience has its limits.

Another duty of the O.D. in World War II was to greet late arrivals for admission to the hospital. When Valley Forge became a center for the blind and for those needing maxillofacial reconstruction, patients would arrive at odd hours from almost anywhere in the world. The appearance of some of these men, eyes gone, and faces practically destroyed were sobering reminders to us of the horrors of war. We had at Valley Forge at that time a marvelous plastic surgeon and maxillofacial team led by the indefatigable and brilliant Lt. Colonel James Barrett Brown of Washington University, St. Louis, Missouri. Colonel Brown was one of the most dedicated surgeons I have ever encountered. When, on my O.D. tour I had occasion to admit a severely wounded patient to his service, I would not hesitate to tell him that our chief of reconstructive surgery was the best in the world and would surely be able to help him. When I could say this, with sincerity, it gave me a sense of relief from having to witness the mayhem of war. When they were well enough, we shared our mess with them. Who can ever forget sitting across the table facing the blind and the disfigured faces of these casualties? I came to know Colonel Brown quite well. He knew more about the mouth and its appendages than anyone I have ever met. He it was who treated and cured my wife's suppurative parotitis secondary to a Stensen's duct stenosis without having to make an external incision that might have left a scar on her beautiful face. In turn, I had the privilege of helping his wife with a medical ailment. Lt. Colonel Brown was one of those held in grade for many months by Colonel Beeuwkes at the time when he rated the full chicken colonel's eagles, which he ultimately did receive. I did a great deal of medical consulting for Colonel Brown, a good bit of it due to the high incidence of malaria among his wounded. As a result I became Valley Forge's expert on malariology. Most of it was vivax malaria in veterans from Guadalcanal, the Solomons, and North Africa, and later in the China-Burma-India (CBI) Theater. Occasionally we were faced with falciparum malaria and rarely with quartan.

Colonel Brown was an unassuming person who bore short shrift with formal military protocol. A story that tickled most of us was that one day, a freshly minted MAC 2nd Lieutenant, Wayne Murphy, dialed Colonel Brown's office asking to speak with him. The person answering the telephone merely said "Hello." Murphy was incensed and proceeded to lecture this individual on military telephone etiquette. "Answer, 'This is Private First Class Jones, Ward Office 5.' Ask Colonel Brown to come to the telephone"; after a slight pause "This is Brown speaking." Murphy later said if he could have found a hole in the floor he would have crawled into it.

Colonel Brown attracted some very talented young medical officers to his staff, eager to learn his skills in plastic and reconstructive surgery. Many of the young men went on to outstanding careers in this specialty. One of the best was Bradford Cannon of Harvard, son of the famous physiologist, Professor Walter Bradford Cannon of Harvard, a teacher of my professors, Wallace O. Fenn and Edward F. Adolph of the University of Rochester. "Brad" had been deferred from military service for some time because of heavy civilian responsibilities in Boston and for some reason had been given only a first lieutenant's commission and allegedly told by someone in the surgeon general's office that this was a "pretty good rank." He was married and had several children and deserved a majority, which he was eventually awarded. Professionally he was very happy to serve under Colonel Brown. While at Valley Forge, his wife gave birth to another child but suffered a postpartum pulmonary embolus, which fortunately was not lethal. She was transferred from a Philadelphia hospital to Valley Forge General Hospital for careful observation on my section where she made a complete recovery. It was for this reason that I was invited to a dinner that Brad and his wife gave for his father and his mother at the Officer's Club. I was delighted to spend an evening with the famous professor who had contributed so much to American and world physiology.

There was another young doctor, Captain Joseph E. Murray, assigned to Colonel Brown's service at Valley Forge in 1944, who had completed a one-year internship in Boston after being graduated from Harvard Medical School and was then assigned to Valley Forge, where he sought every opportunity to work in the plastic-surgery wards. There he saw a great many soldiers with severe burns, "Many of them with so much skin destruction that autografts could not be used. Often, skin grafts were taken from other individuals and used for purposes of a temporary surface cover." Murray became fascinated with the mechanism by which the host could distinguish another person's skin from his own. He discussed the matter with the distinguished plastic surgeon, James Barrett Brown. Brown had postulated that the closer the genetic relationship between a donor and a recipient, the slower the process of rejection. In 1937, he had experimentally crossed skin from a pair of identical twins and documented permanent graft survival in both. It was this experience that ultimately led Murray to study organ transplantation.[9] On 8 October 1990, Reuters announced that the Nobel Prize for Physiology and Medicine of 1990 went to JOSEPH E. MURRAY AND E. DONNAL THOMAS.

Who could have imagined that this young doctor at Valley Forge in 1944 would one day win a Nobel Prize! After finishing his Army tour of duty in 1947, Murray completed his residencies in general and plastic surgery and ultimately became professor and chief plastic surgeon of the Peter Bent Brigham Hospital. In the late 1940s during his residency at the Peter Bent Brigham he joined a team of clinicians and researchers studying end-stage renal disease, including John Merrill

---

9. *The Pharos*, Winter 1992, p. 45; J. Palca, "Overcoming Rejection to Win a Nobel Prize," *Science* 150 (1990), p. 378.

and David Hume.[10] "Then, in late 1954, Richard Herrick turned up at Peter Bent Brigham Hospital with end-stage renal failure. His identical twin brother, Ronald Herrick, was prepared to donate a kidney and Murray reasoned that, since Ronald's healthy kidney would be genetically identical to Richard's diseased kidney, there should be no problem with rejection. The operation, performed on 23 December 1954 was a 'spectacular success,' says Murray."[11] The next decade was devoted to a search for anti-rejection medication. The concluding paragraph of this short essay in *Science* was, "This year's prize sends a useful message, says Emil J. Freireich, director of adult leukemia research at M.D. Anderson Hospital in Dallas. It acknowledges that physicians can do the same kind of high-quality science Ph.D.s can do. And that should give a boost to policy-makers who are worrying about attracting enough physicians into careers in science." Having been a colleague and friend of J. Barrett Brown, I am delighted to have learned that his seminal experiment with skin grafts in identical twins stimulated a gifted young intern, Joseph E. Murray, to pioneer in renal transplantation. Murray joins the list of dedicated practicing physicians and surgeons including Banting, Minot, and Dickinson Richards who have made great contributions to medical progress while continuing to take care of the sick. Caring for the sick is not incompatible with scientific research. Oftentimes the driving force behind a physician's research work is the sick patient with a "hopeless" prognosis. The best physicians, in my experience, have been those who have been able to combine science with the art of medicine in achieving the healing process that is the hallmark of good medical practice.

Today, it is said that these are renaissance men and women, impossible to replicate in today's rush to the narrow and more lucrative procedure-oriented subspecialties. I refuse to accept this popular notion. However, given that the present methods of medical education seem to have failed to provide men and women with these capabilities, I must admit that these individuals are exceptional and scarce in any era, but they are, to my mind, the gold standard toward which we must strive.

My emergence as Valley Forge General Hospital's authority on malaria and other tropical diseases led to some interesting experiences and I was in demand as a speaker on these topics before several County Medical Societies. One was the Lackawanna County Medical

---

10. Ibid.
11. Ibid.

Society in Scranton, Pennsylvania, on 15 May 1944. Shortly before this meeting I was notified by the surgeon general's office that I was not to use the word malaria in my talk, no members of the press would be allowed, all comments were to be off-the-record and the talk was to be labeled "Restricted." Lt. Robert Johnson, assistant chief of laboratory service at Valley Forge General Hospital (who assisted me) and I were amazed at these restrictions and wondered how we could handle the topic and still comply with our Army orders. The reason for the secrecy was that malaria was proving to be a greater adversary in the Pacific Islands than the Japanese. The surgeon general did not wish to publicize this. Of all of the patients with malaria seen by me at Valley Forge General Hospital, the most unusual was a twenty-four-year-old Chinese air force cadet who had been admitted to the locked ward of the Neuro-Psychiatric Service with the diagnosis of dementia praecox, type-paranoid. The note that accompanied the patient read as follows:

> (NMI) CADET, CHINESE AIR FORCE. April 9, 1943
> Age:24
>
> March 20, 1943 this patient, according to the interpreter, has always acted somewhat peculiar but wasn't bad. He would often play and strike his fellow companions but suddenly change mood and become sad and sorrowful. He would at some times attempt sexual perversions as thinking himself a woman and attempt love affairs with other cadets. On March 19, 1943, on a transport en route to New York from Bombay, at 5:00 P.M. he began to act funny and pushed over a visitor in the room. He threw a glass of water on the floor and began to cry. He was asked what the trouble was and he said nothing. He stopped crying and began to laugh and talk incoherently about difficult subjects. He finally went to bed and was guarded overnight. In the morning he still did lots of talking and began to say that he was "Tarzan." He would throw a dart at anyone coming in and brandished his knife. He was persuaded, after much attempt, to be brought up to the sick bay but on the way up he had his knife drawn; one of the cadets took it away from him and a fight started.

He was finally brought to the locked ward. On admission he was very wild, kicking, spitting and screaming, saying that he was "Tarzan." He managed to bite an attendant before being locked up. Morphine sulphate injection and intravenous sodium amytal were administered. Cold-pack treatment was given. After two days he gradually improved and became more rational. On April 3 he was well enough to be put into another room with less restraint. After one day he suddenly became violent again and needed barbiturate medication to keep him under control. Diagnosis: Dementia Praecox, Type-Paranoid. During his admission to Valley Forge General Hospital, medical consultation was obtained. A blood smear was positive for Plasmodium vivax which was treated vigorously. He responded dramatically to anti-malarial therapy and was soon returned to full active duty, cleared of his neuropsychiatric symptoms. Malaria, to this day, remains a mimic of almost any disease, a treacherous field for the novice and unaware. In my Lackawanna Society Lecture of 1944 I said, "We have seen this disease (malaria) manifest itself by psychosis, dysentery, abdominal pain suggesting a perforated viscus, curious anemias, splenic pain, bronchitis, grippe, nasopharyngitis, coma, jaundice, nephritis, liver disease, fever of unknown origin, duodenal ulcer and multiple aches and joint pains. The most important factor in making an accurate diagnosis is the doctor's mental attitude, that is, he must be 'malaria conscious'! Ask the patient whether he has had it! Has he served in malaria country? This may be perfectly obvious but it is amazing how often it is not done. A final caveat, do not assume that malaria is the diagnosis without checking the blood smear."

When the Duke of Windsor and his consort, the Duchess, paid a visit to Valley Forge on 9 June 1943, I was assigned by Colonel Fulton to escort the Duke to the plastic surgery service. I found him to be a warm and appealing person as did our wounded soldiers. He lingered longer than usual at the bedside of one of my patients, who had relapsing malaria. The Duke said in an almost cockney accent that he too had malaria on a trip to Kenya and the two had quite a conversation on the topic, which was interrupted by a message from the rather imperious Duchess ordering him to return to her side as soon as possible. A special dinner in honor of the couple was held in the Officer's Club, where they signed our guest book. Edward signed one page and Wallis the other. Some of our merry-making officers signed the same book as Tom, Dick, or Harry upsetting Colonel Beeuwkes who was somewhat of an Anglophile.

From the sublime to something else was the visit to Valley Forge General Hospital of Fats Waller on a blazing hot summer day. We rolled a grand piano out on the lawn, put a pitcher of ice water on it and cheered Fats Waller on as he played jazz as he alone could play it. His face dripped in sweat and he kept drinking the ice water which we later learned was heavily spiked with Gin. The more he drank, the better he played to the delight of our wounded as well as the staff of our hospital. There were many professional visitors to Valley Forge, including most of the leading doctors of Philadelphia, who lectured and consulted. All in all our professional lives were substantially rewarding but economically deprived by the failure to be given the promotions we had long before deserved.

When Colonel Tom Fitz-Hugh was assigned as the first chief medical consultant of the Third Service Command, he started the ball rolling. He made regular rounds with us, and won our respect, confidence, and affection. We knew we had a superb professor and seasoned clinician at the top of his profession and we learned a great deal from him. Colonel Tom was an Oslerian clinician who was a superb internist and diagnostician with a hobby, hematology. He had already earned an eponym entitling him to enduring fame—The Fitz-Hugh-Curtis syndrome of right-upper-quadrant abdominal pain due to subdiaphragmatic violin-type adhesions caused by gonococcal peritonitis.[12] Before entering military service with the University of Pennsylvania's 20th General Hospital in the CBI Theater, he had taught for many years at the University of Pennsylvania and conducted one of Philadelphia's outstanding private practices. He hit it off very well with Colonel Fulton and, wonders of wonders, was able to deal with our commanding officer with tact, diplomacy, and firmness. He also quickly won the respect of the Third Service Command including the commanding general and, best of all, the command surgeon, Colonel Frank Strome. It was no accident that the Third Service Command was the last of the nine Service Commands to accept a medical consultant. It is no secret that the concept of a civilian consultant with the rank of colonel being assigned to each service command was initially opposed by some, if not all, of the command surgeons as an intrusion on their authority and also viewed as a threat to their autonomy and rank. Colonel Tom quickly won the respect of the hierarchy and was accepted and respected.

By his skill in communication and his tactfulness and persuasiveness, he soon improved the sometimes strained relations between command headquarters and the various hospitals within its jurisdiction. The first thing he set about doing was to sit down with each individual doctor, make rounds, look into his background, and evaluate how he was functioning in his position assignment. He it was who introduced the method of physician evaluation developed by General Hugh Morgan and saw to it that this evaluation was placed in each officer's 201 file as a permanent record and kept up-to-date. He quickly became aware that all of our section chiefs were serving as captains

---

12. T. Fitz-Hugh, Jr., "Acute Gonococcic Peritonitis of the Right Upper Quadrant in Women," *Journal of the American Medical Association* 102 (1934), p. 2094.

when their assignments under our Table of Organization called for their being majors. This would make a substantial difference in their pay and help pay their bills, something Colonel Beeuwkes failed to understand or did not wish to consider.

Finally on 11 August 1944, I received my promotion to major after having served as a captain since 12 December 1942. This was the first promotion to field grade at Valley Forge; the ice jam was broken and other well-deserved promotions followed.

We had a large contingent of enlisted men and WACs at Valley Forge General Hospital who served as corpsmen and corpswomen, and with time, effort, and tight supervision they became indispensable for rendering care to our patients. Nurses were few and far between. Good ones were scarce. When we sought to promote a nurse to first lieutenant it was not easy. For those recommended for captain's bars, we were told that if the individual were promoted to that rank, she would no longer be a head nurse but could be lost to us by being assigned as a supervisor. This came up with our head nurse on the Officers' and Women's Section, First Lieutenant Edith Hyde. I pulled every string I could to move her up to captain without losing her, emphasizing that her work was outstanding and very much needed in the provision and supervision of personal nursing care. We made our point and were happy to see her elevated to the captaincy that she richly deserved, but the Army had the final word. She was made a supervisor and we lost our head nurse. The WACs were rather a mixed bag. Some fitted into hospital work very well and became indispensable for their bedside nursing care. Others simply had to be reassigned to other duties. All of them needed close supervision to assure positive results. This was equally true of the corpsmen. They were only as good as their supervision, discipline, and training. I soon found out that the time spent in teaching and observing the corpsmen and WACs paid enormous dividends. Periodically, especially when a convoy of wounded and ill arrived from overseas, hundreds at one clip, I would give my enlisted men and women a pep talk. This would be reinforced by frequent spot inspections and words of encouragement when something especially good was done for a patient. A two-day pass for work well done could do wonders for morale. A promotion in grade from private to corporal or even sergeant was good for the entire outfit if it were earned and deserved. All in all, in Navy parlance, I ran a happy ship with tight discipline. The corpsmen knew I was there around the clock and did not miss anything of importance. My corpsmen and WACs were so exceptional that we were soon being raided by hospitals going overseas. This would lead to problems in the near future. One of the best WACs was Sergeant Eva Grenier, a mature person who was better than many nurses at rendering bedside care. She came into service as a private and ended up as a highly respected sergeant on my unit.

One of the more difficult roles I had to assume in military service was making judgments as to whether illnesses were feigned or real. The effective doctor in the military cannot serve solely as an advocate for his patients. He must also protect the interests and requirements of the armed service involved. This dual role may be quite confusing and difficult for doctors coming from the usual civilian background where they have been trained to act as patient advocates, often to the neglect of other considerations.

In my work as the director of the personnel medical department of the largest medical center in the world, I learned a great deal about job placement and the physical requirements for a variety of positions. This experience paid off substantial dividends during my military service.

I recall quite vividly how difficult it was to believe that the healthy-looking infantry man who appeared to be running a high fever was a malingerer who had learned to manipulate his rectal thermometer by rubbing his buttocks under the sheets until the thermometer registered 103–104 degrees Fahrenheit. In the days when we did not do blood-alcohol levels, I remember one officer who was drinking Vitalis hair tonic for his highs only to be exposed by my sergeant, who followed him into the lavatory one day and found empty Vitalis bottles in the waste basket. A more subtle example was that of a high-ranking medical officer who had been sent back from England because of a history of biliary colic and non-visualization of his gallbladder, despite repeat examination with a double dose of dye. When I reviewed his x-ray films I became suspicious, because none showed any of the gallbladder dye in the intestine, suggesting that the dye had not been ingested. This led to further questioning and finally the officer admitted he had not taken any of the dye. The real problem was that he had learned from a friend and neighbor that his wife was philandering while he was overseas and he had devised this scheme for getting home. Seeking a large tax-free disability pension, a high-ranking National Guard officer, a lawyer, claimed under oath that he had never had a duodenal ulcer until after his entry on active duty in World War II. After persistent effort we obtained documents from several Veterans' Administration Hospitals revealing that he had been hospitalized on repeated occasions for a duodenal ulcer long before his entry into World War II military service. When confronted with this at the retirement-board proceedings, his comment was to the effect that he had tried and lost in a fair hearing so he bore no malice.

In a less subtle manner, an Army colonel seeking a tax-free pension for hypertensive cardiovascular disease divulged that he had been hypertensive for years. When told that all of his physical examination records over the years had reported his blood pressure to be in the normal range, his pithy comment was that "Do you know what I would have done to my battalion surgeon if he had reported my blood pressure to be high?"

Colonel Fitz-Hugh received his eagles while assigned to the Third Service Command as chief medical consultant and was kind enough to give me two of his silver leaves of his Lt. Colonelcy with the prediction that it would not be long before I would be wearing them. While Colonel Tom was our chief consultant, things ran quite smoothly. When he retired he was succeeded by Colonel Roy Turner of Tulane University, who was a first-rate scholar but whose stay with us was of short duration. I shall never forget his advice on a patient with severe ulcerative colitis whose stool cultures and many tests for ova and parasites, perhaps 20, had all been reported negative. Colonel Turner insisted that we obtain fresh material on sigmoidoscopic examination and that the stool so obtained be studied immediately on a warm stage. The patient had Entamoeba histolytica, the causative agent of amebic dysentery. He responded dramatically to anti-amebic therapy when all else had failed.

Colonel Turner was succeeded by an individual from Washington, D.C., with no academic credentials of any note, who had gained his eagles by National Guard Service. This was a great setback for those of us on the medical service, quite a letdown from the experience with previous consultants who were both university medical-school professors and seasoned consultants and clinicians. We soon found that every time the new consultant made his monthly visit, we would lose an essential medical officer or non-commissioned officer, usually both. We did not look forward to his visits. He also had a little notebook that he kept for notes while we were talking with him and on more than one occasion he would issue a veiled threat that we might all be ordered overseas. I became so incensed over his weaknesses and his prejudices that I almost told him where to go. Running a service being drained of its essential personnel made our work at the hospital more and more difficult. This consultant was hurting us rather than supporting us in our mission.

One consultant who brightened up our days was Colonel Henry W. Brosin, a professor of psychiatry from the University of Chicago, a superb teacher and an excellent liaison between medicine and psychiatry. He visited us on a number of occasions and made excellent teaching rounds. His tour of duty was preceded by Brigadier General

William Menninger of Topeka, Kansas, the chief psychiatric consultant to the surgeon general's office. General Menninger was a down-to-earth renowned psychiatrist whose great message to us was that all of us had to become psychiatrically oriented so that we could deal effectively with many of the psychoneuroses so prevalent in men and women under the stress of war. He stated firmly and unequivocally that there simply were not and never would be enough psychiatrists in the Army to take care of all people with various types of psychiatric disorders. The general medical officer had to be trained and geared to take care of these patients without assigning them to psychiatric wards. This was common sense from a very high source and it influenced us enormously. Remember that most of us in internal medicine had been through training and education stressing the biochemical and physiological aspects of human illness. Those patients not fitting into these concepts of illness were simply cast aside as neurotics, malingerers, psychopaths, or worse. This was a crossroads for many of us in military medicine and it led to a revolution in our attitudes toward psychiatric illness that would carry over into civilian medicine with the end of the war. Psychiatry was entering into a new and exciting era. While at Valley Forge I was very much impressed by the complimentary things the Peter Bent Brighamites had to say about a dynamic teacher and young professor of psychiatry on their staff named John Romano, who was destined for a major role in the teaching of psychiatry in America.

While at Valley Forge I also had the pleasure of being the physician to Captain Theodore Lidz, a talented psychiatrist who had been rotated home after service in the Pacific with the Johns Hopkins unit. I have followed his illustrious career at Yale since then with considerable interest. Colonel Brosin had the knack of telling funny stores. One that I remember described the legendary imperturbability of the British under stress. As I recall it, the story went this way. At the opera in London, the orchestra seats were filled with black-tied and white-tied men with their elegant ladies when a chap in the mezzanine whipped out his penis and began urinating on those below. One of the ladies being sprayed complained to her escort and demanded that he do something about this dastardly act. He did so by crying out "I say old boy, won't you wobble it a bit?"

My professional work at Valley Forge, despite some problems, remained challenging and rewarding. My internship and residency at Duke continued to pay great dividends. One of these was in the field of fungal diseases, a subject that Dr. David T. Smith had taught so well at Duke. The tank divisions, including General George Patton's, were arriving at Indiantown Gap Reservation ready to go overseas for the Normandy Invasion after having trained in the Southwest, including the San Joaquin Valley and the Desert Training Center of California and Arizona. These troops were exposed to coccidioidomycosis and many became ill with it by the time they reached the Gap. Many were sent to Valley Forge General Hospital where we made the diagnosis and had no real weapons to fight the disease. I saw many patients with coccidioidomycosis, most of it confined to the lungs but some with systemic involvement and manifestations. Some were severely ill, often with central-nervous-system dissemination with lethal effect. During this "epidemic," we learned a good deal about the natural history of this disorder. I was quite impressed by a complement-fixation test of the patient's blood done by Dr. Charles Edward Smith in California. He had an uncanny ability, based on this test, to predict which patients would develop systemic coccidioidomycosis and those whose disease would remain confined to the lungs.

To further stimulate our interest in this entity at that time, we learned that Dr. Edward Chamberlin, the professor of radiology at Temple University Medical School, had taken his family on a trip to the San Joaquin Valley in his camper. On returning to their home in Philadelphia, the family cleaned out the dirt from the van and soon most of them came down with coccidioidomycosis from the sand and dust accumulated during the desert stay. Fortunately their illness was mild.

During my assignment at Valley Forge General Hospital I was honored by being asked to give a lecture at the New York Academy of Medicine on small-intestinal disease, a subject that occupied my attention for many years.

In 1944, while at Valley Forge, I was summoned home on an emergency. One of my sisters, Annette, was severely ill at home under the care of a local physician. Hospital beds were at a premium, nurses were almost impossible to obtain, and physicians who made house calls were few and far between. I obtained an emergency leave and drove quickly to New York. I found my sister in critical condition with obvious clinical signs of bilateral extensive bronchopneumonia. I ordered a private ambulance and arranged for her admission to the Columbia-Presbyterian Medical Center and placed her under the care of Dr. Gwendolyn Jones, the doctor who had taken my place as personnel medical director. She was kind enough to arrange consultations with Dr. Robert F. Loeb and Dr. Walter W. Palmer, my professors, as well as others of the staff. It was nip and tuck for many days but by dint of judicious use of sulfadiazine, an oxygen tent, and excellent nursing care and supportive measures, my sister survived. Her husband was engaged in the invasion of Sicily as an artillery man and could not be contacted while she was ill. This was a very close call and I am happy I was able to get to her bedside and made the arrangements that led to saving her life.

As time rolled by Valley Forge became an outstanding hospital and patients streamed in from all quarters of the globe including the Solomons, Guadalcanal, New Hebrides, New Guinea, Australia, North Africa, Liberia, the African Gold Coast, Southern Italy, India, Germany, England, and France, as well as from the Southern and Western United States. The variety of medical disorders we were seeing was enormous and taxed our clinicians to their utmost. Remember that during World War II the general internist or diagnostician was the backbone of the medical service. Subspecialty areas were opening up but really were still in their infancy. We were required to be excellent general clinicians capable of caring for all medical ailments. Inevitably we also developed hobbies in the subspecialties, but many of us resisted being assigned to subspecialties because the most attractive positions and assignments went to general internists, as did the higher grades. When Colonel Fulton was transferred to another general hospital and Major Schnitker became chief of medicine, in addition to my duties as the chief of the Officers' and Women's Section, I became assistant chief of the entire Medical Service and was Valley Forge's expert on tropical diseases and hepatitis. When our gastroenterologist, Major Samuel Morrison, was transferred to another station I also became the gastroenterologist for Valley Forge.

I was rapidly learning more and more about Army administration and its various boards and other institutions, especially the Retiring Boards of Officers. Toward the end of my stay at Valley Forge General Hospital I was devoting a good bit of my time to testifying before Retiring Boards for my officer patients. Some of our doctors disliked these proceedings and some feared the cross-examinations to which they were subjected. I learned early on that to be effective as a witness, it was essential that I be consistent and truthful so that I did not have to remember a lie. The legal guidelines observed were a fairly simple list of Army regulations (A.R.) that were easily memorized and very helpful.

I tried to be as honest and forthright as I could, and soon became known for my presentations to the degree that more and more high-ranking officers were electing to come to Valley Forge General Hospital to seek my professional and administrative services. In the process, I met some very interesting people. General Norman Randolph, commanding general, Third Service Command, sought me out and entered Valley Forge General Hospital on my service. He had a disability for which we retired him. After the war, he would travel to see me in my Park Avenue office from his home in Philadelphia and we became good friends. He was a West Point classmate of General Eisenhower, who was then president of Columbia University and visited him regularly. In fact, he recommended that Ike and Mamie see me in consultation.

In 1945, Colonel Beeuwkes consulted me and became a patient at Valley Forge. Despite our differences, I had always maintained respectful discipline toward him and his position as my commanding officer. I treated him as I would any other patient, giving him the best of care. I appeared on his behalf at the Army Retiring Board and refrained from any adverse comments and emphasized his outstanding World War I service. Shortly after this meeting, he wrote a gracious letter of commendation and appreciation to me that served to heal some of the past experiences. The letter dated 14 March 1945 sent Free Mail, did not reach me until June 1945, when I was with the 303rd General Hospital on Tinian. It read as follows:

March 14, 1945

Major Michael J. Lepore
Valley Forge General Hospital
Phoenixville, PA

My dear Major Lepore:
    I will derive much satisfaction in writing this letter as I wish you to know the great satisfaction I have had in being associated with you and having you on my staff during the last two years. You have done a difficult and outstanding job in caring for our medical officer patients and many letters have been received from these patients expressing satisfaction and gratitude for your interest and your skill. You have thus brought great credit to Valley Forge and to the Army. May I therefore congratulate and thank you for fine general work and also for your service professionally to me and to Mrs. Beeuwkes.

Sincerely yours,
Henry Beeuwkes Col. M.C.

From the perspective of nearly half a century later, and the maturity that has accompanied it, I regret that I did not know more about Colonel Beeuwkes when I served under him at Valley Forge. His outstanding service to his country during and after World War I and in famine relief in Russia under Herbert Hoover, followed by years of work for the Rockefeller Foundation on yellow fever, ensure his place among the heroes of this century. Perhaps those of us who served at

Valley Forge and made it one of the greatest of the Army General Hospitals were a little harsh in our judgment of its first commanding officer.

My tour of duty at Valley Forge was nearing its end. Most of our officers and enlisted personnel were receiving orders assigning them to units preparing to go overseas. The war in Europe was over but we were faced with a cruel and dangerous adversary, the Japanese, who had fully demonstrated their will to destroy us no matter what losses they might suffer. At Valley Forge we had an opportunity to see first-hand what this enemy could and would do to our soldiers who had been POWs. A large number of those who had been prisoners of the Japanese were rotated through Valley Forge for intensive treatment and observation. We were appalled by the malnutrition and pitiful deterioration in physical health manifested by these brave men. They resembled the people of Dachau and the other German prison camps. I shall never forget the appearance of an emaciated young American Army colonel who was in uniform but walking with a cane. I soon realized that this young man was blind, not due to wounds but due to beri-beri caused by the starvation "diet" fed to him for many months by his Japanese captors. I had been taught that beri-beri is a treatable disease, reversed by injections of a B vitamin, Thiamine chloride. The colonel had been made blind by his vitamin-deficient starvation diet, developing bilateral optic neuritis which, unfortunately, was irreversible by the time of his rescue from the enemy. He was permanently blind. Among the POW officers sent to Valley Forge General Hospital for observation, rest, and recuperation was Captain Manon R. (Manny) Lawton of South Carolina, a survivor of the infamous Bataan Death March and three-and-one-half years of mistreatment as a prisoner of war of the Japanese.

As an officer, he was probably assigned to my service, the Officers' and Women's Section of Valley Forge General Hospital, but I must confess that I do not remember him, but I salute his marvelous account of his experiences written in 1984.[13] I was especially interested in his description of how the Japanese tried to punish or kill the prisoners by starving them. Lawton's description of his beri-beri is startlingly accurate. The polyneuritis, edema, weakness, and fatiguability are classical. I was also intrigued by his description of his loss of vision, which fortunately was restored when he obtained some

---

13. Manny Lawton, *Some Survived: An Epic Account of Japanese Captivity During World War II* (Chapel Hill: Algonquin Books of Chapel Hill, 1984).

high-protein food, including canned salmon and sardines. He was luckier than the colonel that I saw at Valley Forge whose loss of vision was irreversible.

For some reason, the story of the mistreatment of prisoners of war by the Japanese has not received the publicity accorded to the Germans for their atrocities at Dachau and Buchenwald. In *The Other Nuremberg—The Untold Story of the Tokyo War Crime Trials*, Arnold C. Brackman examines this issue in considerable detail. He quotes Frederick Mignone of Connecticut, one of the assistant prosecutors, complaining that the American press coverage was skimpy and begrudging. "Perhaps the distance barrier is responsible for lack of interest in this important unveiling of criminality in the Far East."[14] Mignone also observed that "in Japan and in the Orient in general the trial is one of the most important phases of the occupation. It has received wide coverage in the Japanese press and revealed for first time to millions of Japanese the scheming, duplicity and the insatiable desire for power of her entrenched militaristic leaders, writing a much-needed history of events which otherwise would not have been written."[15]

On 3 May 1946 the first public meeting of the International Military Tribunal for the Far East (The Other Nuremberg) was held in Tokyo. At that time I was stationed on Saipan, as chief of medicine of the 148th General Hospital. There I received a letter from my friend, Lt. Colonel Maurice Schnitker, then the medical consultant with General Douglas MacArthur, offering me a key position on his staff with a view to replacing him as consultant in the near future. I had a feeling that if I accepted the assignment I might end up in the Army of Occupation. After some deliberation I wrote Colonel Schnitker, declining the offer with thanks, saying General W. W. Irvine wished me to stay on Saipan.

The receipt of overseas orders was greeted in various ways by our medical officers. Most saw it as their duty and their turn to go to the front lines. A minority became very upset and sought every means to avoid going overseas. My own reaction was that since my turn had come and I was needed for the Pacific War, I would willingly go where I was most needed.

---

14. Arnold B. Brackman, *The Other Nuremberg: The Untold Story of the Tokyo War Crime Trials*, 1st Quill edition (New York: William Morrow, 1987), p. 212.

15. Ibid, pp. 212–213.

My orders came in May 1945, assigning me to the 303rd General Hospital at Camp Shelby, Hattiesburg, Mississippi. I was greatly touched by a parting gift from my staff at Valley Forge and the accompanying card signed by my head nurse, my corpsmen and WACs, and Major Jack Lucas MAC and Major Gordon Mackmull M.C.

Chapter 15
Tinian, 1945

M Y OVERSEAS ORDERS ARRIVED during the last week in May 1945, couched in classical "Army Speak":

TO PHOENIXVILLE 503 FROM HAYES COMMANDING GENERAL 3RD SERVICE COMMAND BALTIMORE, MD. TO COMMANDING OFFICER VALLEY FORGE GENER- AL HOSPITAL, PHOENIXVILLE, PENN. GRNC ORDER ISSUING RELIEVING MAJOR MICHAEL J. LEPORE 0–505–780 FROM ASSIGNMENT THIRTEEN EIGHT SEVEN SERVICE COMMAND YOUR STATION AND ASSIGNING HIM THREE HUNDRED THIRD GENERAL HOSPITAL CAMP SHELBY MISSISSIPPI. STOP LEAVE EN ROUTE AUTHORIZED REPORTING NOT LATER THAN 15 JUNE STOP DIRECT OFFICER PROCEED ACCORDINGLY COPIES OF ORDERS TO BE FOR- WARDED NEW STATION STOP

I was about to embark on one of the most interesting journeys of my life and by far the most hazardous. Perhaps it was just as well that I did not know exactly where I was going. The war in Europe had ended and it did not take a genius to figure out that my destination was the Pacific theater of war, I was pleased to be assigned to a num- bered general hospital, the *crème de la crème* of overseas duty, or so I thought. Thus far, each of my previous assignments had been with general hospitals. Number one was the Army and Navy General Hospital in Hot Springs, Arkansas, for a brief period followed by over three years at the brand new Valley Forge General Hospital, adjacent to the historic valley for which it was named.

The short leave provided a few days of leisure to spend with my wife driving South and visiting with her cousins who lived in Knoxville, Tennessee, nearby a massive, newly built, and mysterious installation called Oak Ridge by some and the Manhattan Project by others.

In Knoxville we were told by friends and relatives that they all knew a secret weapon was being developed at Oak Ridge that would wipe out the Japanese and end the war. It sounded like a Buck Rogers story, but it was nice to hear and seemed consistent with other infor- mation I had acquired during my professional work at Valley Forge.

On reporting to the 303rd General Hospital on 5 June 1945 in Camp Shelby outside of Hattiesburg, Mississippi, I was quickly informed by the C.O., Colonel James W. Howard, that I was the last of his officers to arrive and that I had exactly twelve hours to arrange my affairs because we were departing soon by troop train for the West Coast. This gave me exactly three hours of a business day to find a buyer for my car in a community of strangers. My wife could not drive, so there was no way to get the car back to Philadelphia. There was no time to establish any contacts and I had to be certain that I dealt with a reliable dealer who could pay me by certified check. I located one on the main street in Hattiesburg and accepted his offer, which I knew was about half the amount I could have gotten in Philadelphia, but I had no choice with the clock running fast. Getting a hotel room that night in Hattiesburg and a train ticket home for my wife were rather hair-raising experiences for both of us but we did succeed. Without any fanfare my newly made Southern acquaintances knew I was going overseas and they were glad to help us out even though we were total strangers. The uniform made a difference. So did my beautiful and beloved wife whose southern charm enchanted all who met her.

When I reported for duty early the next morning back at the post it was not too long (18 June 1945) before I was on a troop train headed for the Rocky Mountains and beyond. The train was slow but I enjoyed the countryside. We stopped frequently and were often greeted by the local people, all of them very courteous and supportive.

They all seemed to know where we were heading though we ourselves were not certain. One stop that I enjoyed was in the Rocky Mountains of Montana at a place called Deer Lodge. This was a beautiful, verdant valley, the mountain air crisp and clear, contaminated only by our two coal-burning locomotives. We took a break and walked about. It was so peaceful and quiet that it was hard to believe that there was a war on and that we were heading toward it. Later on, I found out why Deer Lodge was so quiet, peaceful, and unpopulated. It was the site of a large state penitentiary.

We finally learned that we were heading for Fort Lawton, Seattle, Washington, where we arrived on 23 June 1945, five days after leaving Camp Shelby. One of the things I have never forgotten was a barber shop located just outside of the post gate. It had a large sign, "We Fix Army Haircuts," and it seemed to be a very busy place. The sign made a real impression on me and reinforced my belief in the free enterprise system. Once we were ensconced in our quarters on this giant Army base, some genius in our headquarters discovered that I had never been on the infiltration course to qualify for overseas duty by crawling on the ground past obstacles for 100 yards or more, stimulated by exploding charges plus overhead machine-gun fire with live ammunition. What the genius had not discovered in my 201 (Personnel) File was that I was on limited service from the surgeon general's office due to myopia, and should have been exempted from this test. Here I was, getting ready to go overseas, with a completely strange outfit and reluctant to cry chicken at the last minute. I decided to go ahead with the infiltration course test. It was set up for a cold early morning and I found I had to remove my glasses, because the lenses were not shatter proof, and I had to proceed without really being able to see where I was going. I also found that I was going on the course alone, another odd situation, usually a group of men went on the course together. I had purchased a new set of fatigues to protect my uniform and went to the trench and climbed out of it as the machine-guns fired overhead. No one had scoured the terrain for snakes as they were supposed to do. When I came out of the trench, sure enough, there was a snake in front of me. I dropped back into the trench and started out again in a different area. By this time charges were banging away and rocks and sand were falling about me and on me. This seemed to provide entertainment for the enlisted men running the show. Since I could not see much without my glasses, my course was hardly a straight line. It was the longest 100 yards I have ever traveled but I finally made it, having torn up the fatigues to the point that I could never again wear them.

From that point on I knew what I had always suspected; limited service is for the birds because it is almost never enforced in the field. This was no great surprise to me. The next day we found out that we were one of five 2,000-bed general hospitals going overseas on Amphibious Personnel Attack (APA) ships to the same destination. Most of us thought we were headed for the Philippines. We were all brought together in an amphitheater where we were told that we were going on Navy ships that were virtually unarmed except for what looked like pea shooters. No protection for the convoys was possible because most of the Navy combat vessels were in action in forward areas and could not be spared. We were told by a young officer that statistically there was only a small chance of our being attacked by the enemy submarines or other Naval vessels. But in the event that this should happen, we were going to be taught how to abandon ship. This was a real exercise with rope ladders and a simulated abandon-ship maneuver that we somehow managed to complete without killing or injuring some of our companions in the scramble down the side of a cliff-like wall built to resemble a ship. Departure day finally arrived and we left Seattle on a cold gray morning. We were quiet and rather glum, not much was said until the stink of rotting fish on the docks reached our truck convoy. The field grade officers were in the lead truck behind the commanding officer's staff car. One of us was a psychiatrist from Wichita Falls, Texas, who had a great sense of humor and a loud voice. When the stink reached his truck, Major Charlie Brown hollered, "My God, do you smell that? She must be back." The truck load burst into laughter, the gag was passed along to the other trucks and everybody had a belly laugh that broke the gloom. At the docks we were met by two Red Cross ladies who fed us hot coffee and donuts, and we went up the gangplank onto the U.S.S. Telfair, a Navy APA. We were crowded in like sardines and hoped for a short trip.

Someone, I believe the C.O. or his adjutant, came up with a new wrinkle shortly after we put out to sea. He ordered all officers, including field grade, to go down to the hold to observe and communicate with the enlisted personnel who might be frightened or seasick. He assigned each officer to a four-to-six-hour shift with mine starting at 2 A.M. I had never been on a large ship and was not familiar with the layout of this one. As is common off the coast of Washington and California, at about fifty miles out the ocean is often very turbulent and stormy weather may be encountered. I got out of my berth for the 2 A.M. shift, found the decks awash in a turbulent sea, slipped, and nearly fell overboard. Finally, I located the stairs and descended into the hold.

When I got there the floors and stairs were smeared with vomitus and undigested food. The stench was awful. Many of the men were horribly seasick and we had no really effective medication for this ailment. There was nothing we could do to help them. It was not long before I myself was as seasick as most of the others and I barely made it back to my bunk. I tried to get to sleep to no avail. I had a perfectly miserable number of days and could understand why some of my friends who experienced seasickness said they would sooner die in combat. Our convoy of four ships was, of course, blacked out as we advanced across the Pacific following the zig-zag pattern mandated by the naval command. Sailing on an APA crowded to the rails is a far cry from the Queen Mary. There was no place to sit except on your bunk. The deck was full of standees. As we began to get our sea legs, we moved about the ship making new friends. I met an old friend, Dr. John Rearden, who had been on the ob-gyn staff at Columbia-Presbyterian Medical Center before entering naval service. He was now the senior Navy physician in charge of all medical services and was having a busy time with some rather complex medical and surgical cases. Fortunately, he had ample numbers of consultants among the Army hospitals aboard and did not hesitate to call upon them for help. John told me that in the previous voyage he had participated in the Okinawa invasion and before that Iwo Jima. He said Ernie Pyle, famous as the GI's correspondent, had been on our APA and was killed in action when he landed with the marines on Ie Shima during the Okinawa battle. For a fellow who spent most of his professional life delivering babies in a famous medical center, John Rearden was holding up well under very stressful combat conditions. The Navy crew on board seemed very young and unmilitary but full of fun. John assured me that these kids were great in combat. Some had risked their lives, many were wounded, and a few died. Under kamikaze attack at Okinawa, the Telfair shot down three enemy planes and incurred some damage.

Dr. Lewis Thomas of New York was on an Army transport when he participated in the attack on Okinawa that he described so well in *The Youngest Science—Notes of a Medicine Watcher*.[1] He was assigned to NAMRU 2, the Naval Research Unit based on Guam, and ordered to advance under fire on the Okinawa beachhead. His job was to study Japanese encephalitis said to be present on the island. To pursue his research activities, he needed a special breed of white mice for testing. As he went down the rope ladder in the face of enemy fire, he says one of the Marines seeing him carrying a cage full of white mice yelled out "Now I've seen every *f u c k i n* thing."

Meals aboard a Navy ship were quite formal. There were three officers' mess calls, the earliest for the most junior ones, the middle for higher grade, and the last for the highest grades. We were seated at the table clockwise according to rank. Since there were five General Hospital staffs aboard we were loaded with field-grade officers, especially majors, posing some problem for the eating arrangements. The Navy had it all figured out and seated us according to our date of rank. Black crewmen served us. I had not realized how segregated our military forces were until this trip. This was further confirmed when I saw that the port battalions of enlisted men aboard ship were all black except for their white officers.

When my appetite returned and I became interested in food, I noticed that there was very little left by the time the tray had completed the clockwise circle with me at the end of it. No one seemed to give a damn about those seated toward the end. After several episodes of this I got up and said, "Gentlemen, I recommend that the

---

1. Lewis Thomas, *The Youngest Science: Notes of a Medicine Watcher* (New York: Viking Press, 1983), p. 98

serving platter be moved clockwise one man at each meal in order to provide equitable access to all." It worked. At the end of the voyage, after we had disembarked, we learned that the Navy boys had conned the Army officers of one of the general hospitals by charging them for meals aboard ship that should have been supplied without charge. By the time the Army officers learned about the scam it was too late to recover the cash.

The ocean voyage was boring and essentially uneventful. Many of the officers played poker for hours on end, leaving the table only for physiological necessities and meals. One day, while watching the flying fish, some of us noted other ships and land. This turned out to be Eniwetok, an enormous harbor within a narrow horseshoe-shaped rim of coral. I had never seen anything like it. There were at least two aircraft carriers with their planes, several battle cruisers, a number of baby aircraft carriers, many destroyers, and destroyer escorts. That night the lagoon was lit up like Times Square in sharp contrast to the strict black-out we had observed for many days. When I saw this massive armada all lit up and movies being shown aboard ship, I realized the enormous strength we had and the lack of fear of enemy attack. We seemed to be saying come on in and make our day. It felt great to see it and be part of it.

We stayed over in Eniwetok for several days and then resumed our journey. About six miles out of Eniwetok we had the first and only general-quarters alarm of our entire voyage. The alarm went off and the bosun's whistle, followed over the intercom by "Now hear this! Hear this: general quarters, general quarters, assume assigned battle stations." At the time I happened to be in the head (Navy for toilet) emptying my bladder. I also noted that the young infantry lieutenant in charge of a contingent of port battalion troops was in one of the stalls bent over in pain, trying to have a bowel movement. When the alarm went off, he suddenly emptied his bowels and dashed out to be with his troops while I hurried above to my assigned post. When I arrived there, I was still grinning about the experience in the head. Our C.O. said, "What's so funny? This is a serious matter." "Well, Colonel Howard," I said, "I was in the head when the general-quarters alarm was sounded. There was this young Army lieutenant trying to have a bowel movement and in considerable discomfort that was quickly relieved when the alarm went off." We all had a good laugh and we needed it. The alarm was thought to be due to a submarine picked up on sonar. Soon two little destroyer escorts appeared and began dropping depth charges. Best of all a baby aircraft carrier appeared on the horizon and the general quarters was canceled. The next event of any consequence was the announcement over the loudspeaker system that our ships were going to stop for target practice, and we were told that we were within range of Wake Island, still Japanese-held. That Sunday, religious services held on deck were unusually well attended by those of all creeds as well as agnostics and atheists. It has been said there are no atheists in foxholes nor were there any aboard ship that day.

Finally, after twenty days at sea, on 14 July 1945 we made landfall but none of us knew where we were. As we steamed along, it appeared that we were nearing two small islands, one larger than the other and only three to four miles apart. We welcomed the sight of any sort of terra firma. Finally the secret was out. We had reached our destination, Saipan and Tinian in the Mariana Islands. Most of us had never heard of these islands. We had been expecting to go to the Philippines. After a brief stop in Saipan Harbor, the ship turned back toward the smaller island, Tinian, and we prepared to debark on 16 July 1945. Why Tinian? Why was a 10,000-bed general hospital center being set up on this tiny island in the Pacific 10,000 miles away from home? The Mariana Islands are a series of fifteen lush tropical islands built of volcanic and coral formations located in the Western Pacific Ocean 1,500 miles east of the Philippines and stretching 500 miles parallel to the Mariana Trench, a deep cleft in the ocean including the world's deepest spot, 36,198 feet down. They lie between latitudes of 13 and 21 degrees North and are about 1,300 miles from Japan, a distance bringing them well within the round-trip range of the B-29 bombers based on Guam, Tinian, and Saipan.

Discovered in 1521 by Ferdinand Magellan, the Portuguese navigator sailing under the banner of Charles V of Spain, the Marianas were not colonized until 1668 when Jesuit missionaries changed their name from the Ladrones Islands (Thieves' Islands) to honor Mariana of Austria, then regent of Spain. Following the Spanish-American War (1898), Guam was ceded to the United States, becoming an "outlying territory." The Northern Marianas, including Saipan, Tinian, and Rota were sold to Germany. Japan, an ally in WW I, occupied the northern islands in 1914, and after WW I the League of Nations placed them, with the exception of Guam, under a Japanese mandate. Because of its excellent harbor, Guam was kept under U.S. control. The Japanese proceeded to occupy Saipan and Tinian, using them for growing sugar cane as a major crop, settled it with loyal Japanese, and surreptiously fortified the islands. One of the persistent but unconfirmed rumors on Saipan and Tinian during WW II was that Amelia Earhart, flying over the Marianas, had discovered the fortifications, was rescued from the sea by the Japanese when her plane fell, and was killed as a spy by her captors.

On 9 December 1941, two days after Pearl Harbor, 5,000 Japanese troops stormed ashore, or more accurately, walked ashore on Guam. On that day, Guam's only weapons were said to have been four machine guns manned by 153 Marines and 80 Chamorro natives led by marine sergeants. It wasn't only Pearl Harbor that was asleep at the switch. When we arrived, both Tinian and Saipan had been utterly devastated by military action in bloody battles. Nothing of any significance was left standing. Only the Japanese block houses had withstood the naval bombardment, and even these had been pierced and battered by our heavy shelling.

As we landed, we noted a number of unusual things about Tinian. It was a small island with a total land area of 39 square miles, only ten miles long and quite flat. It was roughly the shape of a miniature Manhattan Island, something the Seabees (naval construction battalions) had noticed, inspiring them to plan the roads they were building along the lines of New York's Manhattan. The roads were named and labeled Broadway, 125th Street, Riverside Drive, Fifth Avenue, Eighth Avenue, etc., roughly corresponding to their location in Manhattan. Anyone who knew Manhattan would know his way around on Tinian and might even feel a bit at home.

When the 303rd General Hospital landed on Tinian, it was quickly apparent that this small island was now an enormous airport with little room for anything but the B-29s based there. Philip Morrison, an American physicist who arrived on Tinian to help assemble the Fat Man atomic bomb, described the scene with great accuracy and perception.

> Tinian is a miracle. Here, 6000 miles from San Francisco, the United States armed forces have built the largest airport in the world. A great coral ridge was half leveled to fill a rough plain, and to build six runways, each an excellent 10 lane highway, each almost two miles long. Beside these runways stood in long rows the great silvery airplanes. They were there not by the dozen but by the hundred. From the air this island, smaller than Manhattan, looked like a giant aircraft carrier, its deck loaded with bombers
> . . .
>
> And all these gigantic preparations had a grand and terrible outcome. At sunset some day the field would be loud with the roar of motors. Down the great runways would roll the huge planes, seeming to move slowly because of their size, but far outspeeding the occasional racing jeep. One after another each runway would launch its planes.
>
> Once every 15 seconds another B-29 would become airborne. For an hour and a half this would continue with precision and order. The sun would go below the sea, and the last planes could still be seen in the distance, with running lights still on.

Often a plane would fail to make the takeoff and go skimming horribly into the sea, or into the beach to burn like a huge torch. We came often to sit on the top of the coral ridge and watch the combat strike of the 313th wing in real awe. Most of the planes would return the next morning, standing in a long single line, like beads on a chain, from just overhead to the horizon. You could see 10 or 12 planes at a time, spaced just a couple of miles apart. As fast as the near plane would land, another would appear on the edge of the sky. There were always the same number of planes in sight. The empty field would fill up, and in an hour or two all the planes would have landed.

Our first temporary headquarters for the 303rd General Hospital was in tents already set up by Seabees. Latrines had been dug and filled with lime to kill bacteria and insects. We urinated in public view into open funnels on a long pipe set into the sandy ground near the latrines. Meals were eaten cafeteria style in a mess-hall tent. Utensils, GI issue, were carried by each individual to the mess. Prior to entry, we dipped the utensils in boiling water in large metal drums to assure their cleanliness and to kill bacteria. The water supply was heavily chlorinated and subject to considerable variability in quality, quantity, and safety due to intermittent and unpredictable carbine attacks by Japanese in the adjacent jungle upon the bamboo pipes used to carry water. The enemy would fire into the bamboo pipes with a carbine so that they could fill their own containers and canteens while the pressure fell in our water system and we were left without any until the holes could be plugged and the pipes replaced. The food was K rations, C rations, Spam, powdered eggs, and powdered potatoes. All in all a very unappetizing menu. Nothing tasted right in the oppressive tropical heat. We all lost weight.

The stink of the jungle was all-pervasive. Gecko lizards, snails, rats, snakes, bats, and ants, mosquitos, and other insects abounded. Airplanes regularly flew over the island and sprayed DDT in large amounts, saturating us in the process. We slept under mosquito bars to avoid being bitten at night by insects, bats, and rats, and many of us wore long-sleeved khaki shirts and long trousers despite the enervating heat. We shaved out of our helmets and brushed our teeth from them. At night the helmets served other purposes. Cold showers were obtained, when water was available, from tin pails perforated with holes. It was not unusual to be interrupted while brushing our teeth by an intercom warning to avoid the water because the supply had been contaminated, usually by enemy action involving the bamboo pipes serving as conduits. The opportunity to acquire parasitic tropical diseases was a common hazard. Fortunately malaria was not present on Tinian or Saipan because the Anopheles mosquito that carry the parasites was not indigenous. Dengue, so-called "break-bone fever," was endemic and at times epidemic. The native Chamorros were loaded with parasites, almost universally affected with yaws, and a leper colony flourished on Tinian. There was little or nothing to do. No reading matter was available. The heat and humidity were so oppressive that we had very little desire to exercise or engage in any strenuous activities. A few tried volley ball but not for long. Occasionally a Japanese soldier would emerge from the jungle firing a few rounds at whoever was in sight. Fortunately their aim was not too good and none of our people was hit during our tour. The commanding general at first sent patrols into the jungle hoping to persuade the Japanese to come out of the caves to surrender or, if they refused, be killed. We would end up losing one soldier on patrol, causing the general to cancel the patrols. When and if the enemy came out, the order was to kill them if they did not give up. The hospitals were also ordered to dump K rations or C rations on their outskirts so the Japanese could eat and perhaps cease to disturb the hospital patients and personnel. A canine corps unit helped flush the enemy out of caves. In addition to cemeteries for our troops and the enemy, there was a canine cemetery on Tinian, its wooden crosses topped by silhouettes of police dogs who had fallen in battle.

The only diversion was the "happy hour" before mess call, regularly attended by all officers. General MacArthur's headquarters in WESPAC (Western Pacific Base Command) had decreed that no alcoholic beverages, not even beer, be available for the enlisted men. The officers, on the other hand, had too much booze. My own reaction was that if the rule applied to enlisted men, it should have also been applied to the officers. Officers who paid sixty dollars into a voluntary pool would be entitled to buy at least six or seven bottles of liquor, some of it not great but most of it excellent bourbon and Scotch, at very little cost. Some of the officers would buy multiple shares entitling them to almost unlimited access to hard liquor. Its consumption before dinner, the unappetizing food, and the lack of responsibility and work assignments, coupled with anxiety and boredom, drove some officers into ethanol addiction. Those who had such problems before coming overseas were the first to succumb, but there were some men who might never have become alcoholics in civilian life who became addicted during the conditions of military service. In addition, for those flying the B-29 missions there were added pressures, not the least of which was a memo that I saw from the chief of psychiatry in the Marianas encouraging the men returning from missions over Japan to drink a substantial allocation of bourbon or

Scotch on arrival at home base. Before we had received our allocation of liquor, we noticed that one of our medical officers seemed to be perpetually inebriated and we wondered where he was getting his supplies. When it was too late, we found that he had been stealing from the hospital ethanol supply and putting it into his canteen. We eventually had to send this highly skilled physician home as a chronic alcoholic. His subsequent career was tragically downhill, ending in suicide. I think he was as much a casualty of war as anyone wounded in action, and I felt very sorry for him and his family.

While on this topic, I must add other wounds of war that were not inflicted by enemy action. Separation of men from their families placed many strains on their marriages. I have no statistics on this, but I know of instances of broken marriages, divorces, separations, and mésalliances from the stress of military service. Some marriages, probably most, survived the temptations and stresses but some did not; they were among the real but uncounted casualties of war. To escape the pervasive boredom, many of the officers developed hobbies. Some became quite expert at melting silver coins and making jewelry of them. Others gambled, usually at cards. Some collected sea shells, and woodcarving was popular. What was seriously lacking was any form of organized activity designed to keep these good minds active. There should have been energetic efforts to promote medical education but there were none. Chiefly this was because there was no leadership to pursue this. There was no blueprint for action in any of the manuals. Innovation could have been the answer but there was none of this. Clinical Pathologic Conferences (CPCs) could have been held and even Grand Rounds. If they had, morale of the medical officers would not have fallen as it did.

To compound the evil, medical officers were assigned to non-professional duties such as counting candy bars in the post exchange and the like. Perhaps the silliest of all was an order that all medical officers of field grade don M.P. bands and large revolvers to pull military police (MP) duty to protect 300 female nurses newly arrived on Tinian from the onslaught of hordes of young Air Force officers, many of whom had not seen a white female in two years. I find it hard to believe that this was done, but it was. I came away from that experience feeling that it was the officers who needed to be protected.

The greatest fear expressed by doctors in these isolated areas of the military theater is not that of enemy action. It is fear that because of medical inactivity they may be losing their clinical skills. My solution to this, which I would put to the test, was to institute a vigorous program of teaching and continuing medical education in the Quonsets and prefabs surrounded by the stink of the jungle and the oppressive heat, forgetting those handicaps and promoting medical education. Having said this, in all fairness, I must admit that there were other matters of great importance under study at the highest possible level by the Joint Chiefs of Staff that may have had a great deal to do with the failure of the regional commands to act with greater vigor. These considerations and deliberations were not known to me and my colleagues on Tinian in 1945, but information made available since then has provided startling and revealing insight.

By early 1945, a full-blown assault on Japan seemed the only way to win the war. The planned invasion, code-named Operation Downfall, was to involve the entire U.S. Pacific Fleet, the largest naval force ever assembled, dwarfing the Normandy invasion, including thousands of ships, many thousands of planes and 4.5 million men. General MacArthur estimated there would be one million American casualties. There were to be two separate invasions, the first, code-named Olympic, would attack Kyushu in southern Japan and was scheduled for 1 November 1945, followed by operation Coronet, scheduled for 1 March 1946 attacking Honshu and Tokyo. The Joint Chiefs of Staff had agreed on this in January 1945, but there was disagreement among them as to who should be in command. General MacArthur wanted it because the invasion was primarily a land campaign. Admiral Nimitz was not about to place the Navy under the command of Army Generals and General "Hap" Arnold, who felt that his B-29s could conquer Japan, wanted to retain command of the Army Air Corps. The argument raged for several months, the final decision being for a three-pronged Command staff including all three services. On 24 May 1945 the Joint Chiefs of Staff finally ordered OLYMPIC to proceed. On 18 June 1945 President Truman officially approved the invasion plan, despite some reservations expressed over the enormous casualties anticipated.

Shortly thereafter, the Tinian military staff was notified of the decision and it was not long before the cat was let out of the bag for the troops on Tinian. When we arrived on Tinian we thought that our 10,000-bed Hospital Center was going to be built there and would operate from this base. One look at the island should have told us this could never be. Tinian was small and essentially on a vast airfield loaded with B-29s with no room for a large hospital center. Obviously we were headed for something else. The answer came during the end of July when we were notified that all of us were to be measured for woolen Eisenhower jackets that would be given to us without charge. We had come to the tropics in Khakis and they were giving us woolens. Clearly we were tapped for a trip to the north, about 1,300 miles away—obviously, an invasion of Japan. The dangers were amply clear to us. What had looked like an excellent and relatively safe assignment was going to be a nightmare. Pandemonium reigned but we finally settled down and prepared for the inevitable.

Luis Alvarez, the Nobel Laureate physicist, son of Dr. Walter Alvarez, the distinguished physician and former student of Dr. George Hoyt Whipple, was on Tinian with the 509th Composite Group as an observer. He describes preparations for the projected invasion, including stores of ammunition, supplies, and a large number of wooden caskets. While we waited for further orders, in mid-July 1945 some of our people heard Walter Winchell broadcast "Good Evening Mr. and Mrs. America and all the ships at sea," in his staccato style, saying that an enormous explosion had occurred in a place called Alamogordo, New Mexico, suggesting that a special experimental weapon had been fired. We did not know what to make of this. In retrospect, this had to be Trinity, the first test of a plutonium bomb. A leak had developed in the greatest military secret ever.

At this point in my story, I shall take the liberty of divulging a conversation I had with Brigadier General F. V. H. Kimble, who commanded Tinian in 1945–46. The general had become quite ill with pneumonia and was flown from Tinian to the 148th General Hospital on Saipan where I was the chief of medicine and the senior medical consultant for the Marianas. I was fortunate enough to cure the general and we became good friends, as often happens between doctors and their patients. I asked General Kimble whether he had known anything about the atom bomb prior to its use on Hiroshima. He said that one day at the end of March 1945 Colonel Elmer E. Fitzpatrick, an Army Engineer, arrived on Tinian and asked to inspect the island saying he needed an airfield for a special project. The general replied that Tinian was under his command and nobody could touch it without his permission. Colonel Fitzpatrick produced a set of orders signed by the president that gave him the power to seize anything he needed for a top-secret project. General Kimble said he knew he shouldn't ask any more questions. He gave him clearance. The site chosen was part of North Field, Tinian. The area was promptly cleared by Seabees and encircled by a fence and machine guns with signs indicating that the site was off-limits to all except authorized personnel. One of my hospitals was across the street from this area but I never attempted to enter the compound. Several special B-29s were stationed in the area and pits were dug for some purpose at the loading area. All sorts of people arrived, many of them civilians, including a number of physicists. A sign read that this was the headquarters of the 509th Composite Group. General Kimble told me that he was informed that a cruiser, the *Indianapolis*, former flagship of the Pacific Fifth Fleet, was arriving in Tinian Harbor with a special delivery connected with the North Field project. He was asked to authorize whether the "package" should be delivered under the cover of night darkness or daylight. He decided that it would attract less attention if it were handled as ordinary freight in the daytime and taken to its reception point. It turned out that the package was uranium needed to arm Little Boy, the first atomic bomb. The parcel weighed 300 pounds, 200 of them being lead shielding. When it was being unloaded July 26, 1945, in Tinian Harbor, a crowd gathered around watching the event. The crew bungled the first pass at unloading its cargo onto an LCT (Landing Craft Tank) by using a cable that was six feet too short and they had to repeat the entire maneuver to the crowd's catcalls and jeers. General Kimble told me he felt uneasy because so many individuals witnessed this episode. This discomfort was greatly aggravated when, four days later on the way home near Leyte, the *Indianapolis* was sunk by a Japanese submarine in what has been termed the greatest naval tragedy of WW II, and perhaps the most unnecessary, with the loss of 880 sailors. General Kimble told me that he was so upset by this, suspecting that a Japanese spy had been on Tinian, that he could not sleep. His reassurance came when the submarine commander was captured after the Japanese surrender and testified that he knew nothing about the *Indianapolis* and the atom bomb. It was just an accident of war that led to his meeting with the cruiser and its sinking.

The atomic bombs were stored and assembled on Tinian at 125th Street and Eighth Avenue on North Field under tight security. The unit handling the project was the 509th Composite Group commanded by Lt. Col. Paul W. Tibbets, a seasoned flier and excellent disciplinarian. This organization, unique in many ways, had nothing to match it in our military establishment. It had one goal, to deliver atomic bombs with accuracy and quasi-surgical skill upon the enemy. Each member had been virtually hand picked for his skills. In addition, all were sworn to secrecy and monitored to assure this. Those who failed were summarily dismissed and assigned elsewhere, usually Iceland. We knew the 509th was on Tinian but we knew nothing of its purpose or mission. The other macho B-29 crews flying regular bombing missions over Japan could not understand what the 509th was up to and ridiculed it because it dropped only occasional single practice bombs. Jeers and catcalls accompanied their take-offs from North Field and a ditty made the rounds:

> Into the air the secret rose
> Where they're going nobody knows

Don't ask us about the results or such
Unless you want to get in Dutch
But take it from one who is sure of the score
The 509th is winning the war.

On August 6, 1945, at 2:45 A.M., the Enola Gay, a B-29 named after Col. Tibbetts' mother, based on North Field Tinian and carrying Little Boy, took off for Hiroshima and history. We learned of it on Tinian via an official and supposedly censored Army radio broadcast shortly after the bomb was dropped. I shall never forget that day. The announcer said a new weapon, an atomic bomb of tremendous power, had been delivered onto Hiroshima at 9:15 A.M. destroying that city. He went on to say that the bomb had been flown in from Tinian and he gave some historical information about the bomb. I remember his saying that Colonel Stafford Warren had played a major role in the development of the bomb. Since Colonel Warren had been my professor of radiology at the University of Rochester School of Medicine, I was much impressed but not completely surprised. When the broadcast ended, our C.O., Colonel James W. Howard, said, "Obviously Mr. Truman is using psychological warfare to get the Japanese to surrender. It sounds like a very heavy conventional TNT bomb." At this point, I simply had to differ and I tried to do this with some diplomacy, but I probably was not quite up to it. I said, "Col. Howard, I'm sorry but I must disagree with you. This was a nuclear weapon, an atomic bomb, something never used before." "How do you know so much about it?" "Well, I think I am free to discuss it now in the light of the official radio broadcast we have just heard that named my professor of radiology, Colonel Stafford Warren." I then proceeded to tell him what had tipped me off to the atomic bomb.

In March 1945, while chief of the Officers' and Women's section of the Medical Service of Valley Forge General Hospital in Phoenixville, Pennsylvania, I admitted a patient, Brigadier General James C. Marshall, from the Pacific theater of war who had a severe dermatological condition of his hands diagnosed elsewhere as "jungle-rot." It proved to be a severe eczematoid dermatitis. Our new dermatologist was not board-certified and he had very little training in dermatology. He recommended that radiotherapy be given. I had reservations about this, as did the general, but his were of another nature. He said that if he were to have any form of radiotherapy these three doctors must be called in consultation: Col. Stafford Warren, Oakridge, Tennessee.; Dr. Andrew Dowdy of the University of Rochester School of Medicine; and Dr. Hyman Friedel of Western Reserve Medical School in Cleveland, Ohio.

All of these were eminent radiologists. By this time I had gotten to know General Marshall quite well and he learned that I was a graduate of the University of Rochester School of Medicine. He asked me whether I knew Dr. George Hoyt Whipple and I answered, "Of course, he was my mentor and Dean of the Medical School and Nobel Laureate." "Well," the General said, "I had a rather difficult time with him when I went to see him about getting Dr. Stafford Warren to direct a military project of great importance. Dean Whipple's reaction was very strong. He said he simply couldn't run a medical school in wartime if any more of his faculty were taken from him. He had already lost his professor of medicine, Dr. William S. McCann, to the Navy, and dozens of others. Now he simply could not lose his professor of radiology." When Dr. Whipple finished, General Marshall handed him a slip of paper with three names and telephone numbers one of which was, as I remember it, to the White House. The General said, "I'll come back at two o'clock for your answer." When he came back, Dr. Whipple said, "You may have him." A few days later, while General Marshall was still on my service at Valley Forge General Hospital, I was in the barbershop when my chief NCO Sergeant Levine burst in quite excited and said that a civilian was in my ward office looking at General Marshall's chart. I jumped out of the chair and hurried down the long corridor to my section, opened the office door, saw a short man in civilian clothes with a chart in his hands and shouted, "What the hell are you doing in here?" At that moment I heard a loud chuckle from on high, looked up, recognized my friend and teacher, Colonel Stafford Warren, all 6 feet 7 inches of him, who was responsible for this joke and laughing about it. "Mike," he said, "quiet down. I've just came down here to see this old friend of mine." We went over the problem deciding to forego radiotherapy because I thought it was not needed or indicated. The general had experienced some radiation exposure in the past.

The discussion in General Marshall's room was rather odd. Some comments were made about something they were working on. I do not recall the exact words but I knew very well that something big was being hatched. Most of all I knew I was privy to a top secret that had to be kept that way with no record of it in the general's chart and no mention of it to any of my colleagues or superiors. I also knew that I could not discuss it with my wife. I had the impression that these men were dealing with some sort of Buck Rogers weapon involving radiation but I did not suspect it was a bomb.

As a result of this encounter with a patient during the course of my routine professional work, I had knowledge shared by only a few people. To find myself on a tropical island 10,000 miles from my home in the company of this bomb was something I shall never forget. It is of some significance that the official radio broadcast on the atomic bomb that we heard on Tinian was never again repeated and for at least one very good reason. The enemy now knew whence the bomb had come and was getting ready to do something about it.

The afternoon of August 6, when Colonel Tibbets brought the Enola Gay back to Tinian, there was a wild celebration that continued late into the night and early morning. It was a rainy night and very muddy outdoors. In spite of this the drinking and shouting and singing continued. In our outfit one voice was especially unique and loud crying out in an Oxford accent, "The Bloody War is Over." This was instantly recognized by all of us as that of one of our young doctors, Capt. Adrian Hogben, the son of Lancelot Hogben, the British mathematician. Capt. Hogben, who later emerged as a brilliant physiologist, had the tough luck that night to join a group of merrymakers who decided to dump the adjutant of our hospital from his army cot onto the outside mud. Hogben was blamed for the entire affair because his voice and accent had clearly identified him. The vindictive adjutant had him reassigned to a port battalion on Saipan, from which I was lucky to rescue him several months later.

Following the atomic bomb drop, Tinian, previously declared secure, was again placed on wartime alert and we saw that the black night fighters had been brought back and we were ordered to stay blacked-out. Later on I asked General Kimble why we were put on these precautions and he explained it this way: The Armed Forces Radio Broadcast had been unwise because it gave out too much information, including the site of launching of the atomic bomb. He had information that the Japanese were hoarding their medium-range bombers in northern Japan, hoping for better weather to fly to Wake Island, refuel, and then launch a kamikaze attack on Tinian where this awful weapon had been lodged. Full war alert was declared and precautions taken as we awaited an attack. In the meantime, Admiral Halsey was bombing the devil out of Japan's northern airfields where those medium range bombers were hiding.

Following the atomic attack, we expected the Japanese to surrender unconditionally, but they delayed. Part of this may have been because the Japanese people were not fully informed of the massive destruction of Hiroshima. The militarists and fanatic Japanese loyalists appeared to be in control. There was only one other bomb immediately available for use, plutonium-armed and called the Fat Man because of its shape, but another was nearly ready stateside. After a good deal of deliberation and soul searching at high levels, the decision was made to use the Fat Man on Kokura as the primary target and Nagasaki the secondary. The concerns that Colonel Tibbets and Captain Parsons had experienced and that led them to arm the Little Boy bomb in flight rather than to risk an explosion on takeoff, blowing Tinian and perhaps Saipan to bits, did not apply. The Fat Man was already armed on the ground before takeoff, the detonating devices being too complex to manipulate in flight.

On 9 August 1945, at 0349, B-29 #77, "Bock's Car," named after Capt. Fred Bock, its usual commander but for this mission commanded by Major Charles Sweeney, took off from North Field, Tinian, carrying the five-ton plutonium Fat Man bomb. Special precautions taken during takeoff had been to have no other planes arriving or leaving from North Field and multiple, specially equipped emergency crash teams stationed at key points near but not too close to the runway. While the Hiroshima mission had been technically almost perfect, the Kokura-Nagasaki project was plagued with problems. Visibility over Kokura was poor, leading to the bombing of the secondary target, Nagasaki, with less precision than the Hiroshima drop, but most of all, the mission ran out of fuel and had to make a hazardous emergency landing on Okinawa for refueling before completing the return trip to Tinian. When Bock's Car and its crew returned to Tinian, there was more celebration but still no word of surrender from the Japanese. The war continued, and the B-29s remained on the offensive as we waited for the ultimate word from the enemy.

General Curtis E. LeMay, in command of our B-29s said it best. "Hiroshima brought no instantaneous prostration of the Japanese military; nevertheless it was a startlingly rapid disintegration. Meanwhile we were still piling on incendiaries. Our B-29s went to Yawata on August 8th and burned up 21 percent of the town, and on the same day some other B-29s went to Fukuyama and burned 73.3 percent. Still there wasn't any gasp and collapse when the second nuclear bomb went down above Nagasaki on August 9th. We kept on flying. Went to Kumagaya on August 14th—45 percent of that town. Flew our final mission the same day against Isezaki, when we burned up 17 percent of that target. Then the crews came home to the Marianas and were told that Japan had capitulated."[2] The *New York Times* front-page headlines proclaiming "Japan Surrenders, End of

---

2. General Curtis E. LeMay, with Mackinlay Kantor, *Mission with LeMay: My Story* (Garden City, N.Y.: Doubleday & Company, 1965), p. 388.

War!" were not available to those of us serving on Tinian that day on 15 August 1945, but we lived to see them at a later time.

What now of Life on Tinian? Gone were OPERATION DOWNFALL, OLYMPIC AND CORONET. Saved were hundreds of thousands perhaps millions of lives. Perhaps our own. Gone were the day-to-day perils of war. What next? Who would go home and when? Who would be held for occupational duty in Japan? Would those who had already served their country so well be required to continue to carry the burden while their colleagues who had not entered the fray remained secure, prosperous, and undisturbed in their homes? These were important questions to be answered. There were also many others, not the least being how did it happen that I myself was on Tinian at its greatest moment in history, and what would chance, planning, or something called "fate" next have in store for me?

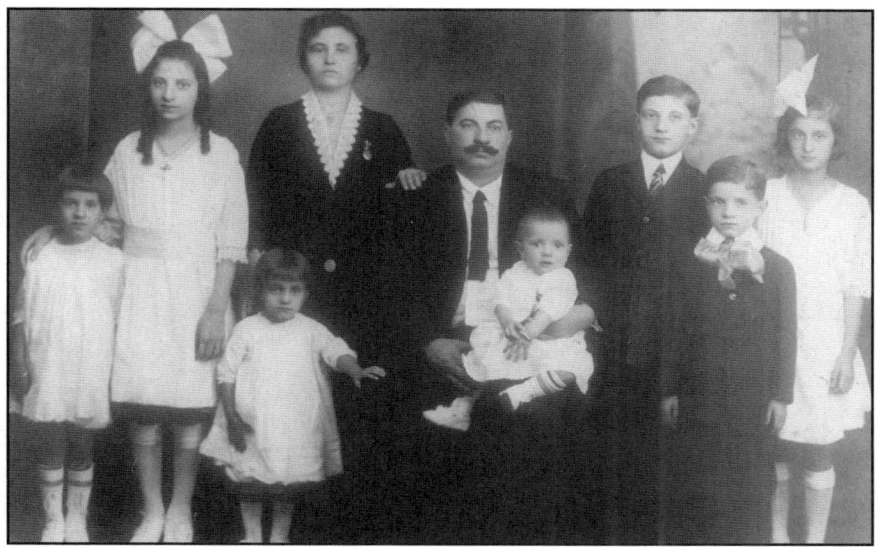

1. The Lepore Family in 1921. *Left to right:* Anna (Donatelle), Millie (Carmella), Phyllis (Filicetta), Filomena (MJL's mother), Giuseppe (MJL's father), Lucille (Lucietta), MJL, Frank (Francis) and Nonnie (Marie Antoinette).

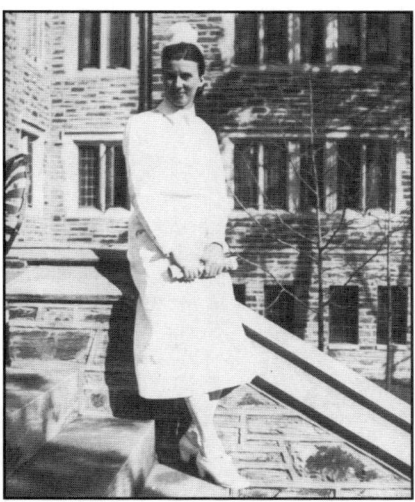

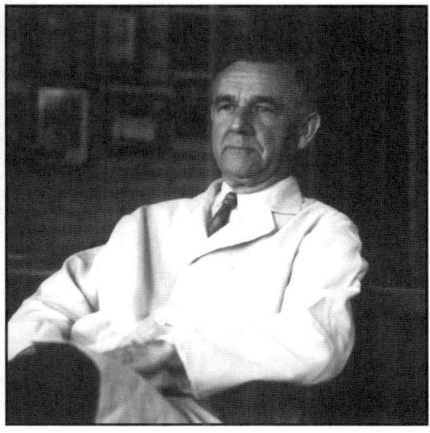

2. MJL's future wife, Ardean Clough Everett, was a Head Nurse at Duke University Medical Center in 1934 when they first met.

3. Dr. George Hoyt Whipple, Nobel Laureate, founding dean of the University of Rochester School of Medicine & Dentistry, and mentor to MJL.

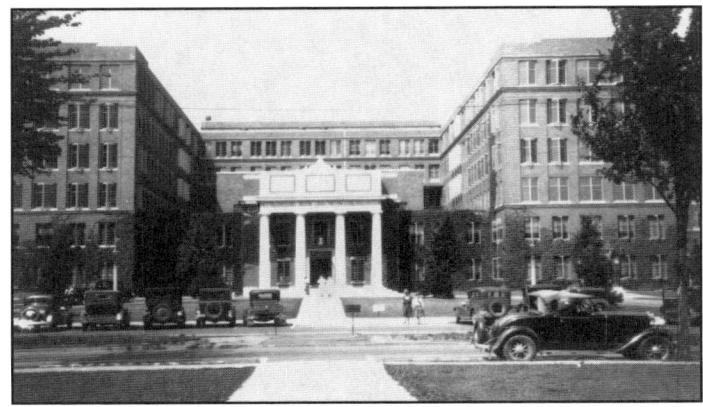

4. Strong Memorial Hospital, 1930s.

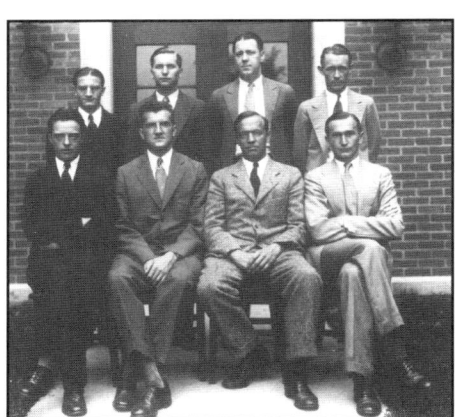

5. The Department of Physiology at the University of Rochester School of Medicine & Dentistry, 1930-1931, when MJL was a Fellow in Physiology. *Seated from left to right:* Charles Wright, Edward F. Adolph, Wallace O. Fenn, and Albert Hegnaver. *Standing from left to right:* Michael J. Lepore, John J. Jares, Milton Nudo, William Latchford.

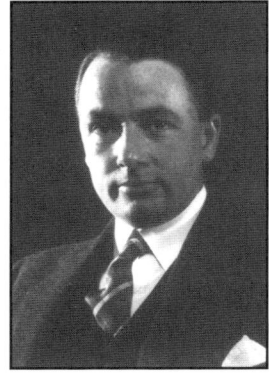

6. Dr. William S. McCann.

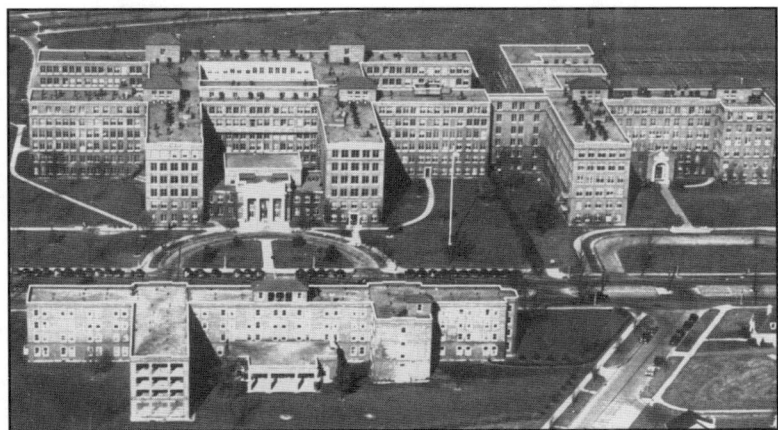

7. University of Rochester Medical Center, 1930s.

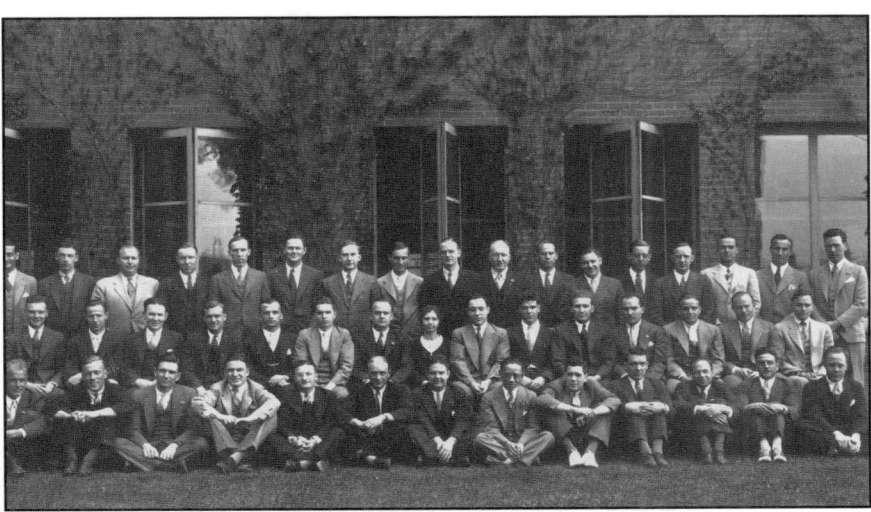

8. University of Rochester School of Medicine and Dentistry—Class of 1934. MJL is seated in the first row, fifth from the left.

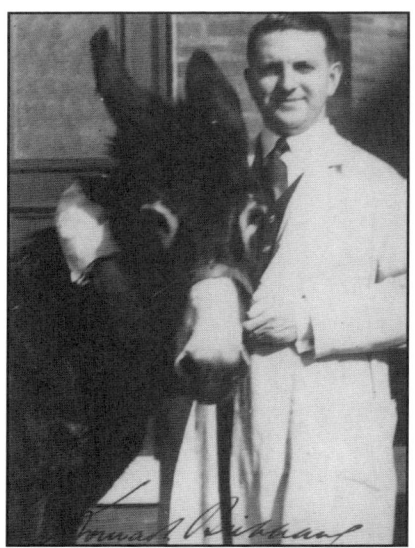

9. Dr. Konrad Birkhaug.

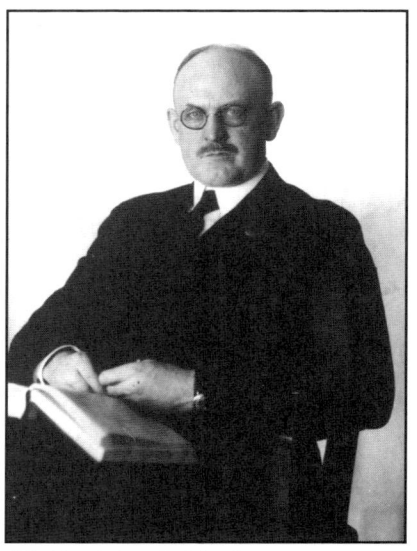

10. Dr. John R. Murlin.

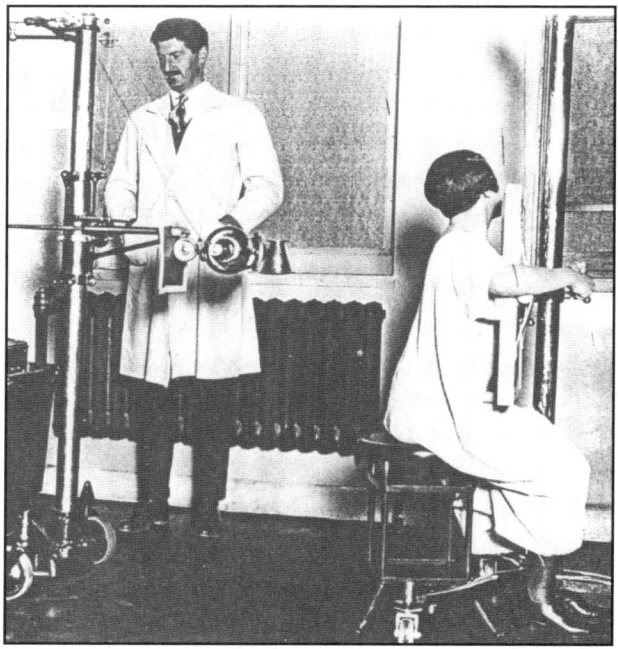

11. Dr. Stafford Warren—Chairman of Radiology at
the University of Rochester School of Medicine &
dentistry, 1926.

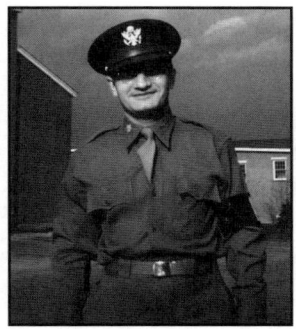

12. *Left:* Major Michael J. Lepore serving as Officer of the Day at Valley Forge General Hospital, August 1944.1

13. *Below:* Map of Tinian Island in 1945.

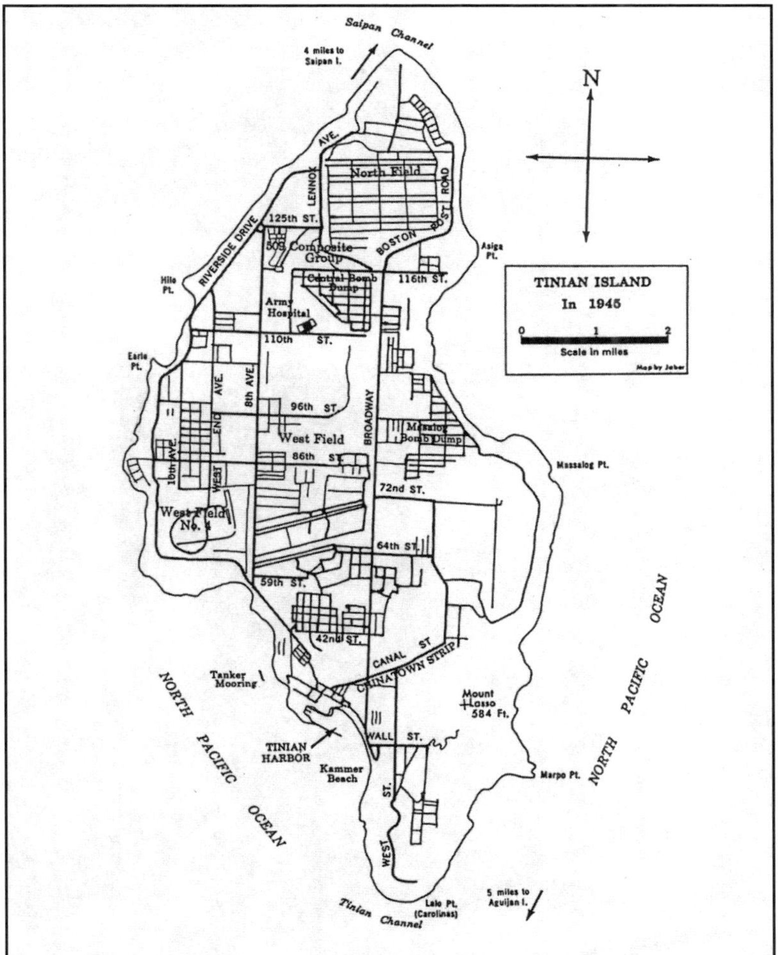

Tinian Island, 1945

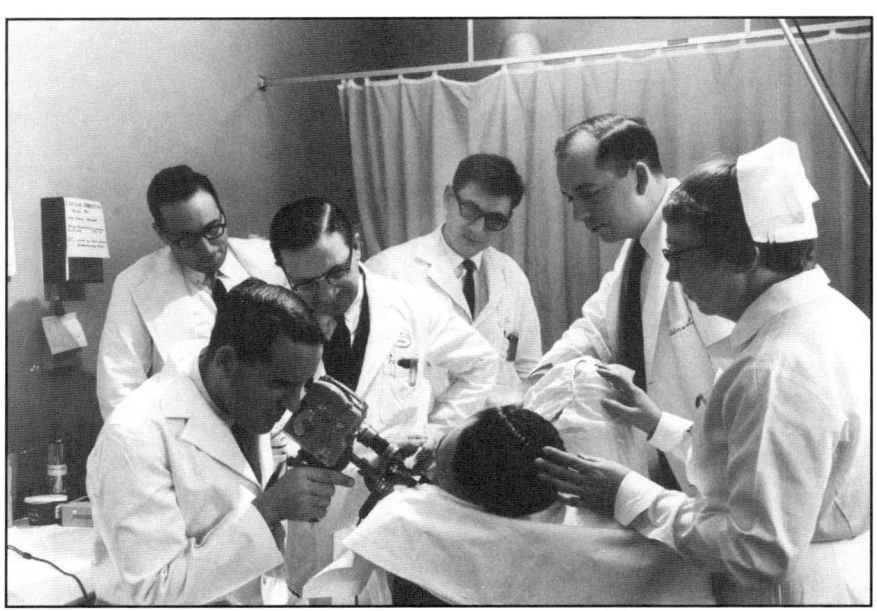

14. Dr. Lepore attends a cine-endoscopy procedure at the Upjohn Gastrointestinal Service, 1964.

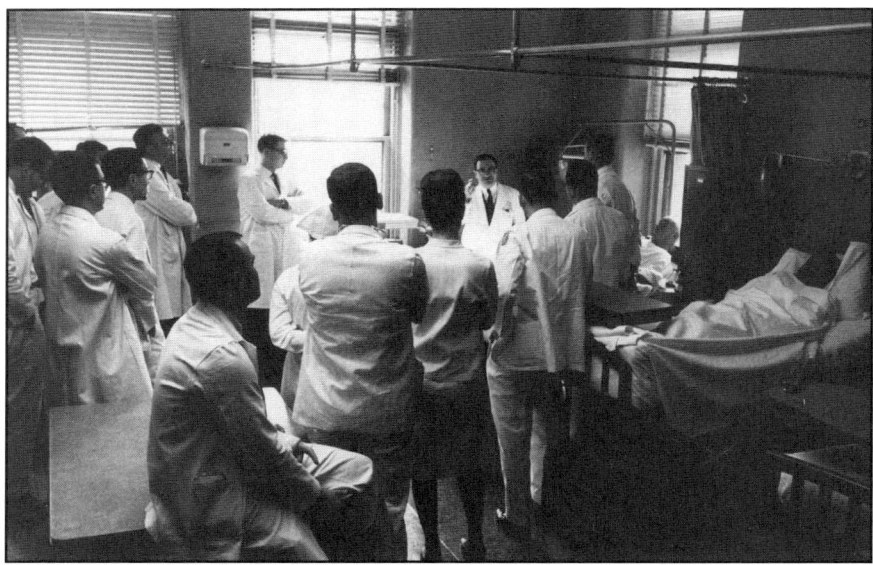

15. Dr. Lepore on teaching rounds at Roosevelt Hospital in New York City in 1964.

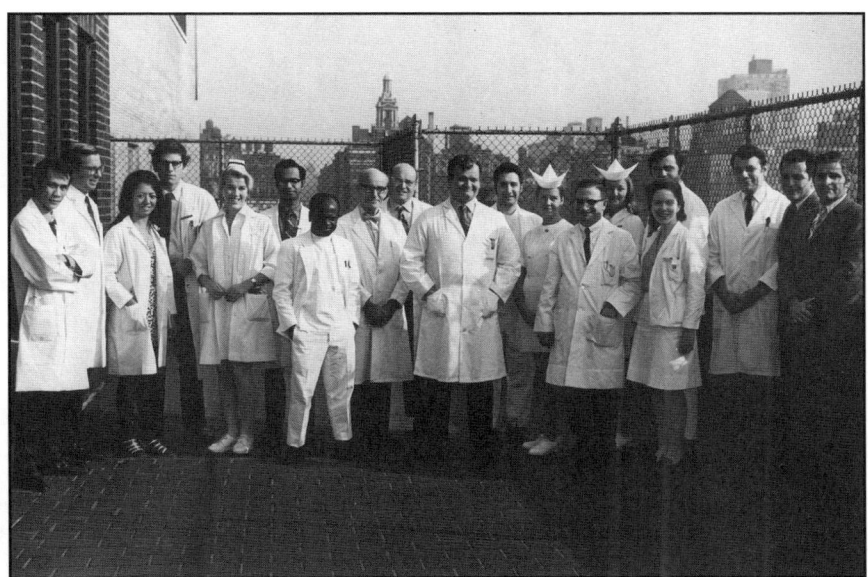

16. The Plasmapheresis Team on the roof of St. Vincent's Hospital and Medical Center of New York, September 1970. MJL is seventh from the left.

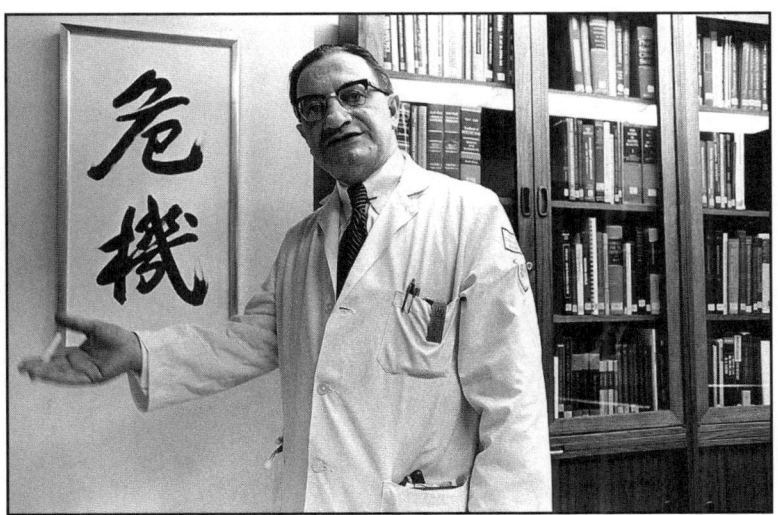

17. Dr. Lepore in front of a Chinese calligraphy for "Crisis" in the Upjohn Gastrointestinal Foundation Library at St. Vincent's Hospital, 1974.

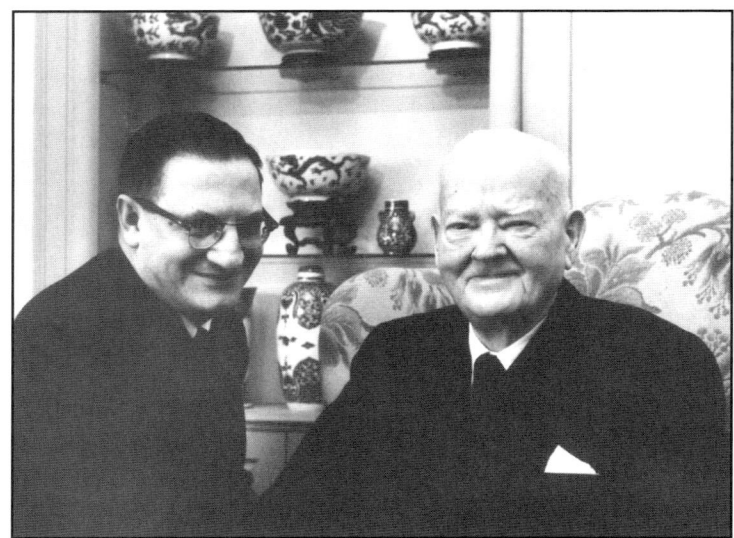

18. Dr. Lepore with his patient, President Herbert C. Hoover, in 1964 at President Hoover's apartment in the Waldorf Towers.

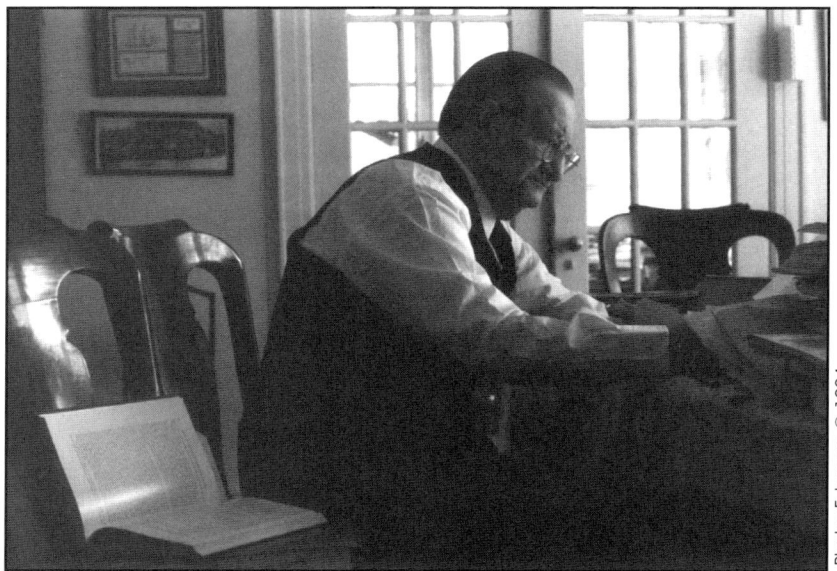

Photo: F. Lepore © 1994

19. Dr. Lepore writing *Life of the Clinician* at the dining room table of his home in Englewood, New Jersey in 1994.

Chapter 16
Saipan, 1945–1946

Now that the war was over everyone wanted to go home, right now. Clearly, this was impossible for many reasons, including lack of transportation. Some of the B-29 units used their airplanes to fly home, but this was stopped after several serious crashes occurred, probably due to inadequate maintenance. It upset us no end to learn that brave men who had eaten with us and enjoyed our company, had completed their wartime bombing missions only to die in an aircraft accident while heading for home. Our commanding general, W. W. Irvine, was equally disturbed and ruled that airplane travel was forbidden except for official business and emergencies. There simply were not enough ships to get the men home in a hurry. Some medical specialists would have to await replacements while others would be needed for occupational duty. A point system was set up to bring equity to the demobilization process. Those with longer periods of military service would be given preference over those with less time in service. But humans being what they are, some sought to escape by having their families enlist the assistance of the Red Cross in obtaining emergency leaves. The "emergencies" were, at times, trumped up. One doctor on Saipan arranged to be called home because his wife had given birth. Another went home because his father had died. There were other such excuses for expediting a quick return. The real problem was that none of these individuals was, to my knowledge, ever returned to his overseas post once the "emergency" was over. Medical officers in scarce categories were locked into their positions by the inability to obtain replacements from the zone of the interior. I recall one poor fellow, a captain M.C. and ENT specialist, who had served in forward areas in the Pacific with combat units for over two years, who was being held because there was no replacement for him. He began to drink heavily and was drunk on duty. The commanding officer was contemplating a court-martial for him and asked me for my advice. I looked into the problem and discovered that the doctor had served well for a number of years and had seen his potential replacements rotated back home on an emergency basis, leaving him holding the bag on Saipan.

I reported to the C.O. that I sympathized with the man and did not feel we should court-martial him. I pointed out to the C.O. that the doctor's replacement had wangled his way home on a flimsy pretext and was never returned to his assignment on Saipan. I had a long talk with the captain and persuaded him to stop drinking during work hours. Being drunk off duty was no crime and a common occurrence. I was also able to see that he soon received orders to head home. All of this was accomplished with confidentiality and tactful diplomacy without the captain's knowledge that I had saved his hide. I do not remember his name and I know he has forgotten mine.

Let me backtrack a little. With the war over, we knew that most of us would be reassigned to other hospitals. With the 303rd General Hospital, I had been assigned on paper to be the chief of gastroenterology because they were loaded with majors who were senior to me and had a priority for being chief of the medical service. I pointed out to Colonel Howard, our C.O., that I wished to be placed in my 3139B MOS classification as the chief of medicine of a general hospital and that my 201 file clearly supported this. With the breakup of the 303rd General Hospital, I became a free agent and was quickly picked up to head the medical service of the 369th Station Hospital, a 2,000-bed installation on Saipan. This was done, I learned later, by Colonel Warren Brown of Yale, its commanding officer. Colonel Brown remembered me from my fellowship at Yale and was delighted to have me on his staff. The Yale unit, stationed on Saipan, had been in the Pacific area for a long time and was being rapidly demobilized. In order to go to Saipan from Tinian, a distance of less than five miles, I had to fly over in a cargo plane because the waters about Tinian and Saipan were loaded with mines. It was my first trip on an airplane. When I arrived at my new station, I found myself chief of medical service with twenty-one medical officers under my command. The hospital was made up of prefabricated buildings and Quonsets. The staff was bored with overseas duty and eager to leave. One night a soldier with dengue, or so-called "break-bone fever," was admitted as an emergency and it developed that none of the medical officers had done a spinal tap in recent years. We needed it to rule out some type of acute meningitis. My sergeant woke me up, I dressed and went over to the infectious-disease Quonset hut and examined the patient. I agreed that a lumbar puncture was indicated and proceeded to do it myself without further ado. The spinal fluid was normal, ruling out meningitis. The next day I held a meeting of my staff and informed them that I was arranging to give them a personally conducted teaching session on how to perform a lumbar puncture using as subjects a number of our soldiers who were under treatment for syphilis and needed the spinal tap to exclude central nervous system involvement.

Every medical officer on my service quickly became competent in performing this simple diagnostic procedure. I was not about to be called to do every spinal tap in my 2,000-bed hospital. The doctors soon realized that I knew what I was doing and was willing to teach them. My weekly Medical Grand Rounds were stimulating and adapted to the needs and material available on Saipan. I made my rounds on my 600-bed medical service by Jeep, communicated regularly with all of my officers, was available to them at any hour of the day or night, and tried to keep the standards of medical practice at the highest level possible in a forward area. I soon noticed that very little routine laboratory work was being done on the hospitalized soldiers. Routine tests such as a complete blood count, urine examinations, and Kahn tests were not being done even though the laboratory equipment for these tests was available. I looked up the chief of laboratories, who turned out to be a pleasant but indolent physician who seemed rather laid back after a long tour of duty in the Pacific. His first comment was to ask for my permission to make rounds on the medical service so that he might maintain his clinical skills. I told him that the first priority was that the laboratory work done in this hospital should be brought up to the standards expected in a 2,000-bed Army installation. I insisted that each patient have certain routine tests performed and reported in the chart. He tried to tell me that the tests were unnecessary in a forward area, but I quickly disabused him of this concept and said it simply was not good medical practice and would no longer be tolerated at the 369th. This also led to a shaking up of his detail of enlisted technicians, who were simply goofing off because of the paucity of requests for laboratory tests. The word soon got about that the new chief of medicine meant business and would tolerate no sloppiness. I kept the chief of laboratory so busy that he did not have the time to make medical rounds. There were a few very good doctors on my staff, but the majority left a great deal to be desired. I spent a good deal of time trying to teach them the rudiments of competent medical practice. Some had been overseas too long and had forgotten their skills. Others were bored and obsessed with getting home as soon as possible. Despite all of this, I persisted in conducting daily rounds and weekly grand rounds as if I were working in one of the large medical centers where I had trained and worked. Very soon the doctors realized that they were learning medicine and recovering some of their lost skills under the stimulus and guidance of a competent teacher. Their morale improved and later I received letters from many of them attesting to the benefit they derived from my teaching program.

The 369th Station Hospital on Saipan was also the hospital that provided medical care and consultation for the Catholic nuns who had been on the island for many years. I had occasion to examine and treat the Mother Superior and her assistant. They were blue-eyed, blonde Spaniards who had managed to convert many of the Chamorros to Christianity, and they had undergone many vicissitudes during the Japanese occupation. Both were ill with conditions that required surgery, one for a badly diseased kidney, the other for gallstones. The Army was not authorized to do anything but emergency surgery on the nuns. They would have to be sent to Oahu for surgery in one of the Catholic hospitals. Transportation to Oahu in wartime was a problem. Special permission had to be sought from General MacArthur. This took several months but finally it arrived and these dedicated and benevolent people were transported by Hospital Ship to Oahu.

Then one day, after having succeeded in raising medical standards at the 369th, *mirabile dictu*, I was requested by Colonel James W. Howard to become the chief of medical service at the 148th General Hospital on Mt. Tapotcho on Saipan, one of the best hospitals on the island.

The staff at the 148th was of high calibre. The chief of surgery, Major George Archer, was a product of the Mayo Clinic, alert and competent. The section chiefs were well qualified and we even had a neurosurgeon. The laboratory chief was Paul Szanto, a Viennese pathologist of considerable eminence and associate of the renowned Dr. Hans Popper. The thoracic surgeon, Captain Robert K. Brown of Denver, Colorado, was a talented specialist who participated actively in our teaching program. After returning home, he had a distinguished career and rose to be a professor of surgery at the University of Colorado. The hospital was well run. Colonel Howard turned out to be an excellent C.O. and administrator. I came to respect him and worked effectively with him.

I was a little uneasy about serving with him because of our argument about my assignment on paper at the 303rd General Hospital. Once we actually started working together, he confessed that had he known me better I would have been his first choice for chief of medicine. He said the tougher the going the better I performed, to the point that in my "201" file he used the term "brilliant" to describe me and said he had never used that term for a medical officer in the past.

Under Colonel Howard's command and his excellent adjutant, Major Daniel Sanchez, the 148th soon became known as the premier general hospital in the Marianas. I plunged into my new assignment with enthusiasm and vigor. Soon we had the WESPAC doctors telling about their interesting cases and things medical and surgical rather than complaining about the weather and the delay in getting home.

Grand Rounds and other conferences were well attended by our own staff, many of the doctors from other units on Saipan, as well as some who flew in from Iwo Jima, Tinian, and Guam. There was always in the audience a contingent of Navy doctors as well as flight surgeons from the B-29 units. Since the Navy was responsible for the medical care of the entire Chamorro population and our hospital had a number of well-qualified specialists, we were often called upon for consultation and responded generously. In the process we saw many interesting patients with all sorts of tropical diseases, including many with yaws, and we included these in our teaching program.

A combined medical-and-surgical-staff conference was held once monthly announced by a bulletin sent out to all of the installations in WESPAC, sample attached:

148th GENERAL HOSPITAL
APO 244

COMBINED MEDICAL & SURGICAL STAFF CONFERENCE

Thursday 20 December 1945

PROGRAM

INTRODUCTORY REMARKS BY
    Col. James W. Howard Commanding Officer   148th General Hospital

1. HAMMAN'S SYNDROME
    Case Presentation   Capt. Joseph B. Bolotin
    X-ray Features   Capt. A.M. McCallen
    Discussion   Major Michael J. Lepore

2. SALIVARY DUCT STONE   Capt. Erich Fischer

3. THORACIC SURGERY CASES   Capt. Robert K. Brown

4. COLOR FILM
    "Decortication of the lung"   Capt. Paul H. Wedin

I still remember the patient with Hamman's syndrome. He was a healthy young soldier who had been scuba diving off a coral reef on Saipan, using rather primitive makeshift equipment. After a prolonged dive, he surfaced, crying for help and complaining of severe chest pain and shortness of breath. He was quickly transported to my hospital, where he was admitted with the diagnosis of a probable acute myocardial infarct. When I saw him on rounds I found he had palpable subcutaneous emphysema and a sub-xiphoid crunching sound along the left sternal border synchronous with his heartbeat. His electrocardiogram was normal. His chest x ray revealed mediastinal emphysema. My diagnosis was Hamman's syndrome with an excellent prognosis. The patient made an uneventful recovery and was returned to full duty after several days in the hospital. I had never seen a patient with mediastinal emphysema, but I had read Dr. Hamman's paper in the *Bulletin of the Johns Hopkins Hospital* of 1939 and have never forgotten the vivid description of what became known as Hamman's Sign or Hamman's Syndrome. This is not the first time nor will it be the last that I have made a diagnosis based upon reading. I have always had the knack of tucking away in my mind information that I can recall, sometimes years later, for solving a problem. I believe this is a very important asset for a clinician, and it seems to improve with experience and longevity. This skill is waning. In the current era of multiple-choice questions and check-off answers, the art of writing has declined to the degree that quasi-illiteracy is encouraged.

Why did I remember Hamman's original paper? Louis Hamman was a consummate clinician at Johns Hopkins, one of its volunteer staff who was much sought after as a diagnostician and consultant. Case 1 in his now classic paper on "Spontaneous Mediastinal Emphysema" puzzled him no end and illustrates how a brilliant clinician goes about his work.

"SPONTANEOUS MEDIASTINAL EMPHYSEMA"

Case 1. On February 12, 1933, Dr. W. Cabell Moore invited me to come to Washington to see a physician, fifty-one years of age, who had symptoms strongly suggesting the occurrence of coronary occlusion. Theretofore he had always been a robust, healthy man busily engaged in carrying on an exacting practice. On the morning of February 8, while shaving, he was suddenly seized with intense pain under the sternum radiating to the left shoulder. The pain lasted about half an hour and then gradually passed. When Dr. Moore examined him two hours later no definite abnormality was found. The heart and lungs were quite normal. The temperature was 98°F; pulse 54 and regular, respirations 20; blood pressure: systolic 110, diastolic 80. An electrocardiogram taken the next day was reported by Dr. J. W. Esler as follows: Regular rhythm, rate 60; T waves upright in all leads; conduction interval normal; maximum QRS potential 9 mm." The blood count was normal, the leukocytes 8,500 per cubic mm. On the morning of February 11, the patient reported to Dr. Moore that during the evening before when lying on the left side, he had heard a curious bubbling, crackling sound synchronous with the heartbeat. His wife, sitting on the bed beside him, had heard the sound very plainly. At this time Dr. Moore could make out no abnormality whatsoever on physical examination. The heart and lungs were quite normal. The temperature was 98°F; pulse 66; respirations 20; blood pressure: systolic 100, diastolic 75. Later in the day Dr. Esler heard the sound and interpreted it to be a pericardial friction. This seemed to confirm the diagnosis of coronary occlusion which, very naturally under the circumstances, had already been proposed. When I saw the patient on that afternoon of the following day he was sitting up in bed laughing and talking, protesting that he felt perfectly well. He certainly was in good spirits and had every appearance of robust health. The temperature, pulse, respirations and blood pressure were all normal as they had been before. I examined the heart and lungs with the greatest care and could detect nothing that was to the least degree abnormal. When I expressed chagrin at my lack of skill, the patient laughingly said that he could easily bring on the sound which had excited so much interest. He turned on his left side and after shifting about for a few moments said, "There it is, I hear it now." I put my stethoscope over the apex of the heart and with each impulse there occurred the most extraordinary crunching, bubbling sound. It is difficult to describe. Crunching is the best adjective I can think of though it is far from apt, especially since crunching has been widely used to describe pleural friction, to which it bore no resemblance. It certainly conveyed the impression of air being churned or squeezed about in the tissues. When the patient turned on his back the sound at once disappeared. The possibility of pneumothorax came to mind. However a second thorough examination of the lungs was quite negative. Still I persisted and suggested that it might be a small localized pneumothorax near the apex of the heart. The following day a roentgenogram was taken with a portable apparatus. Dr. E. M. McPeak's report reads as follows: Examination of the chest shows the bony thorax, heart and great vessels to be normal in appearance. There is slight thickening of the interlobar pleura on the right side with some slight increase in density throughout the right base. The appearance in the right base is probably due to bronchiectasis. There is no other evidence of abnormality except perhaps a very slight widening of the aortic arch and the thoracic aorta.

The extraordinary sound disappeared after a few days. At the end of two weeks the patient was up and about and during the past five years had led an active life and has remained well.

The experience left me greatly puzzled. Although the character and intensity of the pain was like that of coronary occlusion, still, the fact that when the pain had gone, the patient felt perfectly well and had none of the constitutional symptoms and other manifestations of shock, which are such typical features of this condition, convinced me that he did not have coronary occlusion. Moreover, the peculiar sound heard over the heart did not have the distinctive features of a pericardial rub, nor did the patient have the pain and fever which almost certainly would have accompanied a pericarditis sufficiently pronounced to have caused such a decided friction. Therefore, after the symptoms had disappeared, I did not hesitate to advise that the patient be allowed to leave the bed and slowly resume his accustomed activities.

Nonetheless, I could offer no reasonable interpretation of the remarkable sound heard over the heart. Never before had I heard such a sound. It was an unpleasantly bewildering experience and almost daily I revolved the problem in my mind seeking an adequate solution, until four months later, when I heard precisely the same sound over the heart of a boy under circumstances which left no doubt as to the way it was produced, and clearly explained the nature and meaning of the symptoms I had observed in the Washington physician.

The second patient had subcutaneous emphysema "over the front of the neck which extended backward to the trapezius muscle on both sides and downward over the clavicles to about the second rib on the left and to the nipple on the right. When I put my stethoscope over the heart, there was the same systolic crunching sound which had so perplexed me when I heard it over the heart of the Washington physician. . . . [T]he roentgenogram demonstrated the presence of air in the mediastinal tissues between the heart and the anterior wall of the chest and in the subcutaneous tissues of the neck.

What are the lessons taught by Dr. Louis Hamman?

1. He listened not only to the chest and heart but also to his patient and was humble enough to admit that he had his limitations "never before had I heard such a sound."
2. He knew he was hearing and seeing a zebra not a horse.
3. He relied on his five senses and his brain rather than elaborate machines.

He doggedly pursued the diagnosis and inspired others to join him in the hunt. These are the hallmarks of a great clinician and teacher, a dying breed in the current era of excessive dependence upon more and more elaborate machinery and technology.

To brighten up the medical scene, we also had a Saipan Medical Society to promote collegiality among the medical staffs of the various hospitals and dispensaries on the island. Tinian had a similar society.

As chief of medicine, I had more than my share of administrative duties and served as a member of "Boards" convened under Army

Regulations to comply with statutory requirements. I recall driving my jeep to a meeting on Saipan where decisions were to be made on whether certain officers should be rotated home because of disability. I was accompanied by the neuropsychiatrist on our staff, a captain who had been overseas for two years. The morning was beautiful and clear, with a blue sky stretching to the horizon, the greenness of the jungle with its colorful flowers providing a striking view. I remarked to the psychiatrist, whom I had just met, "This is a beautiful morning isn't it"? His surly reply was that anybody who thought anything was beautiful on Saipan must be crazy. I knew then that I was going to have a problem with this chap on the Board. He went on to say he was skeptical of the disability of the officers we were going to see and said, flat out, that no one was going to get off Saipan before he did.

He proved to be quite antagonistic during the Board proceedings and when I returned to headquarters, I told Colonel Howard that I thought our psychiatrist needed some help, like a quick trip home. Nothing was done about this until a few weeks after my meeting when a shot rang out from one of the prefabs occupied by the psychiatrist. When we arrived at the scene, the psychiatrist had his revolver in hand and cried out that someone had come into his room while he was asleep and tried to steal his liquor. We got rid of this man as quickly as possible.

In a stateside Army General Hospital, psychiatry was a separate service with its own chief. Overseas, the NP (Neuropsychiatric) service was under the department of medicine and I, as the chief, was also in charge of psychiatry. This got me involved in a number of unusual situations for which I was not well prepared.

One of these was the trial for murder of a black private from one of the Port Battalions. He was accused of breaking into the Post PX to steal some candy bars when he was challenged by the sentry and responded by shooting and killing him. The young man turned out to be illiterate and from a deprived background in Georgia, with no criminal record or prior disciplinary problems. Our neurologist reviewed the problem and became quite involved in the soldier's defense. He thought that the accused murderer had some sort of psychomotor epilepsy and needed thorough neurological study including an electroencephalogram. We did not have an EEG machine on Saipan, so the neurologist recommended that the man be sent stateside for this test and any others that might be needed. The line officers assigned to this trial thought that the neurologist was overdoing it, and some nasty innuendoes were being circulated that perhaps the trial was racially biased with many of the line officers being from the southern states. The final decision was to comply with the neurologist's recommendation, and orders were issued for the soldier to be accompanied stateside by the neurologist and returned to Saipan after the studies had been completed. This was done, except that for some reason, the neurologist was assigned elsewhere. It was because of the missing neurologist that, I, as chief of medicine and in charge of neuropsychiatry, was ordered to examine the accused and to testify as to whether he knew right from wrong when he was alleged to have committed the crime. I had never before had to do anything like this, but orders were orders and I complied. I felt sorry for the young man and questioned him about his background, using queries suggested by the Judge Advocate. I reached the decision that he knew right from wrong. He was subsequently found guilty but appealed. I am not certain of the final outcome.

Another incident involving the psychiatry service occurred when we had decided to transfer a violent locked-ward patient from the 148th General Hospital to more secure facilities on Guam. He was to be accompanied by his doctor, an obstetrician in civilian life, who was a "90-day wonder" given brief training in psychiatry. Colonel Howard issued the order that they proceed by helicopter to Guam, 170 miles away. The doctor, who had been handling the psychiatric unit effectively, sought me out and nearly wept as he said he simply could not fly to Guam in a helicopter because he feared an accident, especially in a helicopter. I tried to persuade him to comply but he continued to refuse. I discussed it with Colonel Howard and we agreed that the order should stand. Very reluctantly, the doctor complied. The mission was safely accomplished and he returned to Saipan unharmed. I must say that I was relieved, for I would have felt very badly if there had been a crash, a frequent occurrence with helicopters in those days.

Still another psychiatric experience occurred shortly after I was assigned to the 148th General Hospital as chief of medicine. We had 600 beds in a 2,000-bed hospital, each Quonset holding forty patients. It took quite a while for me to see all of the patients and to become familiar with their records. Rounds were made by jeep going from one Quonset to another. In the Quonset for sick officers, I finally became aware of two healthy-looking, robust men, one a warrant officer and the other a second lieutenant, who were there, I was told, for administrative reasons. When I asked what these were, I was told that a rather large file on their cases was in a locked cabinet in my office. When I located the file, I learned that the two were homosexuals who had turned themselves in after the war was over, admitting that they were homosexuals but denying that they had committed any homosexual acts while in military service, but feared that they might succumb and decided to seek a discharge from the Army. They had appeared before an Army Board and been turned down, the opinion being expressed by the line officers that they were damned if they were going to send them home with a pension for life with a psychiatric diagnosis. The matter had been sent to headquarters and finally had reached the surgeon general for review. There was at that time no satisfactory method for dealing with homosexuals in the Army and months had passed while the men spent most of their time playing cards and being housed and fed in Army hospitals. After some weeks the surgeon general gave us directions as to how to proceed with this matter. Discharge from the Army was to be accomplished through special administrative channels without dishonor or medical disability.

My professional activities on Saipan continued to be exciting and interesting. Some of the patients we were seeing were fascinating and I shall discuss a few in detail. We saw a few patients with malaria, most of them from the CBI theater. Malaria was not indigenous to Saipan or Tinian because the mosquito vector, anopheles, was not present. Dengue was endemic on Saipan and at times epidemic.

I learned a great deal about pulmonary and hepatic amebiasis from the flight surgeons who had served in the CBI theater and were very experienced in the appropriate use of emetine-hydrochloride injections for these complications of amebic dysentery. We had several patients with cutaneous diphtheria that was very tricky to diagnose before we had learned to look for it. We had one whole Quonset filled at all times with patients with viral hepatitis of all gradations.

With the end of hostilities, our policy for patients with severe hepatitis was to send them to the mainland for the prolonged convalescence that was needed. I would make rounds in the Quonset housing these patients and approve of their transfer that night when the air transport arrived. On one occasion, as I finished my rounds, I said to the ward officer, "Captain there are thirty-nine patients with viral hepatitis who are to be transferred by airplane tonight and there is one malingerer, the sergeant in the third bed on the right. Send him down to my office and search his duffle bag for Atabrine while he is gone and report your findings to me." Sure enough, he had a bottle of 250 tablets of Atabrine. My suspicions were aroused by the lack of yellow pigment in his conjunctivae and the absence of hepatomegaly or tenderness over the liver. Atabrine stains the skin a yellow color but does not do this to the conjunctivae, whereas bilirubin stains all of the tissues. The sergeant denied faking jaundice claiming, that he was taking the Atabrine to prevent a malarial attack. The large supply, he said was due to his assignment as sergeant to see that all of the men took the prophylactic dose of Atabrine each week to prevent malaria. He had an excellent combat record and planned to study medicine. I decided not to court-martial him, but released him to the pool awaiting deployment home on the condition that he would stay away from my hospital unless he was seriously ill. I also looked him straight in the eye and said "Tell your friends in the pool that there's a major in charge at the 148th General Hospital who can tell Atabrine from hepatitis jaundice. The jig is up." I still wonder how many fakers made it to the states and home sweet home.

Viral pneumonia was a common ailment that fortunately did not cause any deaths on my service. When General Kimble, the commanding general on Tinian, had it, he asked to be flown to the 148th General Hospital to be under my care. He recovered well and we became good friends. The hospital very much appreciated the airplane load of King Papaya from Oahu that he arranged to send us. His role in the atom-bomb saga on Tinian has been described in a previous chapter.

Another patient with viral pneumonia that I will never forget was a civilian who was sent to Saipan after the war was over to build and run a Coca-Cola plant. He was a Californian who had been rejected for military service because of coccidioidomycosis with cavitation of the right upper lobe of his lungs acquired in the San Joaquin valley. The pneumonia attacked the same lobe of the lung and we wondered whether it would cause his coccidioidomycosis to flare up and spread. As his viral pneumonia cleared, it was fascinating to witness the healing process that left the coccidioidomycosis cavity intact and unchanged from his old films. I learned from this patient that all Coca-Colas were not the same. The recipe varies from one area to another in accommodation with regional preferences. I was also startled to learn the salary this man was paid. He was paid more than our commanding general!

Entertainment in the Marianas was limited to radio and movies shown each night in an open-air theater, which we usually attended in our ponchos to ward off the frequent rain squalls. Occasionally we had visits from touring USO shows with well-known performers, but more often than not the performers were hacks who needed the employment and money. One of the female dancers with a troupe became quite ill with severe jaundice, enlarged lymph nodes, fever, and an enlarged tender liver. She was admitted to my hospital with the diagnosis of viral hepatitis. The enlarged lymph nodes made me suspect glandular fever, so-called infectious mononucleosis otherwise known as the "kissing disease" and now known as Epstein-Barr disease. This was a fairly common ailment among the young troops and I saw a great deal of it in military service stateside as well as overseas. Fortunately, we were able to confirm her diagnosis with a heterophile titre, a special blood test using sheep cells. The test was strongly positive and accurately mirrored the progress of her disease. If she had severe viral hepatitis, I had to send her home to recover. This would have pleased a GI but this young lady refused to go home and said she was having the time of her life and saw no reason for going home. In fact, this could mean she would lose her job, be out of work, and lose her source of income; so she fought vigorously any move to send her home.

I decided to take a chance and let her continue with her troupe after a period of convalescence in our hospital. We had to order the sheep cells for her tests from Oahu and finally persuaded the command to give us two sheep to keep us supplied with their red cells. The sheep arrived in due course and were placed in a specially constructed pen on the mountain top. Dr. Paul Szanto was very pleased to have this addition to his armamentarium. This was all destroyed when the sheep were stolen one night and the aroma of barbecued mutton could be smelled for miles around. The perpetrators of this crime were never detected, despite considerable but amateurish effort. We did not attempt to replace the sheep.

Another patient on my service was an infantry soldier, a grunt with an unusual history. He was about twenty years old, a denizen of Washington Heights in Manhattan who had been drafted against his will. He knew something about radios and he was made the radioman for his unit and was ordered overseas, where he participated in the Okinawan campaign. He had a falling out with his captain and was told to shape up or he would be sent into frontline combat. One word led to another and the soldier said he had no fears about combat and demanded that he be allowed to go up front. In wartime, if a soldier volunteered for frontline action, he got it. This New York soldier became the lead scout of his unit, his assignment being to draw the fire of the Japanese machine gunners so that they could be spotted and eliminated. This young man became known as a galloping ghost for his ability to escape being killed. He was written up in *Time* magazine as a bona fide hero and was decorated for his bravery in action. I asked him whether he was scared while he was running as the lead scout. He said of course he was, but he soon learned that the Japanese were short of ammunition and were also not very good at hitting a moving target. Toward the end, he wished they would hit him but they never did. His stay in my hospital was short. He had "jungle rot" of both feet and asked me to get him two pairs of low-cut officer's shoes rather than the old combat boots he was wearing. I arranged this and sent him back to the replacement depot with the warning not to come to our hospital unless he was really sick.

Life on Saipan was not all beer and skittles. There were still enemy soldiers in the jungle who refused to surrender and continued to shoot up our bamboo water conduits. Colonel Howard decided to dump surplus C rations and K rations in areas where the enemy was hiding. Patrols were sent into the jungle using a captured Japanese officer who advised the troops to surrender, usually to no avail. If our soldiers entered the caves in search of the enemy, they encountered booby traps. Some of the young Chamorrans acted as scouts and helped to locate the enemy. In the long run, discouraged by some losses among our troops on patrol, the commanding general stopped sending out the patrols. His instructions were to welcome those who wished to surrender and kill those who took offensive action.

A large contingent of enemy prisoners of war was housed in a compound. Occasionally I was asked to examine a sick prisoner and to decide how to treat him. Our attitude was that the sick would be well cared for whether they were enemies or friends, a position quite different from that of the Japanese. I shall never forget the cemeteries for our soldiers and marines on Tinian and Saipan. They were well maintained and were constant reminders of those who had given their lives so the rest of us would exist in a peaceful world. When I saw the names on the crosses and the Stars of David, I swore I would never forget them and that I would strive all my life to avoid prejudice and bias towards those of other creeds and color. We even had a canine cemetery on Saipan for the marvelous dogs who gave up their lives sniffing out the enemy and their booby traps in the many caves. The white crosses on the little graves had painted on them the black head of German shepherd dogs. There were no names.

The native Chamorrans on Saipan lived in a fenced-in compound under very primitive conditions lacking the amenities of civilized life. The fecal stench could be awful, especially if the wind was blowing out to sea and across the road. On Saipan, if you went for a drive in your jeep, you could go in only two directions, clockwise or counterclockwise. When you zipped past the Chamorran compound, you pressed hard on the accelerator and held your breath until you were well beyond the range of the smell.

On one occasion, General Irvine asked me to clean up a group of Chamorros who could serve with pay as household servants for the officers' families that had arrived on Saipan after the end of the war. I told the general that we could easily cure those who had yaws, but the real problem would be their almost universal infestation with intestinal parasites, including hookworm, amoebae, Giardia, and other pathogens. Even if we cleaned them up, the Chamorros could reacquire their infections when they returned to their compound, where sanitary conditions were, to put it mildly, unacceptable. Periodically, in my teaching program on Saipan, I would put a slide of a stool from one of the natives under the microscope in our laboratory and announce over the loudspeaker that we had an interesting specimen to examine. In a single specimen it was not unusual to find three pathogenic parasites. It was a simple, but in a way, an extremely effective way to teach parasitology.

I knew there was nothing we could do about the conditions in the Chamorros encampment, so I insisted that the natives not be used as food handlers, but should taught the simple elements of personal hygiene to prevent fecal contamination and spread of disease. In other words, I insisted that they wash their hands after defecation, not a simple accomplishment given the lack of water, soap, plumbing, and toilet facilities.

The weather on Tinian and Saipan was, of course, notable for the oppressive heat and humidity, but we adjusted to it. When I was still on Tinian in September 1945, we were hit by a horrendous typhoon that tore our hospital, the 303rd, into bits. We were then occupying tents and the storm began with heavy rain and high winds. I was glad to see that my tent was holding up pretty well and I tried to get to sleep on my little cot. At about 2 or 3 A.M. I realized that this was no ordinary storm. I looked out and saw pieces of equipment and roofs from prefabs in the area flying about like toothpicks and smacking into other buildings.

I dressed and left my tent to find my way to the only building that seemed to be standing. There I found Colonel Howard and several other officers, sitting out the storm. We had had no warning of this typhoon and no preparations had been made to cope with it. I found out later that the Navy units had been warned and had moved into large caves that served as a safe harbor. When dawn arrived, the desolation on Tinian was indescribable. Hospital records had been drenched or destroyed. Fortunately no one was hurt. Emergency measures were initiated and soon we were installed in safer quarters in some sturdy Quonsets that had weathered the storm. We were told that the typhoon was headed north toward Okinawa and warned that it might turn back again in twenty-four to forty-eight hours and hit Tinian once more. We were helpless and felt there was nothing we could do and could not understand why better measures had not been taken to prepare for hurricanes and typhoons. We were told not to worry, typhoons occurred only once in three years. This one hit Okinawa and caused severe damage and inflicted many casualties, but it did not turn around to hit Tinian again. My feeling was one of deep frustration in the face of this terrifying freak of nature. I felt that, having survived a war, what a pity it would be to lose my life because of a major storm. Whoever told us that bull about hurricanes and typhoons coming to the Marianas only once very three years was either lying or very poorly informed, probably a combination of the two. Within six months while I was on Saipan we were hit with an aftermath of a tidal wave and then another typhoon. This time we were adequately warned and made preparations to protect our patients as well as ourselves. When we were on Tinian we were awaiting assignments and had no patients to worry about. This time, General Irvine issued an order to empty out our hospital consisting of forty or more Quonset huts, sending the walking wounded and convalescents to their own units, and housing those remaining in a large concrete Japanese-built blockhouse. On short notice we had to get this bunker set up for patients. With my assistant, Captain "Chuck" Boozan, I drove my jeep through the heavy rain in whistling winds to the blockhouse. I inspected it and set it up with cots and whatever equipment we could scrounge. I also realized that I could not put our sick soldiers into such inadequate quarters without plumbing, electricity, or a water supply. I decided to move only a few to the blockhouse and felt that it would be safer to keep the others in a well-equipped Quonset hut on the hill. The CBs, God bless them, gave us a real helping hand. They brought up enormous ship anchors with heavy chains that they swung over the Quonset at each end and another in the middle. These served to anchor the Quonset so that it could not be blown off its base—or so we thought. I also decided that I would stay with my sick soldiers to see them through the storm. It was a rocky night, the Quonset was lifted up on several occasions by severe gusts of wind but rose up and fell back into place without any injuries. By the next day the storm had abated and we set about putting things into shape to receive patients. Unfortunately the chief of surgery, Major Archer had chosen to send all of his patients out to their units. This led to a nasty repercussion. Many of the discharged soldiers had a great deal of difficulty in getting to their units and complained angrily to headquarters. This led to an article in the *Saipan Target*, the newspaper printed by the troops on the island, criticizing the hospital for its callous attitude. General Irvine was quite upset and chewed out the surgical service for their actions. He let me know how much he appreciated the humane manner with which I had handled the emergency for the medical service. What I learned from this is that a general order of the day may be modified by the officer on the firing line when it seems inappropriate or dangerous to the one responsible for carrying it out.

A Soldier with a Rare and Serious Disease Comes to Saipan for Diagnosis and Treatment

On 13 December 1945 I was notified that a seriously ill patient had been admitted during the night to the medical service of the 148th General Hospital as a formal air transfer from the 232nd General Hospital, APO 86, Iwo Jima, with the diagnosis "1. Ill-defined condition, Hepatic system, Manifested by Hepatic Enlargement, fever, leucocytosis and Anemia. 2. Syphilis, old, late, latent."

I hurried over to see the patient, a thirty-six-year-old white male sergeant assigned as a welder to the 80th Field Artillery Battalion having served the past nine months in the Philippine Islands and nine months prior in New Guinea. I saw at a glance that he was seriously and probably terminally ill and I was angered that he was lying flat on an army cot despite marked orthopnea and dyspnea. He was conscious and recognized me as a major and chief of medicine and pleaded with me to try to get him home in time for Christmas with his family and children. I said I would do my best and proceeded with my examination. He was emaciated, febrile, T 103°F, BP 150/95. His skin was discolored by Atabrine taken for malaria prophylaxis plus paleness due to anemia, the combination producing a ghastly ashen hue. He had bilateral foot and wrist drop, a markedly distended abdomen and generalized abdominal tenderness, partly localized to both lower quadrants. The liver was neither enlarged nor tender. There was 3+ pretibial pitting edema. Emergency laboratory studies: hemoglobin 11.2 gm percent; hematocrit 33; ESR 58; NPN (Nonprotein Nitrogen) 110 milligrams percent; WBC 26250 (P88, L 1). Urine: spec gr. 1.008; albumin 3+; glucose 0. Micro: few RBC, WBC and granular casts, My initial impression was that the patient's multi-system involvement was due to periarteritis nodosa, a diffuse and serious collagen disease affecting many arteries, and I instituted supportive measures. I also took the nurses aside and had a long talk with them about his nursing care, or rather the lack of it. I asked why in Heaven's name this dying man was on a flat army cot when there were four crank-up hospital beds with excellent mattresses in that Quonset occupied by convalescing and robust young soldiers awaiting discharge. I ordered the nurses to assign one of the hospital beds to this patient, shifting a healthy soldier to one of the army cots. I also raised the question of why I had to make this point. "What has happened to Army nursing?" I asked in exasperation. My remarks had the desired effect. From that point on the sergeant was given excellent nursing care, including special nurses around the clock and supportive care including intravenous fluids and insertion of a Miller-Abbott tube into the stomach. Having arranged all of this, I turned my attention to the record of illness that accompanied this patient to our hospital, looking for any leads to confirm my diagnosis. I had never before made the diagnosis of periarteritis nodosa and in those days it was the equivalent of signing a death certificate because there was no cure.

The patient's history was of considerable interest. In mid-October 1945, while he was in a rest camp near Manila, he developed aches and pains in his legs and swelling of the ankles and he began to lose weight. He reported to the dispensary of the 29th Replacement Depot, Manila, and was given tablets that gave him only partial relief. The aching in his legs became progressively worse and in early November he developed frequent nocturia. However, he minimized his symptoms because he did not want to miss the boat for home. When he boarded the transport, it is stated that he was in "very weak condition." (It is not unusual for soldiers eager to go home to deny or fail to declare illness when heading for home. Sometimes their buddies carried them aboard saying they were OK but needed some help getting up the gangplank.) On 11 November 1945 the patient was admitted to the sick bay of the transport, the *S.S. Walter Wellman*, where it was recorded that he looked ill and was walking with some difficulty. Temperature 100, pulse 120, blood pressure 140/90. The general examination was negative except for poor nutrition and three-plus pitting edema of both feet, ankles, and pretibial region. No laboratory tests were available, not even a urine examination. He was diagnosed as having acute nephritis and fever of unknown origin, and on 14 November 1945 he was started on penicillin 25,000 units IM q4h. He failed to respond, his temperature reached 103 degrees each day, the edema of the legs persisted, weight loss and anorexia continued. On 16 December 1945 the sick-bay log read, "Due to very limited facilities aboard with absence of laboratory aids, it is strongly advised that the patient be transferred to shore facilities." On 17 November 1945 the transport was diverted to Iwo Jima harbor and the patient was transferred to the 232nd General Hospital APO 86. There, the provisional diagnoses were: 1. Nephritis, acute, 2. Heart disease, hypertensive or luetic, 3. Hepatitis, acute, 4. Amebiasis with hepatic involvement, 5. Malaria. Laboratory studies revealed a moderate anemia, elevated ESR, leucocytosis, positive Kahn & Wassermann tests, normal NPN. Urine: glucose negative, albumin 3-plus, few RBC and WBC and coarse granular casts.

It is of interest that none of the diagnoses was documented except lues, which had been adequately treated in the past. His therapy was empiric and supportive, including four blood transfusions and a course of intramuscular emetine for a possible amebic hepatic abscess, which he did not have, and penicillin injections. He seemed to improve for a time but relapsed and became critically ill. On 13 December 1945, after twenty-six days in the 232nd General Hospital, he was transferred by air to my service at the 148th General Hospital on Saipan. It was here that I first encountered this severely ill soldier who had been a diagnostic enigma since he first became ill in October 1945.

In my very first note, I stated that his clinical picture with multisystem involvement was consistent with periarteritis nodosa, the first time this diagnosis had been proposed by any of the many physicians who had seen him. If my diagnosis proved to be correct, why had it been missed in a major 2,000-bed Army General Hospital where the patient had spent twenty-six days? Despite our supportive efforts the patient's course was rapidly downhill, consistent with severe disseminated periarteritis nodosa, and he died on 16 December 1945. My final note, photocopied from his hospital chart, read as follows:

Final note 16 December 1700

Patient expired at 1650. Special nurse states that he stopped breathing and became pulseless. No convulsion.

Our final diagnosis is periarteritis nodosa with diffuse involvement of the vascular system especially the renal arteries with uremia. We also feel that there has been involvement of the mesenteric vessels and perhaps the appendiceal artery and left testicular artery. The development of hypotension in the past 24 hours points to adrenal insufficiency, caused by the same process and the low serum chloride is corroborative. The EKG changes also indicate myocardial involvement by the same disease. The foot drop and wrist drop point to peripheral neuropathy. This, too, is accounted for by periarteritis nodosa.

Final Diagnosis: PERIARTERITIS NODOSA, GENERALIZED.

> M. J. LEPORE
> MAJOR M.C. AUS
> CHIEF OF MEDICAL SERVICE
> 148TH GENERAL HOSPITAL
> APO 244 SAIPAN

Permission for an autopsy was obtained and it was performed by Dr. Paul Szanto, an excellent pathologist. The autopsy was attended by most of the physicians of the 148th General Hospital. The clinical diagnosis of periarteritis nodosa affecting multiple organ systems was completely documented. This diagnosis, made initially on purely Oslerian clinical grounds, was rarely made in those days and it created quite a sensation in the Marianas.

The Care of the Drunkard's Tapeworm

I became involved in this case when one of our doctors, a captain from New York, was being court-martialled for being drunk and persuading our sentry to become drunk on duty. This was a serious offense, especially with enemy soldiers still prowling around in the jungle surrounding our hospital. The captain was brought before a Board of Line Officers and came up with an ingenious defense that confounded those who heard it. He claimed that he had become an alcoholic on Tinian and Saipan because he had acquired a tapeworm infection from the Australian beef that he ate in the form of raw hamburger. When the tapeworm moved about, it induced abdominal pain and the only thing that quieted it down was a generous quaff of Scotch whiskey, which he consumed in large quantities throughout the day and sometimes at night. His claim was that the tapeworm, acquired in the line of duty, had made him an alcoholic and had been responsible for his inducing the sentry to drink with him. The line officers called for medical consultation and sought my advice. This officer, who was attached to the 148th General Hospital, had been a thorn in our side because of his erratic performance and unpleasant demeanor. The line officers thought that he was lying to escape punishment. I examined him and confirmed that he had a tapeworm and recommended that we deworm him. I admitted him to the officer's Quonset, where we prepared him for the treatment. The medication recommended for this tapeworm was a resinous compound, oleoresin Aspidium. I went to our post pharmacist who located a dusty, sealed, amber bottle of the drug that had been in stock for many months. Since there was no air conditioning, it had almost certainly been overheated. I opened the bottle and it was clearly a resin but there was always the possibility that it had become dehydrated and concentrated in the heat of the tropics. I decided that we had best give him half the usual dose and follow it with a second dose if indicated. The pharmacist dispensed it and sent it over the officers' Quonset, where it was administered by the nurses to the patient. About one hour after, an emergency call went out over our paging system for Major Lepore to come right away to the officers' Quonset. I hurried over in my jeep and was not surprised to see that it was the captain who had collapsed.

He screamed at me that I had tried to kill him with the medicine and that he was about to die. I recalled that one of the unpleasant complications of the treatment was that shock-like collapse could occur, but that patients usually recovered. One saving grace was that the shock-like complication occurred only if the head of the tapeworm as well as its body were passed. I called for a bedpan and we slid it under the patient's buttocks and he passed an enormous tapeworm with the head attached. He was cured of his tapeworm, but would he survive the treatment?

By this time intravenous fluids were being administered, his blood pressure was normal and his pulse was regular. I thought, how lucky he was that I had given him only half the recommended dose. As any rogue might, he recovered completely and was court-martialled and punished with an official reprimand and fined a substantial amount of pay.

A Sailor with Smallpox

It was shortly after this, on 8 January 1946, that I was informed by my commanding officer, Colonel Howard, that he had recommended my promotion to lieutenant colonel. The papers were being processed, had cleared headquarters and had been signed by Brigadier General W. W. Irvine, commanding general of the Western Pacific Base Command. I was told that I could be wearing the silver leaves of a Lt. Colonel almost any day. Of the many majors that went overseas to Tinian with the 10,000-bed hospital center (821st Hospital Center APO 247), I was the only one nominated for promotion to Lt. Colonel for work in the field. Colonel Howard seemed very happy to be doing this and General Irvine was pleased. I was, of course, delighted, and hastened to write the good news to my wife.

I was also receiving some interesting mail. Several letters arrived from Lt. Colonel Maurice Schnitker, who was now serving as the chief medical consultant with General Douglas MacArthur. He asked me to join him and offered me any position I would like as chief of medicine in a 2,000-bed Army General Hospital in his theater. I thought this was going in the wrong direction toward an indefinite stay in Tokyo with the occupation forces. However, I discussed the offer with Colonel Howard and General Irvine. They both agreed that it was an honor to be sought after by General MacArthur, but they also indicated that I was sorely needed on Saipan. General Irvine said he would greatly appreciate it if I would consider remaining on Saipan until we had finished examining 1,000 Air Force pilots for permanent Regular Army commissions. On completion of this assignment, I would be rotated to Oahu to become the chief of medicine of the Tripler General Hospital. This was in the right direction, I thought. I had enjoyed my work with General Irvine and Colonel Howard and decided to stay on Saipan.

On 27 January 1946 I received a call from Lieutenant Kenneth D. Weeks of the Navy, who asked me to consult on the case of a sailor who was being brought to Saipan by his ship as an emergency because of suspected hemorrhagic smallpox. Dr. Weeks had finished his residency in medicine at Duke Hospital and had attended my rounds on Saipan. The Naval Hospital on Saipan had been closed, leaving a skeleton crew and empty Quonsets. Dr. Weeks had never seen a patient with smallpox and neither had I, but I was willing to do whatever I could to help him. My first suggestion was to isolate the patient by opening up one of their closed Naval Hospital Quonsets, in this way minimizing the threat of spreading this highly contagious disease to military personnel and the native population. I also made myself available for consultation at any time. The following day, 28 January 1946, the patient arrived on Saipan and I examined him with Dr. Weeks. This patient's case history was well reported by Dr. Weeks in the *United States Naval Bulletin* 47: 707-715, 1947, and I shall quote from it:

> C.H., a 20-year-old white male SMSC, was a member of the crew of an LCS that departed Shanghai, China, 21 January 1946 en route to Saipan, Mariana Islands. The ship had been on the China coast for almost 2 months prior to that date and the patient had had liberty on the average of twice a week in Shanghai. At the time of his ship's departure he was and had been feeling quite well and during his visits to Shanghai had not heard or seen any evidence of smallpox. The second day at sea he began to experience dull, aching bilateral costovertebral angle and flank pain, more so on the right than on the left, and had to walk bent over to get relief. There was no radiation of this pain and it was constant, not intermittent. Associated with this, there was frequency of urination which increased to two or three times per hour. The urine was described as being dark and cloudy and there was no dysuria. The following or third day out, the back pain and frequency continued and he began to have chills and fever. He was put to bed and the convoy medical officer was informed. Due to rough seas the doctor was unable at the time to board the patient's ship but made a tentative diagnosis of urinary tract infection and prescribed sulfathiazole, 3 grams immediately, and 1 gram every 4 hours. The patient's temperature at the beginning of treatment was 104°F.
>
> On 25 January (fourth day of illness) an erythematous, macular rash was noted for the first time, on the inner aspect of both

thighs. Thinking the dermatitis might be due to sulfathiazole the drug was discontinued after a total of 5 grams had been given. The following day the skin eruption had spread to involve the trunk, arms, and lower legs. At this time the convoy doctor was able to transfer to the patient's ship and described the patient as being acutely ill, toxic and delirious. The skin lesions had become papular with erythematous bases and were most marked over the leg, thighs, and forearms but were also observed on the abdomen, chest, palms, soles and face. Large ecchymotic, pur- puric extravasation were noted over the buttocks following peni- cillin injections which had been started when the sulfathiazole was discontinued. High fever and delirium continued and the patient began to have hemoptysis with production of grossly blood sputum. The back pain and urinary frequency disappeared and the urine cleared considerably. The patient remained acutely ill and delirious and the skin lesions progressed. Some of the papules became vesicular and over the backs of the hands some of them coalesced to form bullous lesions filled with dark, hem- orrhagic fluid.

Due to the gravity of the situation the patient's ship pro- ceeded alone and arrived at Saipan during the early morning hours of 28 January, which was the patient's seventh day of illness. He was immediately transferred to the Navy Hospital at Saipan in a most critical condition. History of previous immunizations showed that he was vaccinated against smallpox at the ages of 6 and 12 and a third time in November 1943 after entering the Navy. According to his statement none of the three vaccinations produced a noticeable reaction but his health record recorded an "accelerated reaction" in November 1943. Upon further ques- tioning the patient was unable to recall any type of reaction.

Physical examination recorded shortly after admission to the hospital was as follows: temperature 103.8°F, pulse 110, respira- tions 24. blood pressure 120/60. "The patient is an obviously desperately ill and febrile patient, age about 20, white male, with a very striking and marked generalized skin eruption. The skin lesions are most pronounced over the extensor surfaces of arms, hands, legs, feet, chest, and abdomen. The forehead, sides of face and neck are also heavily involved but the upper back has been spared. The buttocks show large ecchymotic extravasation about the sites of entry of previous injections.

The most prominent lesion is a diffuse, dark red, macu- lopapular rash which has become confluent over forearms, hands and lower legs. Superimposed on these lesions and scat- tered generally are large numbers of vesicular lesions in various states of development. Many are small and grayish with little ery- thema. Others are large, darker, reddish-brown with umbilicated, necrotic centers. Still others are much larger and even bullous, containing hemorrhagic fluid. Papular lesions are also seen in the palms and soles. Careful search fails to reveal the presence of a "primary-take" smallpox immunization scar.

Lymphatics: the axillary and inguinal lymph nodes were moderately enlarged but there is no generalized lymphadenopathy.

Head: not remarkable. No lesions noted in scalp.

Eyes: hemorrhagic suffusions are noted in both conjunctivae and sclerae, left more marked than right. Pupils round, react and equal. No apparent weakness of extraocular movements. No nystagmus. Ophthalmoscopic not attempted at this time.

Nose: alae nasi rimmed with blood crusts and both breathing passages partially occluded by blood clots.

Mouth: lips swollen darkly discolored and crusted by hemorrhagic areas and old blood. The tongue and gingivae are peppered by numerous small vesicular papules but at this time there is no bleeding from the gums. There are necrotic, hemorrhagic lesions in the roof of the mouth and in the oral pharynx with clotted blood and active bleeding. Tonsils moderately enlarged and involved in the process just described.

Neck: no signs of meningeal irritation. No palpable abnormalities noted. Trachea in the midline.

Chest: symmetrical with equal expansion, bilaterally. Lung fields resonant to percussion but coarse, moist rales are readily heard at both bases and over the precordium. No friction rubs heard. Breath sounds suppressed at both bases, posteriorly.

Heart: precordium quiet. Rate 110 per minute. No palpable shocks or thrills. Not enlarged to percussion. PMI felt in left fifth interspace within the midclavicular line. Rhythm normal. Heart sounds of good quality, no murmurs heard but pulmonic second sound definitely accentuated and louder than the aortic second sound.

Abdomen: nothing of note.

Back: exquisite tenderness elicited by fist percussion of the right CVA and kidney region.

Genitalia: normal except for purpuric lesions in skin of penis and scrotum. No lesions or scars suggestive of old or recent venereal infection. No urethral discharge.

Rectal: fresh blood is noted about the anal region and on the rectal examining finger but no other abnormalities noted.

Extremities: No edema, clubbing or cyanosis.

Neurological: Normal insofar as the patient could cooperate. During the course of the examination the patient frequently coughed up bloody sputum and on one occasion vomited blood.

Initial laboratory data: hemoglobin 11.5 grams, red blood cells 3,850,000, white blood cells 10,650. Differential: polymorphonuclear leukocytes 78 percent, stab forms 3 percent, large lymphocytes 5 percent, small lymphocytes 14 percent. No abnormal cells were encountered in doing the differential but most of the segmented forms showed toxic granulation and fragmentation of the nuclei. Platelets were very rarely observed during the process of doing the differential. Urinalysis: clear amber; specific gravity 1.020; albumin 1+; sugar, negative. Microscopic examination of sediment: 15–20 red blood cells per HPF, 4–6 white blood cells per HPF. Benzidine test strongly positive. No sulfathiazole crystals seen in sediment.

Blood chemistries: NPN 80 mg percent; BUN 25 mg percent; van den Bergh and alkaline phosphatase within normal limits. Blood sugar normal. Kahn blood test negative.

X-ray of chest report (taken at time of admission): The lower two-thirds of both lung fields are infiltrated by a diffuse, coarse mottling which is in keeping with a diffuse bronchopneumonia. There is no evidence of free fluid in the pleural cavities and the cardiac silhouette is not remarkable for a supine film.

Impression: fulminating hemorrhagic smallpox with hemorrhagic pneumonia and hemoptysis, toxic nephritis and hematuria and bleeding from the gastrointestinal tract.

Since the patient appeared to be at death's door, Dr. Weeks and I decided to treat him with what were then considered massive doses of penicillin, 100,000 units intramuscularly every two hours, to combat beta-hemolytic septicemia and pneumonia, the common cause of death in hemorrhagic smallpox. An oxygen tent, intravenous fluids, and blood transfusions were employed. Most of all, three Navy corpsmen assumed his nursing care around the clock. Response to these measures was slow but positive. His pneumonia cleared, the mouth and skin lesions healed without scarring or secondary infection, and the bleeding stopped. He received a grand total of 26,500,000 units of penicillin intramuscularly over a twenty-day period.

On the forty-first day, or forty-seven days after the onset of his illness, he was discharged from the hospital and evacuated to the States for further convalescence. At this time the skin was completely clear of all lesions and there was no evidence of impaired renal function and x ray of the chest showed the lung fields to be clear. He felt quite well and was rapidly regaining the amount of weight lost during his illness.

A Talented Neurosurgeon Threatens to Go AWOL from Saipan Because He Has Nothing to Do

One of my most difficult nights on Saipan was in 1946 when our neurosurgeon (a Major X), told me he had made plans to go AWOL because there were no neurosurgical cases. The war was over, injuries were few, and the army procedure for rotating specialists home left much to be desired. This talented individual calmly told me that after much deliberation, he was going to sneak aboard a homeward bound plane loaded with wounded and sick GIs. He knew this was in defiance of military orders and could lead to a court-martial, but he said he was tired of just sitting around doing nothing as he had for many months. I pleaded with him not to do anything so rash. His professional and military performance had been excellent thus far. I stressed the harm the action he contemplated would do to his career, not only in the military but in civilian life as an academic neurosurgeon at his prestigious medical center. I seemed to be getting nowhere, but in the late hours of that early morning, I finally persuaded him to let me try to work out his release through proper channels. As luck would have it, the day after our discussion, we admitted the patient with periarteritis nodosa to my service at the 148th general hospital described in the preceding pages. Of course, I asked the neurosurgeon to see this patient in consultation.

It turned out that he had had considerable experience with this disease, having practiced medical neurology and been board-certified in neurology and psychiatry prior to becoming a board-certified neurosurgeon. He agreed with my diagnosis and served on the team that treated this terminally ill sergeant. A few days later, a young enlisted man was admitted to my service complaining bitterly of an extremely severe headache. His neurological examination conducted by our neurosurgeon revealed paralysis of upward gaze (Parinaud's syndrome) and bilateral choked optic discs. A ventriculogram confirmed the major's diagnosis of a pineal tumor. The neurosurgeon operated, found the pinealoma, and excised it. It is said by some in medicine that when you see a rare condition there is a high probability that a similar one will soon appear. Sure enough, shortly after the patient with the pinealoma arrived on Saipan, a second patient appeared with severe headaches, choked optic discs and paralysis of upward gaze, which again suggested Parinaud's syndrome. At operation, he had a third ventricle cyst that was excised by our neurosurgeon. By this time, the neurosurgeon was satisfied that his talents were being well utilized and before long he was on his way home with a distinguished record of performance as the neurosurgeon on Saipan. His future career is of interest. He became the professor of neurology at his university medical center and lived a productive life until his death in his late eighties.

I am happy that I took the time that night on Saipan to persuade this bright man from going AWOL.

To return to more mundane matters, I completed the assignment requested by General Irvine. The promotion to Lt. Colonel was stalled in the bureaucracy and delayed long enough to make me ineligible for promotion by being two weeks shy of a newly passed requirement that I had to be in grade as a major for twenty-four months. Had the papers been sent to headquarters promptly, I would have had my promotion in January. I believe there was some skulduggery in this. A new commanding officer, a Colonel Donald D. Singe, was then in charge. This individual was the C.O. of the 232nd General Hospital on Iwo Jima when the sergeant with periarteritis nodosa was a patient. The knowledge that they had missed the diagnosis that I had made may have upset him.

In addition, when the 232nd General Hospital was closed and Col. Singe was transferred to Saipan, he brought with him a young captain from Nevada who was his chief of laboratory service whom he wished to displace our chief of laboratories, Dr. Paul Szanto, who had been a captain only three months and was outranked by the doctor from Iwo Jima. Dr. Szanto was a very experienced Viennese-educated pathologist, an excellent teacher, and a leader in my teaching program on Saipan. Paul tipped me off to what was planned. I discussed this with Colonel Howard and indicated that I strongly disapproved of this move. Dr. Szanto had all of the credentials, including board certification. The doctor from Nevada had inadequate training to qualify him as the chief of anything and least of all chief of laboratories in a general hospital. The upshot was that Paul Szanto remained in place, but I believe that Colonel Singe stalled my promotion long enough to send it back into the basket for recycling.

According to my 201 file, my promotion to Lt. Colonel was resubmitted 22 March 1946. The remainder of the correspondence has been lost but I finally received my promotion to Lt. Colonel on 7 June 1946. When I look back on the Saipan tour of duty, once I was appropriately assigned to good hospitals where I was in charge of the medical service, the time passed quickly and I knew I was accomplishing something worthwhile. I was able to establish beyond any doubt my capacity to run a 600-bed medical service in a 2,000-bed general hospital without batting an eye. I merely concentrated on those things I did best, i.e., providing strong and decisive leadership, emphasizing good patient care, excellent bedside teaching, and topflight daily rounds and Grand Rounds and conferences. I have never let the machines or the laboratory tests run the show then or now. Rather than being immobilized by the lack of some sophisticated laboratory or diagnostic facilities, I was challenged and proceeded to practice and teach what was essentially Oslerian medicine, emphasizing careful history-taking, meticulous physical examination, and close observation of my patients. What the patient really gets when he is seen by me is an attentive human being using his five senses aided by that marvelous instrument developed by Laennec, the stethoscope, and making the most of some rather simple tests. I learned long ago that medicine is not a science but an art based on scientific principles. The essence of medicine is in the art of diagnosis. I have always been challenged by a diagnostic puzzle and jump at it like a pit bull until I have solved it. Essentially, I have always been a general internist and diagnostician with a hobby in gastroenterology. Many know me as a gastroenterologist but I have never limited my practice to that field. I prefer to be remembered as a diagnostician. What a waste it would have been to have been limited to a narrow subspecialty or even a broad one. This is why I raised hell when I was temporarily assigned as a gastroenterologist in the U.S. Army, even though it was only a paper assignment that was never implemented. Board-certified in internal medicine since 1943, I have never sought certification in gastroenterology because I decided long ago not to limit my practice to a subspecialty.

My goal was to practice Oslerian medicine in the framework of modern advances, inspired by my personal heroes, Dr. William S. McCann of Rochester, Dr. Frederic M. Hanes at Duke, Dr. Walter W. Palmer and Dr. Robert F. Loeb at Columbia Presbyterian, Dr. John P. Peters at Yale, and Col. Thomas Fitz-Hugh and Col. Marshall Fulton in the Army of the United States.

While I was stationed on Tinian and Saipan, I received mail not only from my beloved wife but also from a number of my teachers. Colonel Tom Fitz-Hugh wrote occasionally and sent me a reprint of one of his articles, "Experiences of An Army Medical Officer in India," inscribed "For M.J.L—from T.F.H., Jr. with high regards to one of the U.S. TOP FLIGHT INTERNISTS WHO HAS 'KEPT THE FAITH.'"

Dr. Walter Palmer, my chief at Columbia P&S, wrote encouraging letters to me, reminding me to be sure to come back to P&S. Dr. Edward F. Adolph of Rochester wrote me frequently, keeping me in touch with his work on "Man in the Desert" and his many contributions to the war effort.

Mail call overseas is an essential aspect of military life. With the recent Gulf War we have once again seen how important the mail is to our troops. I am very grateful for a marvelous wife who knew just the right things to say and found time to write frequently despite the demands of her position as assistant directress of nursing at the

Graduate Hospital of the University of Pennsylvania. She saved every piece of our correspondence as I did hers. Little did I know that some day the letters would serve as a diary and accurate reminder of the things that happened on Tinian and Saipan. The letters from my teachers, colleagues, and subordinates were so welcome and made me feel that it was all worthwhile. In this day and age it has become gauche for people to mention their patriotism and love of country, but I still recall with pleasure stopping my jeep on Mt. Tapotcho on Saipan when retreat was being sounded and our revered flag was being lowered. Without a soul to witness it, alone on the mountaintop, I stood at attention beside my jeep and saluted Old Glory giving thanks to God that I was serving under it to the best of my ability, seeing that our fighting men were getting the best of medical care. When you have done this in wartime, thousands of miles from home, the feeling will never leave you that it is great to be an American.

As I refresh my memory by reading the daily letters I wrote to my beloved wife while I was serving my tour of duty on Tinian and Saipan, I recall the pervasive air of uncertainty and indecision that hung over us as we awaited reassignment, redeployment, or, most of all, a quick trip home. When our 303rd General Hospital left for overseas in May 1945, the slogan of the younger officers was "Back to Dix in Forty-Six," while the older and wiser hands spoke of "The Golden Gate in Forty-Eight." At the time we knew little or nothing about the atom bomb. All we knew was that we were heading into a confrontation with a dangerous enemy who would leave no stone unturned and no trick undone in its effort to win the war. With the dropping of the two atomic bombs in August 1945 and the sudden end of the war, a period of euphoria engulfed Tinian and everyone expected to go home for Christmas.

Unknown to most of the doctors was a clause in their presidential appointment to the Army of the United States that stated, "This Commission to continue in force during the pleasure of the President of the United States for the time being and for the duration of the present emergency and for six months thereafter unless sooner terminated." The reason we were not aware of this clause is that the certificates of appointment were not given out until the officers left military service. My certificate was not sent to me until 19 March 1947, long after I returned to civilian life. While we were on Tinian and Saipan we heard rumors about such a clause but we had no facts. There were other factors delaying discharge of doctors from the Army. We were told that the Japanese surrender did not necessarily mean that the "present emergency" was over and we might be held for occupation duty. Then we were told that some doctors were in essential categories and could not be relieved of their assignments until suitable replacements arrived. The air of euphoria soon evaporated and was succeeded by depression, anger, and frustration. In January 1946 the Saipan chief surgeon informed me that I would be getting orders to go home soon, but I took this with a grain of salt. The uncertainty was disturbing and I decided to do everything I could to improve the morale of my staff and myself by continuing a strong program of medical education, journal clubs, and conferences. Since a number of hospitals were closing down, I obtained permission to raid their libraries to strengthen the one at my hospital and succeeded in setting up a pretty good library for my staff to use at the 369th Station Hospital. As a result of my teaching efforts, morale among the staff was good and on the whole we had no serious problems on Saipan while there was a near mutiny among the doctors on Guam, who complained that they were being used for non-medical duties such as counting candy bars in the PX. I enjoyed my work and the fine young people assigned to me. They all called me "The Chief" and some still do. My wife saved the following letter adding the note, "This must be one of your Saipan friends. It is a very nice letter so I thought I would pass it along to you, Dean."

14 May 1946

Dear Mrs. Lepore:

When I left Saipan I promised Major Lepore that I would contact you. Mrs. Smith and I had planned a trip to New York City but we have had to postpone it. I'm sorry that I can't keep my word. . . . Being a civilian is the most wonderful thing that ever happened. I'm pleased to think that very soon you and the Major will be sharing this same happiness.

When I saw the Major last, early in April, he was expecting orders. I hope that by this time you have received some very good news from him, and that your reunion isn't very far off. The Major was one of my instructors in medicine at P&S and I say sincerely that our association for my short stay at the 369th was the grandest thing that happened to me overseas. . . . P.S. Please pass along my very best wishes to the "Chief."

Sincerely
W. C. Smith

"Smitty" became a pediatrician and was highly respected in Worcester, Massachusetts, where he practiced for many years.

My tour of duty in the Marianas was drawing to a close. On 15 April 1946 I received my orders to proceed to Oahu to become the chief of medicine at the Tripler General Hospital. The following day,

I was summoned to General Irvine's headquarters, where we had a long and pleasant conversation and he pinned a decoration, the Army Commendation Ribbon, on my shirt and apologized that it was not a higher award. On Tuesday, 16 April 1946, I wrote to my "beloved wife": "This morning, I called upon General Irvine, the Commanding General out here, to say goodbye. He was extremely cordial and talked quite a bit with me about various problems. He told me that he would miss me very much but he knew Tripler needed me more. Really, he said, I should have been going home but there you are! Then he awarded me the Army Commendation Ribbon and pinned it on me. It is a very pretty light green with white vertical stripes. The citation is on a nice bit of stationery and I am keeping it in my special file until I get home where I can have it framed. There is a medal to go with the ribbon and a special lapel button when it is time to become a civilian. I am enclosing a copy of the citation so that you may see why they gave me the award. I think I told you that it is the equivalent of the Bronze Star except it is for work in peacetime. So now, with Leroy's [Ardean's brother] we have two decorations in the family. Everyone out here was mighty glad to see me get the award and all of the men are congratulating me. In addition, the General intimated that my promotion might come through in the near future. It is now in Washington. Don't bank on it too highly, but there is a real chance for it now." My citation read as follows:

THE COMMANDING GENERAL
WESTERN PACIFIC BASE COMMAND
by Direction of
THE SECRETARY OF WAR
AWARDS
THE ARMY COMMENDATION RIBBON
TO

Major MICHAEL J. LEPORE, 0–505780, MC Army of the
United States

CITATION: For meritorious service rendered as Chief of Medical Service of the 148th General Hospital, APO 244, from 23 November 1945 to 4 February 1946 and as Chief of Medical Service 369th Station Hospital, APO 244, from 6 October 1945 to 22 November 1945 and 5 February 1946 to 20 February 1946. Major LEPORE exhibited outstanding ability in maintaining a superior medical service in a large station hospital and a 2000 bed general hospital during a difficult transition period. When losses of key personnel by readjustment presented extremely difficult problems, Major LEPORE expended more than the expected duty time and effort necessary to overcome obstacles encountered. His superior professional skill and expert leadership were responsible for maintaining without interruption the high standards of medical care by these hospitals.

W. W. IRVINE
Brigadier General, USA
Command

201.22 (0) 16 Apr 46

As I prepared to leave Saipan for my next Army assignment, there is a story I must tell about Amelia Earhart (1897–1937) that was making the military rumor mill in 1945 on Saipan. The conversation would start with "Pst, do you know who is Tokyo Rose?" "No, who is she?" "Amelia Earhart." "Oh, no!" "Yes. She was really a spy, was captured when her plane went down while photographing Japanese fortifications of the Pacific Islands, and taken to Saipan. Later she and her navigator were executed." We all believe this was fantasy, but a recent book by Randall Brink entitled *Lost Star—The Search for Amelia Earhart* has once again raised the question with a rather convincing story. He believes that Amelia Earhart was captured by the Japanese while photographing Japanese military fortifications on the islands of the South Pacific and imprisoned as a United States spy on Saipan. Brink insists that the U.S. government has tried to cover up the truth, saying "In this book, I deal only with the truth about Amelia Earhart's last flight, a truth withheld by our government because of a tenuous peace with Japan in the Pacific and concerns for the national security at home. . . . Those who knew this truth, and held it close, knew that Earhart and Noonan had survived. They believed it was their duty to hide the truth, and so they did. . . . Despite the unsettling behavior of officialdom, however, we must not lose sight of the great courage and patriotism Amelia Earhart displayed in her last flight; government secrecy, in fact, has deprived her of her fair measure of glory as an authentic American hero. A pacifist who may have undergone a profound spiritual struggle before deciding to become involved in a military mission, she pursued two goals in her espionage: the protection of U.S. national security, and the prevention of war in the Pacific. In a very real sense, whatever the details of her fate, she gave her life for her country as did her navigator, Fred Noonan. She would not have regretted taking the risk."[1]

In due time I boarded the *Cape Mendocino* for Oahu and, after a boring but tranquil five-day voyage, reached my destination on 10 May 1946. As we docked, there was a message over the loudspeaker for me. I was being met by a sergeant in a staff car assigned to Colonel Tynes, the commanding officer of Tripler General Hospital. I thought this was a very nice gesture and welcomed the opportunity to have some help with my baggage.

I was taken directly to Colonel Tynes's office in the hospital. He was a tall, handsome, and intelligent man who told me how glad he was to see me. He asked me whether I played golf. I said "No." "Tennis?"—same answer. "Surfing?" "I don't even swim."

"Fishing?" "No, sir." "Well, what do you do?" "I guess I must be a pretty good doctor or you wouldn't want me here." He then tried to talk me into extending my stay in the Army for one year, which I declined with thanks. Next he tried to persuade me to stay for six months. By this time, I realized that, since leaving Saipan, something interesting must have happened having to do with my eligibility for a quick trip home. Sure enough, new regulations had been issued and I was now eligible to go home. Colonel Tynes continued the discussion and said the Army would pay for my wife's fare to Oahu if I would stay on. I knew this was no solution for me or Ardean because her mother was sick with Alzheimer's disease and confined to the Pennsylvania Hospital with substantial bills being paid out of my pay-check and Ardean's. I needed to go home to resume my private prac-tice to meet my obligations and secure our future. I did not tell Colonel Tynes about my mother-in-law's illness, but I indicated to him that I had entered the Army as a volunteer, had served effectively, and now was ready to return to my professional career as a civilian. We talked a little more and I agreed to stay at Tripler for two weeks as professional consultant, making rounds and seeing a few special patients in consultation. I later found out that the news had been spread to the large number of retired officers in Oahu that a new and highly qualified professional consultant in medicine and diagnostician had been assigned to Tripler General Hospital. As a result, a number of interesting people sought me out for advice. One of the most unusual was Major General Bryant Wells, retired commander of the Hawaiian command. General Wells was a pleasant, alert man in his eighties who consulted me because of hypertension and backache of several years' standing. He was robust and active, appearing younger than his stated age. Except for essential hypertension of moderate degree I found little of note in his general physical examination. His electrocardiogram and blood-chemistry values were normal, though

---

1. Randall Brink, *Lost Star: The Search for Amelia Earhart* (New York and London: W. W. Norton & Company, 1994).

he had hematologic findings of mild primary Addisonian anemia. His electrocardiogram was normal as was his chest x-ray. A film of his lower back turned up a surprise, a large lead bullet in his left buttock. When I next saw him, I asked whether he had ever been wounded and he answered "Yes. On San Juan Hill as a second lieutenant, infantry, following Teddy Roosevelt. I did what most inexperienced second lieutenants did, kept my rump too high while I was going up the hill and I was hit in my left buttock. But how did you detect this? My battalion surgeon told me he removed the bullet." I informed the General that the x-ray showed a large lead bullet of the type used in the Spanish-American War in his buttock. In those days the bullets were very large but did not have the velocity of current ordnance. The general then said "Let's remove the bullet." I explained to him that his backache was due to osteoarthritis and not to the bullet. I had discussed the problem with the Army surgeon, who advised against removing the bullet because it was not responsible for the General's backache. General Wells was the uncle of Dr. Lawrence Wells Sloan and the brother of Dr. Sloan's mother. Dr. Sloan and I were good friends at P&S where he was a professor of surgery. The general knew I was leaving for home soon and would return to the Harkness Pavilion staff. He said, "Tell my nephew Larry that the Army doctors have lost their nerve. If he will operate, I will come to Harkness Pavilion to have him do it." I did show the films to Dr Sloan, who agreed that the bullet did not need to be removed.

Colonel Tynes showed me through the brand new Tripler Army Hospital nearing completion on a hill looking down on Pearl Harbor. He was very proud of the building and had played a role in its development and construction. I believe he had some training in architecture and construction. Old Tripler Hospital was wearing out and consisted of wooden two-story buildings that were not fireproof or earthquake-proof. New Tripler was a magnificent permanent structure, fireproof and earthquake-proof with all of the state-of-the-art equipment of a modern medical center of that era. Colonel Tynes told me that the cost overrun in its construction was enormous, many millions, and Congress was raising Cain over the enormous costs and demanding an investigation. I told Colonel Tynes that any physician who had served in the Western Pacific Theater could testify that it was essential to have a top-flight permanent hospital center for the forward areas. In fact, I told him that, if necessary, I would be glad to testify before Congress to that effect. The criticism quieted down. The money spent on new Tripler was a fraction of what it would cost today to build a similar medical center. It was a great investment in the future.

True to his word, when I had finished my short tour as professional consultant at Tripler, Colonel Tynes issued orders for me to head for home. My trip home on the *Marine Devil* to the Golden Gate was uneventful and followed by a long and dreary troop train ride from the West Coast to Fort Dix in New Jersey, where I was discharged and authorized to wear the silver leaves of Lt. Colonel given to me by Colonel Thomas Fitz-Hugh.

Chapter 17

Return to Columbia-Presbyterian, 1946

WORDS FAIL ME TO ADEQUATELY DESCRIBE what it was like to return to my beloved wife after a separation of more than a year. To see her beautiful face, to hear her lovely voice, and to hold her close was an incredible reward for the many days and months of separation and living apart. Our first days were spent trying to make up for all that had been lost. Soon we had to come down to earth to face the realities of the day. We disposed of our Philadelphia apartment by turning it over to Ardean's close friend and associate Helen Hawthorne, the directress of nurses at the Graduate Hospital of the University of Pennsylvania. Getting an automobile proved very frustrating. It was routine for auto salesmen to demand cash under the table for a new car, and I had decided I would not pay these bastards any of my hard-earned money as a bribe. This left me with few options. New cars were out of the question. Those who had not gone to war had long before been placed on priority lists for new cars when the manufacturers resumed making them. For shame on the major automobile makers, there was no preference given to doctors or returning war veterans. The automobile agencies we had dealt with before WW II had long since gone out of business. The situation was especially bad in New York City. In Philadelphia, through the intervention of my brother-in-law Leroy, who had returned to his position as vice president of a small bank and was doing business with a Buick agency, I was able to obtain a well-used Buick sedan for $1,200 without any bribes being passed. Ardean and I now had a means of transportation and we set out for New York. Here we found the housing situation in an unbelievable mess. Nothing was available for returning veterans no matter what they might be willing to pay. Finally, a good friend of ours, Miss Martha Swensson, came to our rescue by subletting a modest one-room studio in Greenwich Village on Carmine Street. Each morning, Ardean and I would scan the *New York Times* looking for an apartment to rent, to no avail. The doctors'-office situation was equally bad, except that the Columbia-Presbyterian Medical Center had built some new doctors' offices in Harkness Pavilion expressly for returning veterans. I was given special dispensation by being allocated time in a large and beautiful office on the main floor of Harkness Pavilion.

There was also the problem of finding a permanent place to live. After several months of indecision, we found an advertisement in the *New York Times* of a house for lease in West Englewood, New Jersey. We called to find out whether it was available and much to our surprise it was. We canceled all other appointments and drove to the address in New Jersey. There we found the street cluttered with automobiles, centering about a modest and neat two-story brick house. Inside was a mélange of people milling around. We located the owners, a high school teacher and his wife, who were taking a leave of absence for one year. They seemed quite baffled by the large number of people who wanted the house. Their dog, a Manchester Terrier named Tippy, nosed up to me and, since I like animals, we were soon communicating very well with each other. This was noted by the teacher who chatted with me and my wife and after a bit asked whether we would take care of the dog while they were in Florida for a year. We said of course we would be glad to do this. Needless to say, we were given the lease for the house. We jumped at the opportunity to be living in a house all to ourselves and welcomed Tippy as our guest—or perhaps it was the other way around. I had some reservations as to how well it would work out for me to practice in New York and live in New Jersey. Before the war I had lived in New York City near the Medical Center and I wondered how this new arrangement would work out as my practice increased. Since I had little or no choice, I resigned myself to the inevitable, as did many other doctors on our staff. The adjustment was not difficult and it led to my permanent residence in New Jersey, using the George Washington Bridge each day to commute to my professional headquarters.

When I returned to Columbia-Presbyterian from military service, it was assumed by most that I would return to my salaried position as director of the personnel medical department and continue my prewar teaching activities, clinical investigation, and private practice. Being on geographic full time would facilitate these activities and present many advantages over having an outside office. There were also some disadvantages and problems. After a good deal of thought, I had decided not to return to the personnel medicine position. I felt that my professional future lay in further development of my career as a teacher, clinical investigator and Oslerian-type physician. During my tour of duty in the Army, I had matured in many ways. I knew I could be at the top of any organization with which I was associated. I had earned my spurs or my silver leaves by performing Army service equivalent to that of a clinical professor in charge of a large department. I had the energy and the drive to move ahead and lead where others had faltered. I did not wish to become a full-time academician. I wanted to be a full-time clinician and an expert in the diagnosis and management of complex diseases and dealing with interesting people. I had no desire to be known as an industrial doctor or primarily as an administrator. Was general internal medicine what I wanted to pursue, or would further opportunity be in my development as a subspecialist? These were questions to which I had dedicated much time and thought. Now, after four years in military service, I felt I was in the position to make some interesting moves. Because I had played such a key role in developing the personnel medical department, heavy pressure was placed upon me to resume that post. This included a substantial increase in salary, pension, insurance, and other perks, plus increased budget and space. In addition, it was indicated that soon there would be rationing of office space in Harkness Pavilion. As personnel medical director, I would be entitled to all the hours I needed in a permanent office in Harkness Pavilion for my private practice. If I refused the directorship, my Harkness hours would be reduced. Despite the pressures I decided not to return to the personnel medical department. I felt I had done my job, paid my dues, and was now ready to move ahead with my professional growth along the lines I personally preferred. This meant I was passing up the financial and economic security guaranteed by the position of director of the personnel medical department. Once again, as I did when I left Duke, I was taking the less-traveled path, the lonesome road, the hard way to achieve my career goals. Now I had my beloved wife by my side, encouraging me and supporting my efforts. We were young, unafraid, and confident that we could achieve anything and everything that we sought. I often recalled Dean Whipple's advice to me that success in achieving my goals would depend upon "how I used my leisure time." How right he was!

Let us return to the Vanderbilt Clinic of 1946. It was required of all attending physicians on the staff at Columbia-Presbyterian to teach medical students and give at least two afternoons a week to the Vanderbilt Clinic. After a brief vacation I resumed work at the Columbia-Presbyterian Medical Center and Harkness Pavilion and returned to my two afternoon sessions weekly in the Vanderbilt Clinic. The come-down from high positions in the military where some, like myself, had been in charge of large general-hospital medical services but were now reduced to teaching one medical student two afternoons a week, was humiliating for some, resented by a few, and seen as a challenge by others. Most of us were now board-certified specialists, a relatively new phenomenon for rating professional competence. We had made the grade in stiff competition and we expected recognition for this in the hierarchy of academic medicine.

I was one of the last attending physicians to return to P&S from military service and very few were aware of my outstanding record at Valley Forge and overseas. The medical service at Valley Forge General Hospital where I served for over three years as chief of the 100-bed Officers' and Womens' Section under Colonel Marshall N. Fulton, a distinguished Harvard Medical School professor, a Peter Bent Brigham attending and former Rhodes Scholar and Oslerian, was an unforgettable professional and personal experience. That staff at Valley Forge was easily as good as that of any major university medical school and better than many. We were now, without our silver leaves, ribbons, and medals, merely civilians busy trying to rebuild our practices, pay our bills, work for free in the clinics and wards—re-entering the competition for academic and professional recognition that is the heart's blood of all university medical centers. Columbia University's College of Physicians and Surgeons, like many of the other prestigious medical schools, was niggardly in granting academic recognition to its voluntary staff, holding accomplished and dedicated men and women for years at incredibly low levels with advances at a snail's pace, while salaried full timers, by comparison, were moved up rapidly. Sooner or later these inequities would have to be addressed. One of the reasons that Mt. Sinai Hospital, a superb affiliate of Columbia University College of Physicians and Surgeons, broke away from its parent institution and started its own medical school was the inadequate academic recognition of its teaching staff, most of it consisting of volunteers who were in private practice. I recall quite vividly Dr. Hans Popper's story of the disaffiliation and his interview with Dean Houston Merritt of P&S. Dean Merritt was aware that one of the reasons Mt. Sinai was breaking away was because it had been shabbily treated in its allotment of academic titles. He advised Dr. Popper not to start a new medical school and offered to allocate an increased number of clinical professorships to the Mt. Sinai staff. Dr. Popper listened impatiently and when the Dean had finished, his Viennese-accented reply was, "Dean Merritt, your offer is egzatically tsen years tzoo late." The medical school was started and Dr. Popper, a great pathologist and a marvelous human being, was its first Dean.

Similar problems with respect to the academic recognition of the voluntary teaching staff have arisen in many other centers, not the least of which was Johns Hopkins. There the attack was focused on the use of the title "clinical professor" for the voluntary staff and "professor" for the clinical salaried staff. This was unacceptable to the volunteers, who argued that all of the men and women involved were clinicians, so that the use of "clinical" was redundant. They made their point. The word "clinical" was deleted from the titles and a "professor" is a professor at Johns Hopkins. I have rather mixed feelings about this and wonder if anything has been gained by this change. With the increased emphasis on research and administration and the decline in clinical skills of many academic physicians, perhaps we shall see the day when the title "clinical professor" will be reinstated and regarded as the honor it was originally intended to be.

In keeping with the Flexnerian concept that the university medical center should not be too deeply involved in its surrounding community, Columbia-Presbyterian has never had an on-call ambulance service for the general public. In case of emergency, people of Washington Heights had to depend on the ambulance service of a small and poorly equipped institution, Mother Cabrini Hospital on Edgecomb Avenue. Those who could afford a private ambulance and had a doctor on the staff of the Medical Center could arrange to go there if there was a bed. This was one way to limit access to the Medical Center by sick people with run-of-the-mill ailments deemed unsuitable for the ward teaching service.

A poignant example of this policy in action was brought home to me while I was at Valley Forge. In March 1943 I received a black-bordered letter from my friend Bill Warren. It speaks for itself:

> Dear Michael: As you have doubtless judged from the stationery, mama has passed away. There is little more I can say. She just "sat down" in our hallway two weeks ago and came up with a broken hip (upper left femur). After four hours I finally got a doctor. Of course, little could be done but hospitalization. Unfortunately, no Medical Center connections and Mother Cabrini refused on "age grounds." Result—Morrisania Hospital. As you perhaps anticipated her sclerosis condition which had steadily grown worse, was fatal. She passed away at 8:40 P.M. on March 6th, 1943. Services are being held from the Henry J. Meyer Funeral Chapel at 459 W. 145 Street, N.Y.C. on Tuesday, March 9th and interment will be at Freehold, N.J. We know that you will be with us in spirit. Good luck. Bill.

"Mamma," as he called his grandmother, that great lady who had raised Bill from infancy, and had been so good to me when we were growing up, was gone under circumstances beyond my control. By the time Bill's letter reached me at Valley Forge, delayed by being sent to the Army and Navy General Hospital in Arkansas, the funeral had been consummated and she was laid to rest in the family plot in Freehold, New Jersey, that already held her husband and her son, Uncle Sam Warren. Perhaps it was just as well that I was spared the agony of her terminal illness. Bill and I had lost the only grandmother either one of us had known. I shall never forget her. After the war was over and I had returned to the staff of the Columbia-Presbyterian Medical Center with my office in Harkness Pavilion, I had occasion to examine Bill Warren because of hoarseness. Suspecting the worst, I admitted him to our hospital, where we found he had carcinoma of the larynx requiring laryngectomy. Metastases followed and I said good-by to my friend after several months of illness. It was the end of an era for us. But, at least, this time I was there to comfort him and to see that his terminal illness was as painless as possible in a fine medical center. I had in some measure repaid my debt to "mamma." Among my treasured memories is Bill Warren's black-bordered letter of our bereavement.

As I write this story, tears well up in my eyes and there is suppressed anger in my heart for a system of medical care that served my friends, the Warrens, so poorly during WW II when Mrs. Warren suffered the hip fracture. They were then living only a few city blocks from the Medical Center where she wished to be admitted and she ended up in an overcrowded, understaffed city hospital in the Bronx, miles away from her family and friends. Why hasn't there ever been a municipal hospital in Washington Heights? As one who grew up in that section, actively practiced there, and made house calls, I know that the area needed a large general municipal hospital designed to meet the burgeoning demands of the community. Building Francis Delafield Hospital on Medical Center property was not the answer, for it was limited to cancer patients. What was needed was a second Bellevue with an ambulance service.

I have documented elsewhere that in the original planning for the Columbia-Presbyterian Medical Center there had been no provision for private patients. When Mr. Harkness' attention was directed to this, as an afterthought, Harkness Pavilion for private patients was added to the plans. This pavilion contained single-occupancy private rooms where, in the early days, a nice room cost only seven dollars a day. A few semiprivate rooms were added to the ward floors, also as an afterthought.

During WW II, the Medical Center Administration realized that a large number of low-cost semi-private rooms would be needed. We received a letter overseas advising us that a semiprivate pavilion would be added to the Medical Center in the space between Harkness and the Eye Institute. This promise was never kept. There were several reasons for this, perhaps the chief being the retirement of key administrators and department heads and their replacement by a new team. To complicate matters, a hospital-administrative-faculty committee concluded that the present clinical attending staff was larger than necessary for the educational and patient needs of the Medical Center and that there should be a gradual reduction in the overall clinical staff. You may well imagine how this report was greeted by the medical staff, only recently returned from military service, who felt that they had been betrayed. Instead of providing more beds to meet the urgent demands of sick people, the plan was to reduce admissions by getting rid of some of the staff. I believe that this report, coupled with some unfortunate choices of new department heads and administrators, was the beginning of a downhill slide for the Columbia-Presbyterian Medical Center, from which it has only recently begun to recover.

I have known several medical-school Deans in my lifetime. The best ones wore tan laboratory coats or white coats and continued to teach medical students despite heavy administrative demands. Founding Dean George H. Whipple of the University of Rochester School of Medicine taught us pathology and managed to win a Nobel Prize while building and administrating a great and new medical center. He wore a tan laboratory coat. Another famous Founding Dean, Wilburt C. Davison of Duke, worked in his shirt sleeves without a necktie and taught pediatrics in addition to all of his other duties. Dean Rappleye wore a business suit and, to the best of my knowledge, did not teach medical students.

To my mind the greatest Dean the Columbia University College of Physicians and Surgeons has ever had was Samuel Waldron Lambert, who was appointed to this position in 1904. He is credited with revolutionizing medical educational at P&S by reducing didactic lectures and class size and instituting recitation classes with active student participation, introducing the system of clinical clerks, and bringing medical students into the wards of some New York hospitals when most hospital administrators opposed it.

I did not have the privilege of knowing Dean Lambert, but his son Sam Jr. was my first chief of service in the Vanderbilt Clinic, where he was very helpful and supportive. In an interview in 1976 he said of his father's great record, "And all this was achieved by one Dean, who also maintained a very extensive medical (and obstetrical) practice, and made house calls, and by one secretary, Miss Wheeler, a most remarkable woman."[1] Dr. Albert R. Lamb, who knew the Dean very well and was, in fact, his personal physician, describes him as a

---

1. S. W. Lambert, Jr., *P & S Quarterly*, Winter 1976, p. 11.

marvelous human being and a Dickensian character with an earthy, robust manner, hearty laugh, and a very keen and alert mind.[2] An avid disciple of Izaak Walton and a scholarly bibliophile and an avid anti-Prohibitionist, he believed as did Robert Louis Stevenson that it is the natural act of a sturdy man to inveigh. His friends and colleagues, Henry S. Paterson and Foster Kennedy, said: "He barked often, but he never bit. He defined in himself the notion of a gentleman as being a man who never hurt another man—unintentionally. He reorganized education in medicine. He taught medicine in clear light, without half shadows. He could smell a sham at 100 yards. He added to our knowledge, to our gaiety, to our culture, to our pride."[3]

Another colleague, Edward L. Keyes, said "The most characteristic yarn about him tells how a patient in the Presbyterian Hospital begged that Dr. Lambert come to her room and when he came, said 'Doctor, I had to see you. For days I have listened to you swear so beautifully at the patient in the next room that I just had to have you in to swear at me a little, I do so need to be cheered up.'"[4]

The concept of reducing the staff to cut down the admission of patients was completely out of touch with the real problem, the paucity of beds in an era of great demand. Whoever made that decision was completely out of touch with the realities of the practice of medicine. Service to the sick should have been at the top of the list rather than the bottom. The small but powerful cadre of full timers appeared to have taken over complete control.

When news of this Faculty Committee's recommendations leaked to those of us on the staff, it was interpreted, and I believe correctly, as a blow against the voluntary staff, many of whom were veterans of WW II. Instead of expanding the number of beds as had been promised, they were going to reduce the staff and use private office space in the Medical Center as a weapon for enforcing demands upon the voluntary staff. Within months of their return from active military service in WW II, many of the voluntary staff were called in by newly appointed department directors and advised to reduce their office

---

2. A. R. Lamb, *Presbyterian Hospital and Columbia-Presbyterian Medical Center, 1868-1943* (New York: Columbia University Press, 1955), p. 151.

3. Henry S. Patterson and Foster Kennedy, "Samuel Waldron Lambert (1859–1942)," read before the Charaka Club, April 15, 1942, p. 133.

4. Edward L. Keyes, "For Sam Lambert", read before the Chanaka Club, April 16, 1942, p. 135.

hours in Harkness and to seek non-existent office space in downtown Manhattan. The staff felt that their needs were not being addressed and that promises made to the returning veterans were not being kept. Instead of expanding to cope with the heavy demands being made for the care of the sick who were flocking to our doors, we were being told to get out to make place for the next wave of newly minted residents. Waiting lists for admission became longer and longer. Some of the doctors sought and obtained privileges in other hospitals, making it difficult for them to fulfill their duties at Columbia-Presbyterian. Many began to question the sincerity of Columbia-Presbyterian in their dealings with private practitioners-volunteers. There was much grumbling, but no rebellion because of fear of loss of privileges. Most of all, there was no organization representing the voluntary staff and championing their cause.

Shortly after my return to the Vanderbilt Clinic, renovations of the physical plant were undertaken and some new concepts introduced. The General Medical Clinic was now called the Group Clinic, a term that seemed attractive to the powers that be; the only new thing about it was that when consultants were needed, they could be summoned to the Group Clinic where the students and the attendings would present the case and discuss further management. This was believed by the supporters of the change to mimic how the real world deals with consultations and ambulatory patients. An obvious objection to this was that facilities for specialty examinations were limited, for example for pelvic examinations and Pap smears, ENT and Eye examinations, etc. These were dismissed as minor objections, the goal being to show the medical student how a real doctor in practice solves a problem and calls upon his colleagues for assistance.

The truth of the matter is that in the real world, except for emergencies, the consultant's opinion has to be arranged for another day in his office. We were willing to give the Group Clinic concept a fair trial, but initially we had some reservations.

I soon realized that our medical students were getting a rather mixed bag of teaching from the attendings in the Vanderbilt Clinic. Some of the attendings were highly qualified if not over-qualified for their assignments and some were not. Some were meticulous and prompt in attendance and others were careless or harassed by heavy outside-practice commitments. Some were energetic and superb teachers while others needed re-education and supervision. Theoretically all of us could attend Team Rounds and Grand Rounds, but the pressures and demands of private practice often made attendance at these exercises impractical or impossible. The medical students, through their underground, quickly became aware of the best teachers and sought every device to be assigned to them. For example, if the assigned attending were late, the student could be assigned to a substitute, usually an attending who had already reviewed the one case assigned to him. If he agreed to take on an extra patient, his "reward" would be that the patient be added on to his own patient load and not assigned to the attending who had failed to show up. Over the months and years this could add up to quite an additional caseload for the most dedicated and able attendings. An alert chief of clinic could have prevented this by merely ruling that the extra patient would return to the attending originally assigned.

It did not take a genius to figure out that all attendings are not equal and that some sort of supervision was needed to ensure an acceptable level of patient care in the outpatient setting. Since we were seeing and treating sicker elderly people in the ambulatory setting, I felt that a greater effort should be made to utilize ambulatory patients in our teaching program for their benefit as well as for the medical students and the attending staff. I decided to propose that we have outpatient Team Rounds once weekly at the end of the clinic session at 5 P.M., patterned on the Team Rounds held once each week for the inpatient service. The case presentation would be by the medical student to whom the patient was assigned. The discussion would be initiated by the attending of record and opened to the audience at large. Two cases would be presented.

Freshly returned from military service, I prepared a typewritten memorandum describing the above and sent it through channels to the chief of clinic and awaited his answer.

> Dr. Frederick Randolph Bailey
> Presbyterian Hospital
>
> Dear Dr. Bailey:
>   I would like to take the liberty of making a suggestion regarding the Group Clinic. As you know, the scarcity of hospital beds, the increased demand for diagnostic services and other factors have resulted in the appearance in the Group Clinic of many interesting patients with unusual diseases. Many of these patients, in other times, would have been admitted to the hospital for diagnosis and treatment and some would probably have been presented at Team Rounds. As it now stands, an interesting case may be seen by a relatively small group of men and others who might be interested are not aware that such a patient is being seen in the clinic.
>   Without dwelling upon this at any great length, I would like to suggest that outpatient "Team Rounds" be held once weekly.

This conference could function just as the inpatient Team Rounds with the exception that 1. The fourth-year medical student present his case. 2. The attending who examined the patient would participate in the discussion and 3. The Chief of Clinic would preside.

This program would be of excellent teaching value to the student for it would enlist his active participation and bring to his attention many ailments seen in the clinic and not in the hospital. In addition, diagnostic and therapeutic outpatient problems could be presented for review. This would be of excellent educational value for the attendings and might result in greater uniformity of management of individual cases. Finally, I believe supervision of this sort would result in an even level of medical practice in the Vanderbilt Clinic.

Respectfully yours,
Michael J. Lepore, M.D.

I never received a written answer or explanation. I think there was some fear that the Outpatient Team Rounds might be in competition with Medical Grand Rounds. In addition there were those who felt that it would simply add to their workload. Others felt that the care of ambulatory patients was second-class work and a boring necessity. Some felt threatened by the possible exposure of their weaknesses in teaching. Nothing was really done about this suggestion except that I was assigned additional responsibilities for consultations in gastroenterology. This memorandum was sent in April 1947, only a few weeks before Dr. Palmer retired at the mandatory age of 65 years. Perhaps it was regarded as something that his successor as Bard professor, Dr. Robert F. Loeb, should address.

It was about this time that Dr. Palmer dropped into his Harkness office, where I was seeing my patients, and had a chat with me. We knew he was due to retire but we hoped that he could have an extension. He told me that he was required to accept mandatory retirement at sixty-five, no exception being made. He also indicated that he would have to start private practice, since his pension was grossly inadequate to cover his needs. He still had children to educate. I felt very sad to hear this because it seemed to me that the full-time system that he had served so faithfully had failed to provide him with a pension adequate for his needs. I know he had suffered an acute myocardial infarct some years before and doubted that he had a long period of life ahead. I could not help but wonder why this magnificent teacher, administrator, and man of wisdom was not given a position worthy of his superb capabilities. What kind of a system is this?, I asked myself. His last words to me I have never forgotten. "Lepore," he said, "no matter what they offer you here take my advice, in addition to a few office hours here in Harkness Pavilion, get yourself a downtown office where you can be your own boss when you reach 65." I can assure you that I soon began looking for downtown office space. I also swore that I would never accept a full-time salaried position or be dominated by an institution, a university, a hospital, a corporation, an HMO, or a government agency. A few weeks later, I learned that Dr. Palmer had been appointed director of the Public Health Research Institute in New York with a salary. Unfortunately, Dr. Palmer died in 1950, less than three years after occupying his new position. I had lost a mentor and warm friend who had kept the faith. I shall never forget the encouraging handwritten letters he sent to me when I was ten thousand miles away on Tinian and Saipan.

Chapter 18

The Changing of the Guard at the Medical Center

ON 1 JULY 1947, ONE YEAR after most of the veterans had returned from military service, Dr. Walter W. Palmer accepted mandatory retirement at age 65. He was succeeded as the Bard professor and chairman of the department of medicine by the brilliant and dynamic Dr. Robert F. Loeb, who had been standing in the wings for some years and had turned down many offers to go elsewhere. Dr. Loeb was probably the member of our staff most committed to the policy of full time in the clinical chairs. In fact, it was said of him that he believed that the personal practice of medicine was all right so long as there was no payment involved. If any money changed hands, it was prostitution. Loeb was the only one of the original full-time clinical faculty of 1921 in medicine at P&S who remained on full time when all of the others defected to geographic full time because of the inadequate full-time salaries that were offered. Among those who defected was Dana W. Atchley, a close friend and collaborator of Loeb's. It was common knowledge at P.H. that Loeb would not let the opportunity pass for ribbing Dana Atchley about his prosperous private practice. On one occasion, on meeting Dr. Atchley in the hall, Loeb is said to have jingled some change in his pocket and said "Dana, how much money did you make today?" Loeb could have some very strong opinions and he had few reservations about expressing them. He did not like surgeons and expressed the view that an important function of an internist was to keep the patient out of the surgeons' hands. He also did not like to see young attending staff owning luxury automobiles, and did not hesitate to criticize them. He took a fairly dim view of psychiatrists and the highest compliment he could pay a newly appointed head of psychiatry at P&S was to say he "did not look like a psychiatrist." Loeb was completely committed to Flexnerian full time while Dr. Palmer had taken a middle-of-the-road position, saying in his farewell address of 1947 that he was proud to have brought together a "goodly company of full-time men combined with sympathetic and cooperative men in practice affording wide flexibility in organization."[1]

My personal belief is that Dr. Loeb should have been awarded a Nobel Prize for his work in Addison's Disease. Dr. Loeb was a

Renaissance man, probably the most effective bedside teacher of modern medicine I have ever met, with an amazing grasp of scientific concepts applicable to solving clinical problems. He ran a tight ship and made every effort to spur his house staff, students, and attending staff to achieve higher and higher standards. All papers published from the department of medicine during his tenure had to be cleared and critiqued by Dr. Loeb. In those days when we used to have a sign-in sheet in the doctors' locker room of Presbyterian Hospital, he was always the first to sign in, bright and early. His daily sunrise sessions with his house staff were never to be forgotten and served to keep the entire house staff on its toes and in touch with all of the interesting developments on the medical service and, on occasion, the world outside. It was not long after he was appointed Bard professor that he set aside time for individual interviews with most of the attending staff regarding their aspirations and needs as well as what the department expected of them. He was determined to reallocate the hours and space used by the voluntary staff in the doctors' private offices in Harkness Pavilion, where rooms had been expressly built to accommodate returning veterans. What he wished to do was to displace the veterans so that he could install newly appointed men who had just completed their residencies and needed to start private practice to pay their bills. Of course, this led to some hard feelings among those who had served in the war, especially since the real difficulty was that outside office space was in very short supply and very expensive. Some complained that the hospital had failed to keep its promises. The trouble was that those who had made the promises were either dead or retired. Loeb, a Flexnerian to the core, did not believe that service to the surrounding community should be a high priority for a tertiary-care university center. Carried to an extreme, this could lead to isolation of the Medical Center from its immediate neighbors, planting the seeds of future dissension and hostility. Other changes were taking place in the Medical Center that were causing some concern. During Dr. Palmer's reign, the general internist was king. The subspecialties were relatively unimportant and undeveloped. This tradition prevailed through Dr. Loeb's term of office and Dr. Loeb himself was the epitome of the general internist. Those of us who had been in military service where the medical services were divided into subspecialty sections had adjusted to that system and liked it.

We had learned to work efficiently and harmoniously with our surgical colleagues in an atmosphere of mutual respect. The lessons

---

1. Lepore, *Death of the Clinician: Requiem or Reveille?*, p. 212.

learned would soon be manifest in our day-to-day activities at Columbia-Presbyterian. My practice in general internal medicine was flourishing, and so was my workload in the Vanderbilt Clinic. In fact, as the years passed, the demands being made upon me for service in the Vanderbilt Clinic, largely of my own making, were getting out of hand. Through my interest in sprue, I joined forces with my friend, Dr. Paul di Sant'Agnese, a talented pediatrician and researcher on the full-time Babies' Hospital staff who, with Dr. Dorothy Andersen was an authority on celiac disease of children and cystic fibrosis. I started a celiac-sprue clinic for adults with the disease as well as for children who had outgrown the pediatric clinic age. On another day, I would see and follow adult patients with cystic fibrosis and other pancreatic ailments. In those days children with cystic fibrosis seldom survived into adulthood, so the number being followed in the clinic was small. When broad-spectrum antibiotics became available, the number of survivors increased to the point that I was following twenty-one sick patients. The antibiotics were supplied without charge by various pharmaceutical firms in limited amounts, and our patients were constantly running out of supplies and attempting to stretch out the remaining amounts by reducing the daily dose. One of the most distressing things for me to witness was the abject poverty of the families of those afflicted with the disease, sometimes with several children involved. The sick children would be warmly clothed in the winter while their normal siblings wore castoff and threadbare clothing. Clearly, what these children needed was more than antibiotics and medical care. They were in need of better housing, better food and nutrition, and other supportive measures, something our clinic, no matter how well disposed it might be, could not provide. I discussed this with Dr. di Sant'Agnese and Dr. Andersen on several occasions, and we finally came up with the idea that we should find a way to declare the children to be handicapped and eligible for state aid. This was before we had Medicaid. It was not until the administration of Governor Nelson Rockefeller that our goal was achieved. We breathed a sigh of relief when this assistance was made available to the families of patients with cystic fibrosis in New York. Research in the field was primitive by today's standards, and funds for it were quite limited. With the advent of major funding from the N.I.H., a great stimulus was given to research efforts. It has been a joy to witness the recent identification of the abnormal gene responsible for cystic fibrosis and to look forward to therapeutic approaches to curing the disease. *Mirabile dictu!*

It was not long before I was conducting seven different clinics in the Vanderbilt Clinic and enjoying every minute of it. I soon realized that the era of the general internist as king at Columbia-Presbyterian Medical Center, as in most academic institutions, was headed for oblivion. The subspecialties were undergoing major changes and gaining in power and influence. It was clear that, where the general internist ruled the roost in the era of Walter W. Palmer and Robert F. Loeb, that period was ending and great changes were inevitable. With the growth of the subspecialties, capable men and women would no longer flock to general internal medicine. They would seek to enter the subspecialties, where the economic and academic rewards were more substantial. I have indicated in a previous chapter that I myself resisted vigorously the attempt to be classified as a gastroenterologist in WW II and insisted on my listing and assignment as a general internist as chief of medicine of a 2,000-bed Army general hospital. Since then many changes had occurred and I had to reconsider my career goals.

In civilian practice, I was attracted by the field of gastroenterology first by sprue, then by the inflammatory bowel diseases and pancreatic and liver disease. My beloved wife suffered with a chronic duodenal ulcer and I made sure that I knew all that could be learned in that field. I found my general background in physiology and biochemistry, nutrition and metabolic disease, and general internal medicine, great assets, indispensable in advancing knowledge in this subspecialty. My Army experience in psychiatry and so-called psychosomatic medicine, and tropical medicine could be applied with significant benefit in gastroenterology. Another attraction was the paucity of people competent in this field at P&S. In common with most of the major medical schools, there was no formal division or section in gastroenterology at P&S nor was there one at Rochester, Duke, or Yale. There were no fellowships or residencies in this field and no N.I.H. training grants. Most of the doctors already in this specialty were self-taught. Because radiology was a lucrative specialty, many of the gastroenterologists of the day performed their own diagnostic radiologic studies. Soon they were spending most of their time in the darkroom rather than in the clinics, at the bedside, in the open air of the ward, or at clinic teaching services. With the passage of time, I became more and more attracted to gastroenterology and saw in this subspecialty the golden opportunity that I had long sought to apply to the practice of medicine the basic science principles and the biochemical, nutritional, and physiologic concepts I had spent so much of my life studying and developing.

With the retirement of the former head of the rather primitive and mediocre gastrointestinal clinic at Presbyterian Hospital in 1947, I decided to discuss my future career with Dr. Robert F. Loeb, then the

Bard professor and chairman of the department of medicine. We had a very frank discussion during which he acknowledged that he was interested in my career and would assist me in achieving my goals. I indicated that I was willing to join forces with my colleague and senior by six years, Dr. Charles Flood, who had been appointed head of the gastrointestinal clinic, such as it was. I had one condition that I insisted upon, the assignment to me of a separate room where I could see my patients. This may seem to be a small matter but in those days, with the scarcity of space in the Vanderbilt Clinic, rooms were hard to come by. Dr. Loeb was sure there would be no difficulty in arranging this concession, especially after I had described to him the undesirable state of affairs in the existing GI clinic where there was no privacy for the patients and little or no provision for adequate examining facilities. All I was asking for was the same working conditions in vogue in the rest of the Vanderbilt Clinic where I was seeing my other patients. The next day, Dr. Flood called me and welcomed me to the GI clinic and promised to provide a room for my exclusive use. The first day I arrived in the clinic, my room was occupied by a young surgeon. I objected to this firmly, asserted my turf rights, and was never again challenged about this. It should be added that Dr. Loeb insisted that I continue to give two afternoons a week to the General Medical Group Clinic in addition to my new assignment to the GI clinic.

Soon after my return to Columbia-Presbyterian Medical Center, I admitted a young woman to Harkness Pavilion with severe ulcerative colitis of a fulminating type. She failed to respond to the medical measures then available. We had penicillin and sulfa drugs but no other antibiotics. Cortisone and ACTH had not yet been discovered. Surgical and medical consultations were obtained. Surgery, i.e., colectomy with ileostomy, was refused. The surgical staff at Harkness was ultra-conservative and reluctant to operate. One reason was that in the early days of the Medical Center, a young woman who had undergone colectomy with ileostomy had committed suicide by leaping from a window in Presbyterian Hospital because the ileostomy was unmanageable with the bulky Rutzen bags and the malfunctioning stoma so common in those days. Despite all of our efforts, my patient died of the disease. I felt very badly at her loss and knew that something simply had to be done to improve the care and surgery for patients with ulcerative colitis. I discussed the problem with one of the surgical attendings, Dr. John S. Lockwood, a brilliant young surgeon who was in charge of surgical research. He had consulted on this patient and followed her illness with me and he agreed that this was a disease that deserved further study, one that could be devastating and lethal, its etiology unknown, its medical management grossly inadequate, and its surgical management controversial and unsatisfactory. His approach was to organize a team consisting of selected individuals on our staff from medicine, surgery, psychiatry, proctology, and biochemistry. He said he wanted this group to be approved by the executive committee of the medical board, and to meet regularly to organize and provide medical and surgical care for patients with ulcerative colitis in the hospital and also in the Vanderbilt Clinic. He proceeded to obtain the needed administrative approval and the Ulcerative Colitis Study Group was organized. The initial members were, as I recall, Dr. Charles Flood and Dr. Michael Lepore from medicine, Dr. John Lockwood, Dr. Robert Hiatt and Dr. John Prudden from surgery, Dr. C. A. Burt from proctology, Drs. George Daniels and Aaron Karush from psychiatry, and Dr. Karl Meyer from biochemistry. Later we would be joined by additional psychiatrists including Drs. Robert Weiss, Robert Senescu, Bernard Holland, Leon Moses, and John O'Connor. There was quite a turnover in the psychiatrists, several of whom left after relatively short terms to accept professorships in major institutions. I was pleased to have an opportunity to work together with talented psychiatrists in a general hospital setting. The arrangements were beneficial for all of the participants, including our patients.

I continued to be a very active member of this group from its inception in 1947 until I left Columbia-Presbyterian in 1962 to organize and direct the Upjohn Gastrointestinal Service at Roosevelt Hospital. In addition to serving in the Ulcerative Colitis outpatient clinic, I was eventually called for consultation on many of those who were admitted to the ward service of the Presbyterian Hospital. This liaison function proved to be very important because it gave me the opportunity to communicate freely with the house staff. I soon found that many members of the house staff disliked having patients with ulcerative colitis on their wards because they were very anxious and constantly demanding attention for what were judged by house staff and attending doctors to be trivial matters. This attitude would ultimately spread to the nursing staff and aides who needed to be better informed about the disease, its management, and the patients who suffered with it. The disease is found in all age groups, including infants and the elderly, but the most severely affected are young people in what should have been the best years of their lives. The etiology of the disease was and still remains an enigma. The treatment when we started the clinic was mainly supportive and symptomatic. Without Paregoric or Tincture of Opium, we could never have managed our large clinic. Sulfonamides and penicillin were the only antibiotics available. ACTH and cortisone were about to be discovered but were not yet available for experimental trial. The frightening aspect of the disease was that its course was unpredictable and it could be fatal. One of the reasons we had a biochemist in the group was that a new theory that ulcerative colitis might be due to excessive lysozyme production had been proposed. Dr. Karl Meyer was doing research on lysozyme in eye diseases and agreed to work with us. To further stimulate this study, it had been reported that a substance called Nisulfazole could block the action of lysozyme. One of the members of our group studied the effect of retention enemas of Nisulfazole in patients with ulcerative colitis. What initially appeared to be a positive response to this agent turned out to be a placebo effect of the treatment and encouragement given by therapists. We soon abandoned this approach.

The clinic grew by leaps and bounds for a variety of reasons. Most doctors of that era were not only willing but very happy to send their patients with this disease to a clinic staffed by university specialists serving without a fee. In fact, I still remember a telephone conversation I had with a doctor from Long Island who wished to refer one of his sick patients to our clinic. He said "this patient is diarrhea-poor." "What is that?" I asked. He replied that she had already used up all her money trying for a cure to no avail. Needless to say, we accepted the patient as we had many before. Our group was soon following in the neighborhood of five hundred patients with inflammatory-bowel disease. The psychiatrists were having an interesting time of it, working with us as a team. Soon it became quite apparent that their real function was to teach the physicians and surgeons in the group the rudiments and more of the psychiatrists' approach to sick people. For the first time in the clinics and wards of Columbia-Presbyterian we were seeing how well-trained psychiatrists could function as a liaison with the medical staff in applying their skills to the treatment of some very sick people with multiple complaints. Our patients could be very sick with a life-threatening form of the disease and some would die. Others would have to undergo major, risky, and mutilating abdominal surgery. Unfortunately, the after-effects of surgery—chiefly in the early days, ileostomy malfunction—were deemed by many patients to be worse than the original disease. Both internists and surgeons involved in their care were uncertain as to when to intervene surgically, and it would be several years before acceptable guidelines for decision-making could be established.

A formal report of the experience and findings of the psychiatrists in our group was published in 1977, *Psychotherapy in Chronic Ulcerative Colitis*, by Aaron Karush, et al., published by W. F. Saunders Company, Philadelphia. I quote Dr. Karush's concluding paragraph:

The contribution of psychiatry to a fuller understanding and to a more successful treatment of both ulcerative colitis and granulomatous disease of the colon remains controversial in some medical circles. We believe that the stubborn refusal to consider mental etiological factors exposes colitis sufferers to serious and needless risks. It is perhaps the unfortunate result of a tendency of some medical practitioners to treat patients' organs mechanically. As do other humanist physicians the psychiatrist who works with somatic illness tries to view the patient as a whole and to see his illness as an outcome of many operant pathogenic factors. We can only hope that the work and theories of psychodynamics and of psychotherapy described here will advance that viewpoint. Without sacrificing the important pharmacological and surgical contributions to treatment, a more deliberate and more prolonged use of dynamic psychotherapy can only help the colitis patient and reduce his burden of disability. (p. 140)

It would be even better if we could, in Lewis Thomas's eloquent terminology, discard the "half-way technology" of today by finding the etiology of ulcerative colitis and ultimately its cure.[2] In the meantime, we must continue to follow the old French admonition, *"Guerir Quelquefois, Soulager Souvent, Consoler Toujours."*

In retrospect, all of us who participated in this study of ulcerative colitis benefitted in many ways as did our patients. We built an environment at Columbia-Presbyterian where these patients were welcomed and given competent and reliable support.

The surgical staff became very knowledgeable in the field of ulcerative colitis. The major advance was in the introduction of the Brooke-type of ileostomy that proved much easier to manage and freer of complications than any of those used in the past.[3] The bulky Rutzen bags were replaced by many ingenious types of disposable plastic appliances. Nurses were trained as enterostomal specialists who were a great help to those who needed them. With the advent of ACTH and adreno-cortical steroids, a major therapeutic advance appeared on the scene. We had a great deal to learn about their application, but we did not falter in pressing forward. The flame photometer was developed and it did not take us long to learn how to use this information in the care of sick patients. What a joy it was to be

---

2. Lewis Thomas, *The Lives of a Cell* (New York: Viking Press, 1974), pp. 32–36.

3. B. N. Brooke, "The Management of an Ileostomy Including Its Complications," *Lancet* 2 (1952), pp. 102–104.

able to measure serum sodium and serum potassium in a matter of minutes, as compared with the three days it used to take to do serum electrolytes by gravimetric techniques and with less accuracy. Soon the house staff's reluctance to care for patients with ulcerative colitis was overcome and they found themselves learning at the cutting edge of medicine. The surgical house staff was challenged by what was happening and interested in new approaches being tried by their attending surgeons.

The mortality rate for fulminant ulcerative colitis in our hospital was remarkably reduced. Ileoanal anastomoses were tried to eliminate an ileostomy, but they failed because of loss of rectal-sphincter control and severe incontinence. This problem would have to await the development of new surgical procedures including the construction of rectal reservoirs. For a time a small number of our patients with ulcerative colitis were subjected to truncal vagotomy. Two of my patients with severe ulcerative colitis who underwent truncal vagotomy went into prolonged clinical remission, but promising initial reports from other centers failed to continue and we soon abandoned this approach without giving it an adequate trial. One factor that influenced this decision was the death of Dr. John Lockwood, the charismatic head of surgical research. John had suffered a severe myocardial infarct in his late thirties and succumbed to another in his early forties. What a blow to us! I remember my last conversation with him in his office when he wanted to know how several patients of his were getting along, including one who had undergone truncal vagotomy with an excellent clinical remission that persisted long after Dr. Lockwood had died.

As interest in gastroenterology at Columbia-Presbyterian increased there were demands for a bi-weekly GI radiology conference. Some attendings felt that there were already too many conferences and opposed adding to them. I pursued the matter with Dr. Loeb, who helped me by giving permission to go ahead but qualified it in his inimitable way by saying, "Mike, try it for six months. If it works, continue, if not, don't feel badly if you have to discontinue them." I proceeded to organize this new conference as a combined medical-surgical and radiologic GI conference with Dr. Ralph Schlaeger from radiology, myself from medicine and Dr. Milton Porter from surgery in charge. It was held in the Babies' Hospital auditorium and soon became one of the most popular conferences in the medical center. We found that a good title might be the best way to ensure attendance and participation. I recall one in which we discussed ileostomy in ulcerative colitis. Our title was "Ileostomy—A Cure or a Disease." You can rest assured that we attracted many of the surgeons with that one and the discussion was brisk and at times heated, making for what we called "good, clean fun" and excellent teaching.

This combined type of conference was new to our medical center. I have always been very comfortable in working with my surgical colleagues for the benefit of our patients and never did share Dr. Loeb's antipathy for the surgeons. As a matter of fact, two of the best chief residents in surgery asked to work with me on research projects in gastroenterology. The two were Dr. Keith Reemtsma and Dr. James Malm, both of whom have had stellar careers, the first rising to the chairmanship of the department of surgery at P&S and the second to chief of cardiac surgery at P&S. They approached me one evening at my supper table in the Presbyterian Hospital cafeteria where I usually ate after finishing my work in the Vanderbilt Clinic and was fortifying myself for inpatient rounds in Presbyterian Hospital and Harkness Pavilion. Some of my friends nicknamed these sessions the "Lepore supper club." We conducted a good deal of business and communicated informally with the surgical and medical house staff and learned about interesting patients on various services. At that time (1957), while pursuing my interest in sprue, I had read a report from England that Margot Shiner[4] had succeeded in modifying the Wood gastric-biopsy tube so that it could be used to endorally biopsy the small bowel, thereby avoiding an abdominal operation. Shortly thereafter Crosby and Kugler introduced the Crosby capsule for endoral biopsy of the small bowel.[5] The reason I was so interested in small-bowel biopsies was that, at the time, all of the small-bowel histologic studies in sprue had been made on material obtained at autopsy and were subject to criticism that the changes might be due to postmortem autolysis.

Fresh material obtained by endoral sampling appealed to me as a marvelous source of material for study. I discussed these reports with Dr. di Sant'Agnese, who arranged to purchase a Crosby capsule from his celiac research fund. When the capsule arrived, we discussed its use with Dr. Loeb, who told us that he would not permit its use on the medical service unless the surgical staff accepted responsibility for it. This meant we had to persuade the surgical residents to assemble and pass the Crosby capsule each time it was used.

---

4. M. D. Doniach and M. Shiner, "Duodenal and Jejunal Biopsies," *Gastroenterology* 33 (1957), p. 17.

5. W. H. Crosby and H. W. Dugler, "Intraluminal Biopsy Capsule," *Amer J Dig Dis* 2 (1957), p. 216.

What should have been a relatively simple procedure was being converted into a complex matter involving a team of people. Fortunately, Dr. Reemtsma and Dr. Malm were more than equal to the task and we were soon collecting endoral biopsies with success. The next step was to enlist the cooperation of the surgical pathologists in our project. The specimens were small, we knew little about how to orient them for sectioning, and the pathologists had limited experience with the special techniques that were needed. Again we were fortunate enough to arouse the interest of Dr. Raffale Lattes, a superb surgical pathologist in Dr. Arthur Purdy Stout's department. Soon we were at the cutting edge of inquiring into the pathology of celiac-sprue, the main finding being severe atrophy of the small-bowel mucosa. With the major discovery by Dicke of Holland that the cereal grains of wheat, rye, oats, and barley contained a harmful substance that was toxic for the small-bowel mucosa a milestone was reached.[6]

By eliminating these cereal grains from the celiac-sprue patients' diet, the disease and the pathologic changes in the small bowel could be reversed and the malabsorption, diarrhea, and vitamin deficiencies corrected. Later the toxic factor was found to be gliadin. It was exciting to be in the forefront of clinical investigators in this field despite little or nothing in the way of funds or institutional support. We were really pioneering on our own on a shoestring. We did not have a division status, there was no money for gastroenterology; there were no fellows or residents assigned to us. General internal medicine was the dominant force in the teaching and training programs. We were required to carry heavy responsibilities for patient care and teaching medical students general medicine. Anything we did in the subspecialties was merely another add-on insofar as academic recognition was concerned. In addition, all of this was done without receiving any pay. We did not object to this. We felt that this was what was expected of us as the sons of Hippocrates. We gave more than we took. We were on the whole a very happy, collegial group united in the effort to make our medical center and our students and house staff the best in the world.

On October 30, 1991, I was asked to speak on "The Death of the Clinician—Requiem or Resurrection" at the Annual Meeting of the New York Region Vascular Society. I was introduced by the society's

---

6. W. K. Dicke, "Coeliac Disease: An investigation of the Harmful Effects of Certain Types of Cereal on Patients with Coeliac Disease," doctoral thesis (Netherlands: University of Utrecht, 1950).

president, Dr. Julius H. Jacobson II, the chief of vascular surgery at Mt. Sinai Hospital in New York. Although I had not seen him for many years, he said, "When I arrived to start my internship in surgery at the Presbyterian Hospital in 1952 fresh from Johns Hopkins, I had little or no exposure to gastroenterology because there was no formal teaching program in this field at Hopkins. At Columbia-Presbyterian I met Dr. Michael Lepore, this evening's speaker, and he made gastroenterology come alive and I have never forgotten his superb teaching at the bedside, in the clinics and the wards. Our house staff regarded him as our leading teacher of gastroenterology and I have never forgotten him." This tribute, nearly forty years later, warmed the cockles of my heart.

One of my papers that attracted a great deal of interest was "Long-term or Maintenance Adrenal Steroid Therapy in Nontropical Sprue."[7] When I was questioned by Dr. Loeb as to the mechanism responsible for the beneficial effects of adrenal steroids in sprue, I was unable to give him a satisfactory answer but I speculated that it might be by blocking an allergic response to the cereal grains. The matter is still poorly understood, but recent evidence appears to favor an autoimmune response initiated by gliadin in susceptible individuals. In June 1950 Dr. Thomas Almy asked me to see, in consultation, a patient in New York Hospital, a nurse with severe non-tropical sprue, unresponsive to therapy then in vogue. I examined her on teaching rounds and suggested that he try ACTH. There was a dramatic response. This was the first case of sprue treated with ACTH.[8]

In the early days of our work with sprue, there was always an emaciated patient with intractable sprue on the wards, totally incapacitated and subject to many complications, including hypocalcemic tetany, hypoprothrombinemia with hemorrhage or hematuria or purpura, hypoalbuminemia with edema and multiple vitamin deficiencies. They resembled residents of Dachau. Long-term hospitalizations running into several months at a time were common occurrences. With the advent of the gluten-free diet and adrenal-corticoid therapy we now seldom see patients with sprue occupying ward or private beds. Truly a miracle of modern medicine and research has occurred.

In addition to working with me on the sprue project, Dr. Reemtsma and Dr. Malm studied pancreatic malabsorption with me

---

7. *American Journal of Medicine* 25, no. 3 (September 1958), pp. 381–390.

8. T. P. Almy, "A Refractory Case of Idiopathic Steatorrhea (Nontropical Sprue) with Observations on the Therapeutic Effects of Salt Poor Human Albumin and of Adrenocorticotropic Hormone," *Ann Int Med* 34 (1951), pp. 1041–1048.

using radioisotopes of oleic acid and neutral fats and demonstrated clearly that these tests were useful in measuring fat absorption following pancreatitis or pancreatic surgery, including total pancreatectomy, and on patients who had undergone a Whipple operation, the latter named after the brilliant chairman of surgery, Dr. Allen O. Whipple, a pioneer in pancreatic surgery among his many other achievements. In pancreatogenic malabsorption, the neutral fats were malabsorbed while the tagged fatty acids were normally absorbed, consistent with surgery or due to inflammation of the pancreas or cystic fibrosis. In sprue, both neutral fats and fatty acids were poorly absorbed, consistent with villous atrophy of the small intestine, the hallmark of this disease.

Dr. Frank Gump was another excellent surgical intern and resident who asked to work with me on regional enteritis. We wrote several papers on the subject. He, too, went on to a fine career and became a professor of surgery at P&S. These young men, despite the heavy demands of a surgical residency, somehow found the time, really overtime, to perform significant clinical research. I am proud to have been their associate. *"Discipuli victoria, magistri est gloria."*

One afternoon while I was working in the Vanderbilt Clinic, I received a call from Dean Houston Merritt's office from his secretary who asked me to consult on the case of her sixty-six-year-old aunt who was seriously ill in Holy Name Hospital, Teaneck, New Jersey, and was scheduled to have her stomach removed the following day because of a bleeding gastric ulcer. I was just finishing a gruelling session in the clinic, and had patients to see in Harkness Pavilion. Heavy pressure was put upon me to see the patient who had already been examined by many consultants. I finally arrived at the hospital at about 9 P.M. that evening. The patient's internist had been annoyed by the flood of consultants and failed to meet me at the hospital. This did not make me very happy. I reviewed the chart and immediately smelled a rat. The records showed that this patient's blood count and hematocrit values had been stable for the preceding three days without requiring transfusion. The disturbing feature was that the private-duty nurses, assigned around the clock, were reporting black tarry stools despite repeated enemas. The assumption was that the patient was still actively bleeding. Her vital signs were stable. Toward the end of my examination, following Sir William Osler's aphorism that it is the duty of the consultant to perform a rectal examination, I called for a rubber glove and, as I had suspected, found a large black fecal impaction that had not been removed by the enemas. The black enema returns were due to old blood in the rectum. No one had done a rectal examination during the previous three days. My diagnosis was that the bleeding had ceased at least three days before and that she did not need an operation for the tiny gastric ulcer demonstrated on the x-ray films. This really created quite a stir, especially with her physician who rather pointedly asserted that I was out of line with all of the other consultants and asked if I would accept the responsibility if she bled during the night. My answer was "of course I will," and I gave him my home telephone number. The patient never bled again and lived another ten years, succumbing to hypertensive cardiovascular disease. Some time after her death, her husband made a gift to me that equipped the first Gastrointestinal Endoscopy Unit at St. Vincent's Hospital and Medical Center, a living memorial to a wonderful woman whom I shall never forget.

In December 1952, I was asked to see a patient in the Gastrointestinal Clinic with the radiologic diagnosis of terminal cancer of the stomach. I was not happy at the thought of having to give the patient such bad news. Grasping at any straw, I reviewed his past history very carefully and again I smelled a rat. This thirty-five-year-old bank clerk had been operated upon nearly two years before for carcinoma of the stomach invading the head of the pancreas. He underwent subtotal gastrectomy, duodenectomy, partial pancreatectomy, gastrojejunostomy, (Hofmeister type), choledochojejunostomy and pancreaticojejunostomy. He recovered well from his surgery, regaining the weight he had lost and resuming all of his activities. On 12–9–52, almost two years after his operation, he started having diarrhea and lost weight. By 5–12–53 he had lost a total of 18 pounds and described his stools as bulky and fatty, two or three times daily. A GI series on 5–28–53 at the Vanderbilt Clinic was interpreted by a radiologist as showing evidence of recurrent carcinoma of the gastric remnant. He was referred to me in the Gastrointestinal Clinic on 6–1–53 and by this time weighed only 118 pounds, twenty pounds below his normal weight. There was nothing of note on physical examination except for the weight loss. There were no abdominal masses or hepatomegaly. Rectal examination failed to reveal any evidence of a Blumer shelf or other signs of metastatic cancer. There was foul, fatty, guaiac negative stool resembling rancid butter. Stool microscopic fat content was 4+ and a large amount of unabsorbed starch was also present. The urine was positive for 2 plus glucose. The serum carotene level was zero while the serum Vitamin A level was 86 units per 100 cc. His glucose tolerance curve was diabetic, fasting 128 mg percent, ½ hr 313, 1 hr 392, 2 hr 202, 3 hr 173. I reviewed his GI series with Dr. Ross Golden, who did not agree with the diagnosis of recurrent carcinoma but diagnosed postgastrectomy gastritis with enlarged folds. My diagnosis was that the patient had closed off his pancreatic anastomosis resulting in pancreatic exocrine insufficiency due to lack of delivery of enzymes to the jejunum. I started him on a diet of carbohydrate 250 gm, protein 125 gm and fat 100 gm in six feedings. Pancreatic extract two teaspoonsful TID was prescribed and NPH insulin 10 units qAM, progressing to 25 units. His response was dramatic. The diarrhea stopped within forty-eight hours and he gained weight rapidly, recovering all of his loss. I followed his progress for three more years and at the last visit, five years after his operation, his weight was 141½ pounds and he had no complaints. Dr. Milton Porter and I felt this syndrome should be called the post-pancreatico-duodenectomy syndrome or the post-Whipple operation syndrome, perhaps worthy of an eponym.[9]

One morning when I was busily working in the Ulcerative Colitis Clinic, I was called to the telephone. It was from a well-known woman pediatrician from Bellevue Hospital who started to berate me for having proctoscoped and biopsied a rectal mass in a teenaged girl with cerebral palsy. The pediatrician had referred the patient to the clinic of Dr. Frank Stinchfield, our renowned orthopedic surgeon, for a reconstructive operation on a flail left foot. Dr. Stinchfield had examined the patient and noted a past history of childhood ulcerative colitis and referred the patient to my clinic for evaluation before proceeding with the operation. When I examined her, I was dismayed to find a large rectal mass that proved on biopsy to be a highly malignant adenocarcinoma. The final comment to me by the patient's pediatrician was a complaint that she had sent the patient to Columbia-Presbyterian for a small operation on her foot and we were putting her through many unnecessary tests before clearing her for the orthopedic service. After the pediatrician had vented her spleen on me I said "Doctor, I have the report of the biopsy and I shall read it to you." This I did and there was a gasp from the other end of the line and a weak "I'm sorry" followed by a click. My next move was to explain all of this to the patient's family. Not a very pleasant morning's work.

After I returned from military service and was on geographic full time at Harkness Pavilion, I was asked each summer to take over the practice of Dr. Louis Bauman, a senior internist and biochemist specializing in metabolic diseases, obesity, diabetes, and pancreatic disorders. His appointment was in the department of surgery under Dr.

9. Michael J. Lepore, "Nutritional Management Following Gastrointestinal Operations," *Surgical Clinics of North America* 36(April 1956), pp. 507–517.

Allan O. Whipple, the chairman. I learned a great deal about Dr. Bauman's management of patients with diseases within his realm of interest. I also happened to be in my office in Harkness Pavilion across the hall from Dr. Bauman's when I was summoned to see him in an emergency because of acute chest pain with collapse. I quickly diagnosed an acute myocardial infarct, administered Demerol for pain and nasal oxygen, summoned a stretcher, and escorted him up to a Harkness room. By the time his cardiologist, the renowned Robert L. Levy, arrived, everything was under control. Dr. Bauman made an excellent recovery. During his absence for several months, I took care of his practice with the help of his devoted secretary, Mrs. Huysoon. Through Dr. Bauman I had occasion to review the medical records and course of the original small group of patients who had under-gone the first Whipple operations for cancer of the pancreas. Following the retirement of Dr. Allan O. Whipple, his work in pan-creatic surgery was turned over to one of his finest residents, Dr. Milton Porter. Dr. Porter and I became good friends and collabora-tors and we saw many interesting patients together.

One night, one of my patients from Rockland County called me because she was having severe left-lower-quadrant pain. Knowing that we had no available empty beds on the medical service, I advised the family to arrange transportation to our emergency division where I would meet her. She was in severe pain and on examination had signs of peritoneal irritation in her left lower quadrant with a tender mass in the left adnexal region that we thought was due to an ovarian cyst. Since there were no private beds, she was admitted to the gynecolog-ical ward where it was agreed that she should be immediately explored. I was in the O.R. when she was operated upon. The find-ings by the resident were that she had an ovarian abscess adherent to her sigmoid colon He requested emergency consultation with the sur-gical resident on call. The latter scrubbed and examined the patient and then decided to call the surgical attending on service. He was in his home in Nyack and advised the resident not to try to resect the mass but to drop it back into the abdomen and place the patient on antibiotic therapy. He did not offer to come in even though he was on call. I knew this surgeon quite well and I knew that abdominal surgery was not his forte. The patient was under general anesthesia. Her fam-ily had returned home trusting me to make the decisions. I was unhappy with this turn of events. My patient was entitled to have the surgeon of her own choice but because of the lack of a semiprivate or private room, she was at the mercy of the house staff. Or was she really? I objected to the decision that nothing be done except to place the patient on antibiotic therapy. I was especially upset that the on-call attending surgeon who should have been in the hospital or nearby was miles away. I told the residents that I was not satisfied and asked them to call Dr. Milton Porter at his home and request his advice. Dr. Porter lived across the George Washington Bridge in Englewood, New Jersey. He said he would come over right away. In a matter of minutes he was in the operating room, scrubbing. He advised the resident to perform a transverse colostomy with excision of the ovarian mass with his help.

The patient's postoperative course was smooth. The ovarian mass was caused by an ovarian abscess that was adherent to the sigmoid colon, the site of multiple diverticula. A pure culture of E. Coli was obtained from the abscess, indicating that the primary source was the sigmoid colon. I know I upset the first surgeon who was on call, but it did not worry me. As I have always tried to do, I placed my patient's welfare above all other considerations. The good physician must be his patient's fearless advocate, no matter what! It was neither the first time nor the last that I intervened in the interest of my patient's welfare.

In reviews of malpractice cases against doctors conducted for educational purposes under the auspices of the Medical Liability Insurance Company, I have been impressed by the frequency with which a successful suit was instituted when the defendant physician or surgeon gave advice over the telephone to house staff without coming in to see the patient in person. I have practiced medicine in New York City for over fifty years and I have never admitted a patient to any of my hospitals as an emergency without being there in person. I have never deviated from this rule of conduct and I deplore the trend to neglect this basic tenet of good medical practice. Another of my rules of conduct is that the personal physician of the patient undergoing a major operation should make every effort to be present in the operating room at some stage of the operation. On the ward or teaching service, the next time you review the chart of a patient referred for major surgery, ask the medical resident when he last visited the operating room. The answer may shock you.

Chapter 19

❦

An Internist-Diagnostician Rebuilds His Practice

I WAS PLEASANTLY SURPRISED by how quickly I was able to rebuild my practice on my return to New York. Many of my former patients sought me out, providing a solid base for reconstruction. I was on call and available seven days a week around the clock. This was the way I was trained at Duke in my internship where we were on the Johns Hopkins' system for twenty-four-hour call. I did not consider this a hardship, I thought it was how a real doctor should function. My patients, old and new, were greatly relieved that they had a doctor they could call at any time. What a change from the wartime days when doctors were next to impossible to find. I made my share of house calls when I thought they were indicated and I enjoyed them. I soon realized that my on-call schedule was unusual and the newly minted young assistants in medicine at Columbia-Presbyterian Medical Center seldom made house calls and were hard to find after office hours and on weekends or holidays. Sooner or later this attitude would earn the Medical Center the reputation of being an ivory tower, uninterested in its surrounding community. Focusing on tertiary care was a legitimate goal of the Medical Center, but this should not have been to the neglect of primary care. The nearly five years of practice I had before entering military service had taught me many things that cannot be learned in medical school or in an internship or residency. Scientific training is important, but commitment to service and the care of the patient is paramount in the personal practice of medicine.

Self-referrals were common and some very interesting patients came to Harkness Pavilion from near and far. South American and Central American patients sought out the Medical Center because of its excellent reputation as a clinical center. Many but not all of these patients were well-to-do. Some had been going to the Mayo Clinic in Rochester, Minnesota, or the Ochsner Clinic in New Orleans. They liked to visit New York City and occupied rooms in many of its fine hotels. The city was attractive, clean, and safe. The Medical Center area was safe, clean, and impressive. The patients were especially happy that experienced clinicians, not fellows or residents in training, were the first to see them. Unless they had to be admitted to the hospital, they dealt only with seasoned attending physicians and surgeons.

They told us that at large clinics they felt they were just a number, that much of their care was impersonal, and that the diagnostic workup was relegated to residents or fellows. Dr. Walter W. Palmer and Allen O. Whipple, the renowned Valentine Mott professor of surgery, were never in favor of a Mayo Clinic-type approach to medical practice at Columbia-Presbyterian. Their feeling was that a personal physician or surgeon was essential for provision of the best care. Latin American patients as well as others were voting for this with their feet. While my spoken Spanish was halting, I could understand it quite well and it was not long before I had quite an impressive Latin American following made up of some of the leading families in Colombia, Venezuela, and San Salvador, with occasional Peruvians, Argentineans, and Brazilians. Since I was one of the few clinicians in Harkness who had excellent training and experience in tropical diseases and knowledge of what we now call geographic medicine, many referrals were made to me. My military experience in this area of medicine, added to my internship and residency at Duke, paid off substantial dividends. Through my previous years as director of the personnel medical department, I had become very familiar with the most effective and able surgeons, physicians, and radiologists at the Medical Center and I knew where to turn to for help. I knew how to use the Medical Center's facilities and staff efficiently and skillfully. I knew the weak spots and the strengths and the people to avoid. From the beginning I was guided by the maxim that my job was to get the best possible care for those who came to see me. This was bound to succeed and soon I became one of the most sought-after physicians on staff. My consultants were chosen for their competence, skill, availability, and commitment to rendering the best of care to all of my patients, rich or poor, common or uncommon, without regard to race, color, or creed. Because I was able to spot outstanding doctors early in their careers, my patients invariably had the best of the consultants at Columbia-Presbyterian. In the process I learned a great deal from my consultants. Dr. Lawrence W. Sloan of the surgical staff was a tower of strength and wisdom who served my patients well and taught me a great deal. Dr. Milton Porter, a superb surgeon, and I shared many difficult problems together. Dr. Daniel C. Baker of the ENT service and a bronchoscopist of considerable skill became a great specialist and never let it go to his head. In orthopedics, Dr. Frank Stinchfield added a new dimension to that specialty at Columbia-Presbyterian when he came there like a breath of fresh air from Northwestern. Dr. C. T. Vicale, the marvelous neurologist made the most difficult neurologic diagnosis look easy. Dr. George Cahill and later, Dr. John K. Lattimer, brought great distinction to the department of urology and served as consultants to many of my patients. Dr. Anthony D'Esopo was the outstanding gynecologist and obstetrician of the Medical Center in that era and should have been the chairman of the department after Dr. Benjamin Watson retired. As Dr. D'Esopo's beloved wife once said to me when speaking of her husband's career, "He was always the prime minister but never the king."

These were the great stars and it was my pleasure to work together with them and to enjoy their growth and development. In the selection of my consultants, I had one cardinal rule: the consultant was seldom called for window-dressing purposes; he or she had to carry a share of the load and lighten mine or else risk not being called again. Most of my consultants achieved high status as they aged. Some did not or could not and I simply had to drop them from my list, which led to some awkward moments.

Because I was demanding and meticulous in the selection of my consultants, my own reputation grew and the volume of work being referred to me was expanding rapidly. One group of patients that I derived much satisfaction in caring for were the Presbyterian and Methodist foreign missionaries, especially those from India and China. I never sent them a bill for my services but, like the poor, they were the best payers, because the Lord paid their bills.

I met some of the most dedicated, selfless, and idealistic persons in the world from this group during my twenty-five years at Harkness Pavilion. One I shall never forget was Dr. Goheen, the uncle of the former president of Princeton University who had been a Presbyterian missionary in India where he had postponed his return to the United States for an operation on his kidney because there was no one available to replace him. By the time he arrived at Harkness Pavilion it was too late, and he became a martyr to his way of life. I developed great affection for these individuals and admiration for what they were doing in the "developing world."

Shortly after returning from overseas, I was asked to see in consultation the "richest man in the world," T. V. Soong, brother of Madame Chiang Kai-shek and who had a liver ailment caused by Clonorchis Sinensis, the oriental liver fluke. He had tried many medications without benefit and had sought further advice at Harkness Pavilion, where his sister had occupied a floor during WW II as a patient of Dr. Robert F. Loeb. I examined the patient thoroughly and reviewed his laboratory findings and told the patient that a relatively new medication, Chloroquine (Aralen), might help get rid of the parasite. I had used this drug for amebiasis and malaria, but at the time we had no data on its use in Clonorchiasis. We knew that the drug was effective against amebic liver abscess and malaria and that it was worth a trial. We now know that it may cure the disease in some patients. With the patient's informed consent, we gave him a course of the medication which he tolerated quite well. I was told by his doctor that the treatment had been effective. This was in 1948 and I lost track of Dr. Soong, but I heard he was quite well. In April 1971, when he was 77 years of age, at a dinner party in his honor in his San Francisco home, he choked on food that obstructed his airway and died before medical help could be summoned.[1]

Another source of referrals was the Lederle Pharmaceutical Company and American Cyanamid in Pearl River, New York. Two very talented physicians from Duke were working there in varied capacities. One was Dr. James Ruegsegger, who had been chief resident in medicine at Duke when I was an intern. The other was Austin (Pop) Joyner, who had been one of my students at Duke in 1934. Everyone called him "Pop" because he was older than the other students, married, which was unusual for a medical student in those days, and apt to be acerbic in his comments. He was also very talented and was doing research on staphylococcus toxoid. Pop called me one day and said he wanted me to admit one of the Lederle employees, who was acutely ill with chills and fever and severe backache. He was in a small "hospital" in Spring Valley where the doctors had placed him in a plaster cast for the backache. Pop took a dim view of this approach and I shared it. I also knew that I had rescued another Lederle employee from the same rather primitive hospital, a converted old mansion. I recall Pop's conversation verbatim. Beds in Harkness were in short supply, especially on the medical service, and I wondered whether the patient should be admitted to one of the orthopedists. Pop said "M.J. (my nickname from Duke days), I don't give a damn what area you're specializing in now, but the man needs a good doctor and diagnostician. I'm going to put him in an ambulance and send him down to you!" The patient was rushed to Harkness Pavilion, where I saw him immediately on arrival, accompanied by Dr. John Wood, the intern assigned to that floor. John, who was one of our finest interns and subsequently became a highly respected internist and cardiologist and clinical professor at P&S, also wondered what I was doing with a patient in a cast. I quickly examined the patient and decided that the first thing we would do was to remove the plaster spica cast enveloping his lumbar spine and extending to the mid-thighs. The patient had an elevated temperature and was having chills.

---

1. Sterling Seagrave, *The Soong Dynasty* (New York: Harper & Row, 1985), p. 456.

As I proceeded with my examination, everything was normal until I reached the patient's left groin where there was an area of ecchymosis, induration, and tenderness. Listening over this area, I elicited a bruit. I immediately suspected that this was an arteriovenous fistula infected with bacteria producing chills and fever mimicking subacute bacterial endocarditis. But how had this occurred in a previously healthy forty-year-old executive with a normal heart?

When I questioned the patient he told me that two weeks before, while in Colorado on Lederle business, he had filled an emergency order for medication and packed it himself in a heavy corrugated cardboard container using a large and sharp-pointed pair of scissors. At the very end of the process the scissors that he had placed on a high work table slipped off striking him in the left groin causing brisk bleeding. Pressure bandages were applied and he was taken to a doctor. By the time he reached the doctor, the bleeding had stopped. He was advised to continue with the sterile pressure dressing. No further bleeding occurred and he resumed his normal duties and returned to his home base. After several days he developed chills and fever and backache and sought attention at Lederle. This story, plus my physical findings, added up to my diagnosis of traumatic arteriovenous fistula between the left femoral artery and vein with sepsis due to endophlebitis and vegetation on the aneurysm wall. We took blood cultures and waited for the report. Within less than twenty-four hours the laboratory reported that the patient had streptococcus viridans with a high colony count in his bloodstream. He was started on penicillin and sulfadiazine; the response was dramatic. I called Dr. Arthur Blakemore, our vascular surgeon in consultation. He congratulated me on my diagnosis and operated upon the patient, resecting the lesion and reconstructing the femoral artery and vein. The patient made an uneventful and full recovery. You can bet your bottom dollar that this patient made both Medical and Surgical Grand Rounds and so did I. Home runs like this are important if you want to succeed in the major league of medicine. It also helps with further referrals.

Another key patient was a young man discharged from the Army because of severe viral hepatitis. He had been sent to a Veterans' Administration hospital where he failed to improve. His father brought him to Harkness Pavilion where he was told that I was an expert in liver disease, having seen and treated hundreds of patients with it overseas in the Pacific and stateside. This was true, but little or nothing was known about the cause of the disease and there was no specific treatment.

When I saw this six-foot-tall skeleton of a young man with yellow skin and conjunctivae I knew I had a challenge on my hands and arranged immediate admission to a room in Harkness Pavilion. We quickly confirmed the diagnosis of viral hepatitis and I instituted a vigorous program to combat his malnutrition. I wrote the orders but I did not stop there. I personally saw to it that they were followed and that the patient complied to the best of his ability. From my work as the personnel medical director, I had become known to most of our nonprofessional staff as a friend and almost their family doctor and I had done many favors for them. In order to get the right diet to the patient we needed the dietitian's help and most of all the help of the nursing aide on the floor. Here I struck oil. I had spent considerable time with the nutrition department under Mrs. Nelda Ross, its head, because of my teaching efforts and research in vitaminology and nutrition. Their cooperation was assured. The nurses' aide was a pleasant, cheerful, and unflappable Irish matron who mothered her patients and was able to cajole even the most difficult person into taking nourishment and medications. I spent some time with her, advising her about my program for Mr. F. and why it was important to follow it to the letter. In those days the kitchens in Harkness Pavilion could actually be used to cook food. None of the central-supply system for serving cold, unappetizing food to the patients! I had learned a lot about this at Valley Forge during the war when we had to get the administration to stop using a central-food-supply system for feeding our wounded. By vigorous action we forced administration to open up the kitchens that were situated on each floor but never used. I was amazed to see how much better our soldiers ate when the food was freshly prepared, piping hot, and selected from a menu.

Our nurses' aide filled the bill to a T. She managed to get young F. to eat frequently and to take ample calories. Slowly and steadily he improved to the point that several weeks later he was well enough to go home to continue his convalescence. To this day, I know that the nurses' aide on that floor did more to get him well than I did.

In the intervening years I have seen Mr. F. through a variety of ailments. I am thankful that his liver has held up wonderfully well for the forty-four years since I first met him.

In 1948, on a Saturday, I was asked to see a young professor on the staff of CCNY. This young man had been interested in trying to improve health-care delivery and was advising Mayor Fiorello LaGuardia on the possible solutions, including the pros and cons of starting the HIP Group. The professor disagreed with the mayor about HIP, saying it promised too much. The professor joined Group Health, Inc., instead. He had as his physician a very talented person who became a leader in the field of psychosomatic medicine. The professor had been ill for several months with aches and pains in all of his extremities, headaches, and weight loss. One of his friends, who was a patient of mine, begged me to see him on a Saturday as a personal favor and I agreed to do so. The minute I saw the patient I knew he was quite sick. After taking his history, I proceeded with the physical examination and confirmed the worst of my fears. He had multiple tender nodules along the course of the arteries of both arms and legs. I knew he had polyarteritis nodosa and that nothing could be done for him. I told him and his friend what I thought was wrong and arranged his admission to a semiprivate room at Columbia-Presbyterian. There, a biopsy confirmed the diagnosis but, as I knew, there was no effective therapy. It was heartrending to see this brilliant young man suffer and to know that there was nothing we could do to arrest the course of the disease. Especially disturbing was the sight of his five-year-old son playing in his room unaware that some day his father would be gone. Nowadays, we have adrenal steroids, ACTH and Interferon, and other agents that may stem the disease, but in 1948 they were not yet on the scene. The professor died in his room at Columbia-Presbyterian weeks after his admission. He left me his library on the economics of medical care. I never sent him a bill. As I write this, I am still saddened by the loss of this wonderful young man who had so much to live for.

One day I received a call that the sixty-year-old brother of one of my patients was passing black stools but had no other complaint. I arranged for an emergency visit and proceeded with my history and complete physical. He was clearly bleeding from his upper GI tract. His blood pressure and pulse rate were normal and he was not having any pain. On his general examination, I picked up a firm mass in his left breast that he had never noticed. My diagnosis was duodenal ulcer with hemorrhage and unrelated adenocarcinoma of the breast. I admitted him for his bleeding ulcer, which healed quickly with medical therapy. The breast lesion was an adenocarcinoma. He and his brother had Klinefelter's syndrome, an ailment characterized by hypogonadism and infertility and a female chromatic blood pattern. He entered the hospital with a bleeding ulcer and ended up with a modified radical mastectomy for an adenocarcinoma that he had never noticed. This was one time when a bleeding ulcer led to a life-saving diagnosis of carcinoma of the breast.

Another patient consulted me because of fever of unknown origin. He had seen several doctors and undergone many studies to no avail. He was a healthy thirty-year-old man with no other complaints. I checked his history with great care and performed a thorough physical examination, all with negative or normal results. I took blood for a series of special tests but I was puzzled. There was something in his history that intrigued me. Each attack of chills and fever had come out of the blue at night, cleared within twenty-four hours and was not accompanied by any sore throat or upper-respiratory or urinary symptoms. I asked, "What were you doing on the night before each episode of fever?" He replied nothing in particular, but on further questioning, he admitted that he, usually a teetotaler, had had two drinks with some friends. "What did you drink?" I asked. "Oh," he said, "only gin and tonic each time." On a hunch I said, "I have just examined you and I can find nothing wrong. I would like you to drink two gin and tonics tonight. I believe this may be a reaction to quinine," I added, and "don't call me in the middle of the night but call me tomorrow morning." I received the call. Mystery solved. It was the quinine in the gin and tonic. Very happy patient and doctor.

In October 1952 I was asked to see in consultation a patient on the ward service at Presbyterian Hospital who had been diagnosed by the ward house staff and attending staff as having nontropical sprue but was not responding to gluten restriction. He was a fifty-six-year-old married French baker with the chief complaint of weight loss and diarrhea that began two weeks before admission while he was on a trip to France. His illness began suddenly without prodromata, with up to six copious, fluid, foul, light-yellow stools containing no gross blood or mucus. Loss of appetite and periumbilical discomfort without cramps developed. Paregoric seemed to help. One week later he developed night sweats and fever ranging between 100–101°F and an occasional chilly sensation. He had had a chronic mild non-productive cough for many years. In 1948 he had experienced bouts of migratory polyarthritis lasting two to three days, clearing spontaneously without deformity and recurring at one- to three-week intervals. His physician thought these were bouts of palindromic rheumatism.

His general physical examination revealed an alert but chronically ill man whose skin appeared tanned. There was evidence of recent weight loss but nothing else of significance. His tongue appeared normal and showed no evidence of glossitis or ulceration. The pertinent laboratory findings were listed as follows:

Erythrocyte sedimentation rate	105 mm in 1 hr
Hemoglobin	9.5 gm/100 cc
Red blood count	3.12 million/cu mm
Hematocrit	31 percent$\frac{1}{2}$
Serum cholesterol	102 mg/100 cc
Serum cholesterol esters	63 mg/100 cc

Oral glucose tolerance test:

Fasting blood sugar	88 mg%
½ hr	94 mg%
1 hr	98 mg%
2 hr	89 mg%
3 hr	91 mg%
Intravenous glucose tolerance test	Normal
Stool guaiac	Intermittently 1+ to 4+, at times negative
Stool microscopic fat	.4+ fatty acid crystals

Serum carotene	0
Serum vitam A level	62 units/100 cc

Small intestine x-ray study	Disturbed motor physiology without demonstrable organic disease.

The significant findings were steatorrhea manifested by numerous fatty-acid crystals in the stool, no detectable serum carotene, and a low serum Vitamin A level and anemia. With the findings of a flat oral-glucose-tolerance curve and a normal intravenous-glucose curve, and an abnormal small-bowel pattern, the diagnosis of sprue was suggested by one of the junior attending staff and I was called in consultation. I disagreed with the diagnosis of sprue for the following reasons. A red-cell sedimentation rate of 105 mm Westergren is unheard of in uncomplicated sprue, the febrile course is unusual, and polyarthritis uncommon. I also did not feel that the small-bowel pattern on x-ray examination was that seen in sprue. I wrote a short note on the chart and underlined my conclusions. "I believe this patient has Whipple's disease described in 1907 in the Bulletin of the Johns Hopkins Hospital, Volume 18, pp. 382–391, by Dr. George Hoyt Whipple. I recommend that the patient undergo laparotomy with biopsy of mesenteric nodes and excision of a wedge of small bowel." Dr. Charles Ragan, who was the attending on service, thought this was indicated but ran into an obstacle when Dr. Robert F. Loeb, the Bard professor, saw the patient on rounds. I could not get to the ward rounds but I learned from reliable sources that Dr. Loeb listened to the history, examined the patient and saw my note. His comment to Dr. Ragan was, "Tell Dr. Lepore that we do not explore people on this service in order to make a diagnosis." This was a caustic remark from a brilliant man but in keeping with one of his chief aphorisms, "Keep the patient out of the surgeons' hands." The patient was subsequently discharged to my follow-up clinic. When I learned what had happened, I was displeased and I felt that a serious error had occurred. In 1952 there was no other way to diagnose Whipple's disease. The

Crosby capsule, the Rubin tube, and fiberoptic endoscopes for small-bowel biopsies had not yet been invented. Laparotomy was the only option we had. After some thought, and guided solely by my concern for the patient, I decided to bypass Dr. Loeb by referring this patient to the surgeons. This was taking quite a risk, but I was prepared to accept the consequences. The surgical staff agreed with me and arranged the patient's admission. At exploration of the abdomen on 12 November 1952, the findings were those of classic Whipple's disease manifested by mesenteric lymphadenopathy with individual nodes varying from 1 cm to 6 cm in diameter. Two nodes were excised for study. The final diagnosis by Dr. Raffaele Lattes, surgical pathologist, was Whipple's intestinal lipodystrophy, the first case diagnosed at Columbia-Presbyterian and one of the first to ever to be diagnosed in a living patient. To top it off, it was done by a student and protégé of Dean Whipple. My fears that Dr. Loeb might try to punish me for referring the patient to the surgeons did not materialize. I was asked to discuss my patient at Medical Grand Rounds, which I did with restraint and considerable pleasure. When Dr. Loeb asked me from his front row seat in the amphitheater how I came to make the diagnosis of Whipple's disease, I reminded him that I was one of Dean Whipple's students and I just happened to have under my arm Volume 18 of the *Bulletin of the Johns Hopkins Hospital* of 1907 containing Dean Whipple's article. I also had the pleasure of presenting the case report at the alumni reunion of the University of Rochester School of Medicine on 23 October 1953 with Dean Whipple in the front row. He rewarded me by sending me a rare reprint of his original paper of 1907, autographed, "To Michael Lepore from his teacher and friend. G. H. WHIPPLE" *Discipuli victoria magistri est gloria.*

I wonder what might have happened to me if my diagnosis had been in error. In my report of this case in the 1954 issue of the *American Journal of Medicine*, pp. 160–64, I thought that the remissions in the patient's illness were induced by adrenal steroids and ACTH. In retrospect, the remission may have been due in fact to antibiotics given for severe respiratory-tract infections. At the time, Whipple's disease, a rarity, was uniformly fatal. This patient died of it two years after its onset. We now know that it is caused by a microbe that responds to prolonged courses of antibiotics and is no longer a death sentence.

Chapter 20

The Upjohn Grand Rounds

*How would you like to teach 20,000 doctors in
one evening on closed-circuit television?*

—Steve Schwartz, 1955

ARLY IN 1955, WHILE WORKING IN THE VANDERBILT CLINIC, I
received a telephone call from a Mr. Stephen Schwartz, a total
stranger, who introduced himself as a friend of Dr. Marianne
Wolff, a former medical student of mine who was an outstanding
young attending on the surgical pathology staff of P&S. Dr. Wolff
had suggested that he get in touch with me regarding an important
innovation in medical education. He quickly came to the point, asking, "How would you like to teach 20,000 doctors in one evening on
closed-circuit television?" I was a little staggered by this proposal but
managed to blurt out, "Tell me more." He proceeded to outline his
plan, saying that he had major financial support for the project. What
he had in mind was using the format of Grand Rounds with case presentations of live patients before a panel of renowned experts under
the guidance of a seasoned clinician-moderator. To enhance the suspense, the panelists would have no prior knowledge of the actual
diagnosis of the patients being presented. The aim was to demonstrate
to an audience of doctors how world-renowned clinicians go about
diagnosing and managing patients they are seeing for the first time.

In 1955 television was in its infancy and subject to considerable
censorship. To preserve privacy of the patients and panelists and to
avoid upsetting some viewers, closed-circuit television would be
employed on channels unavailable to the public at large. Mr. Schwartz
assured me that nothing would be spared in bringing together the very
best men and women in the world of medicine. There would be a
minimal or no sales pitch for pharmaceuticals but the sponsor would,
of course, be credited with supporting the program. Approval had
already been obtained from a number of organizations, including the
AMA and specialty societies. Steve's next question was, "What topic
would you select for the first Grand Rounds?. My answer was "The
Acute Abdomen," a title I felt would bring in doctors in droves
because of its universal appeal and practical significance for most

practicing physicians and surgeons. Steve's next question was, "How would you go about getting this done?" My first proposal was to start with an ambulance ride in response to an emergency call to the home of a patient with severe abdominal pain. Having made many of these calls by automobile in my early days of practice in the Bronx and Manhattan, before the 911 system was installed, I knew from personal experience what it was like to be called out in the middle of the night to see strangers in distress and to have to make important decisions without laboratory or x-ray help, quickly and without a committee to advise me on what to do.

As Steve and I kept talking, I agreed that it would be well-nigh impossible in 1955 to get a mobile television crew involved. We finally compromised on stationing a television crew in the emergency room of a busy hospital filming patients with abdominal pain from the moment of arrival in the emergency room. Steve Schwartz was very pleased with my suggestions and arranged for a series of meetings with him and his staff at the William Douglas McAdams Advertising Agency, where he was head of its radio and television department. This agency had as a major client the Upjohn Pharmaceutical Company. I learned later that the McAdams Agency was controlled by two talented Drs. Sackler, brother psychiatrists with a wide range of very successful enterprises in medical communications. Through Steve, I was introduced to the world of television and met some very interesting people. I made sure I was not carried away by the atmosphere and excitement of this new medium.

As was true of much of my work at that time, for example, my teaching in the Vanderbilt Clinic, I received no pay for my participation. My busy life as a clinician, practitioner, and educator at P&S continued to occupy most of my time. Steve asked me to be the moderator of the first Grand Rounds that were to be held in Boston at the Tufts New England Medical Center, where Steve's brilliant brother, Bill, was a professor of medicine and chief of nephrology and a rising star. Through his intercession the active cooperation of Dr. Samuel Proger, chairman of the department of medicine at Tufts, was secured as well as that of G. Gardner Child III, chairman of surgery. Since my affiliation with Columbia-Presbyterian would be listed in the prebroadcast publicity, I sought and obtained Dr. Robert F. Loeb's permission to accept this assignment. He seemed pleased that I had been asked to do this and encouraged me to continue with it. Later, I would learn that he himself disliked public speaking and avoided it like the plague.

The television project proved to be a major enterprise, involving a host of lay persons and enormous amounts of equipment and

major expenditures. It was estimated that the fees paid to the telephone companies for outlets and lines to the various cities selected as
reception sites for the Grand Rounds closed-circuit programs reached
one-quarter of a million dollars for each show. Modest honoraria and
travel expenses were paid to the participating doctors, but they were
peanuts compared to the telephone-line fees and the advertising-
agency and filming and productions costs of the operation.

The sponsor for the Grand Rounds was the Upjohn
Pharmaceutical Company of Kalamazoo, Michigan, a well-regarded
ethical firm with a genuine interest in continuing medical education.
They not only paid the bills, they encouraged us to innovate and
cheered us on from the very first program to the last. The shows were
quite appropriately named *The Upjohn Grand Rounds*. In addition to the
closed-circuit sessions, each show was placed on kinescope, the forerunner of today's videotapes, which were supplied without charge by
Upjohn to teaching institutions around the world as well as to U.S.
military installations. Translations in various foreign languages were
also made available. The kinescopes are still being shown, their historical interest enhanced with the passage of the years as mementos
of the famous physicians and surgeons who participated.

The invitation to participate in this exciting and novel approach to
medical education arrived in 1955 at a special time in my life. I was
then forty-five years old, at the peak of my powers, inspiring the
growth of gastroenterology at Columbia-Presbyterian, and eager to
do more teaching in this rapidly expanding field of medicine. I felt
that my talents were not being adequately employed at this institution
in the teaching program. This was especially galling after having risen
in WW II from captain to lieutenant colonel in the Army Medical
Corps, in command of a 600-bed medical service in 2,000-bed Army
general hospitals where I was decorated for my teaching, leadership,
administrative and patient care services, and offered a career opportunity in the Regular Army.

I had also received several offers to re-enter academic medicine
on a full-time basis. Colonel Tom Fitz-Hugh invited me to join him in
private practice in Philadelphia. I turned down these offers because I
wished to be with my large and devoted family in New York, where I
was sorely needed. On my return from military service I became only
one of an army of private practitioners and clinicians serving without
pay on the teaching service of the great medical center at Columbia-
Presbyterian. I wanted no part of full-time medicine.

I had made this decision for sound reasons in 1937 when I left
Duke to enter private practice in New York and I had no reason to
change my mind. What I sought to do was to teach students and

house staff, do clinical investigation, and continue with the personal care of the people who, of their own volition, sought me out. With the unexpected advent of the Upjohn Grand Rounds, I saw an opportunity to put my teaching and clinical interests and capabilities to the test of a medical school without walls with the world as my audience. I saw in this endeavor the opportunity to bring continuing medical education to thousands of doctors and, in the process, improve the diagnosis and care of many thousands of people I would never see in person. This is what led me to devote so much time and effort to the Upjohn Grand Rounds.

Once again, I gave more than I took, an essential factor of my life creed. It took almost a year from the time of my first talk with Steve before the first Grand Rounds telecast was held. Steve had arranged to send a television crew to the emergency room of the Boston City Hospital, where it remained for two weeks, filming cases as they appeared. To Steve's horror, for the first four days of their stay, the Boston City Hospital established the unheard-of record of not admitting a single patient with an acute abdominal emergency.

Fortunately, things picked up and soon an ample sample of cases had been placed on film for review in New York. Three patients were selected for the show. The technique we developed was to start photographing the patients immediately on arrival in the emergency room where the admitting resident or intern did the initial questioning and examination and ordered appropriate x rays and laboratory tests and discussed the diagnosis and management with the attending surgeon or physician.

On the actual Grand Rounds telecast, we would break from the emergency room to question the assembled panelists regarding their diagnoses and decision management. If there were differences of opinion, the moderator would identify them and encourage brief rebuttals during which many pearls might be dropped. If an operation were needed, the camera switched to the operating room for further dialogue and questions for the panelists. Throughout, an atmosphere of spontaneity, professionalism, and some degree of anxiety was maintained that served to keep the panelists on their toes.

I was told that spectators who attended the shows sat on the edge of their chairs and some even clapped and cheered the panelists with whom they agreed. I pioneered as the first moderator of the Upjohn Grand Rounds Number One telecast on the evening of 15 January 1956 in Boston at the Tufts New England Medical Center. The panel consisted of the following renowned teachers:

BOSTON
CHARLES GARDNER CHILD III
Professor of Surgery, Tufts University School of medicine

DR. ORVAR SWENSON
Clinical professor, Pediatric Surgery
Tufts University School of Medicine

CHICAGO
DR. WALTER L. PALMER
Professor of Medicine, University of Chicago School of
Medicine

MINNESOTA
DR. LEO G. RIGLER
Professor and Chief of Radiology and Physical Therapy
University of Minnesota Medical School

DR. OWEN H. WANGENSTEEN
Professor and Chief of Department of Surgery
University of Minnesota Medical School
Surgeon-in-Chief Surgical Service
University of Minnesota Hospital

Formal invitations had been sent to 100,000 physicians and surgeons in the United States:

THE UPJOHN COMPANY
Requests the pleasure of Your Company
at "GRAND ROUNDS" on the occasion of the opening
of a new series of live closed-circuit television
presentations of actual bedside medicine on
Wednesday, January 18, 1956

Subject:

Diagnosis and Management of
ACUTE ABDOMINAL PROBLEMS

Steve Schwartz later described the enormous amount of work that had to be done to produce the show. "Ten thousand feet of medical film in six cases was the net result and back in New York this meant the beginning of a massive job of screening, cutting, decision-making. A series of meetings were held which brought together key clinicians from the first telecast including Dr. George W. Dana, Dr.

Charles G. Child of Boston and Michael J. Lepore from New York. Three cases were eventually selected and the upshot of two weeks of shooting was eleven minutes of finally edited film."[1] Of course the films were an essential feature of the telecast, for they brought the patient to the Grand Rounds from the arrival in the emergency room to the scenes and the action in the operating room. By questioning the panelists at various stages of the telecast, I was able to elicit differences of opinion, controversy, and constructive criticism with each of them on his mettle before a nationwide audience. Steve Schwartz summarized it well, saying, "Now, through a bold but natural step, the traditional hospital staff meeting held in the privacy of a conference room or amphitheater, where frank give-and-take may prevail, was thrown open to doctors in every corner of the country."

The telecast reached 20,000 doctors that night in more than fifty cities across the nation. The incoming mail was laudatory and enthusiastic, requesting more of the telecasts. We learned that audience reaction at the various sites was extremely warm. Many letters of thanks were sent in to the Upjohn Company. I was greatly touched by letters and telegrams sent in by doctors and county medical societies in small and sometimes isolated areas requesting that we continue the programs to help them keep abreast of the latest in medical and surgical thought. One example was a letter from the Jackson County Medical Society in Medford, Oregon, signed by all of its members, saying, in part, "We that live here in the Rogue River Valley, no longer feel isolated from the medical centers of the world. You are certainly to be highly commended for the work and organization which we know had to go into this production."

I received personal letters from numerous individuals, led by Dr. E. Gifford Upjohn, president of the Upjohn Company, who wrote, "There is no doubt in our minds that our 'experiment' was a huge success. Naturally we are delighted with the outcome and deeply grateful to those who took part in Grand Rounds. I want to personally congratulate you and to thank you not only for the important contribution which you made but also for your willingness to cooperate with us in this venture. We are proud to have had the privilege of being associated with you in this. I can't help feeling that both of us have had a part in introducing an important innovation in medical education." Earl L. Burbidge, M.D., medical director of the Upjohn

---

1. Stephen W. Schwartz, "Medical Education and Television," *Medical Annals of the District of Columbia* 26, no. 1 (August 3, 1957), pp. 29–31.

Company, wrote, "Of course, we all had the extreme pleasure of seeing the program and frankly, were pleased and amazed that it was so exciting and interesting. I am sure that you will be pleased to know, also, that we have had hundreds of enthusiastic letters from physicians who saw the performance, the chief comment being the unrehearsed spontaneous presentation, with additional comments that they hoped we continue such outstanding presentations. We are very happy indeed that you consented to participate in the Grand Rounds and this is merely a note to thank you for a job well done." Finally there was a nice note from Steve Schwartz, producer of the Grand Rounds: "I have just seen the complete kinescope of the program that you so ably moderated, and it was a real thrill. Viewing the program as a whole is quite different from observing it on a series of monitors in the control truck and the richness of the content was evident. It was evident as well to physicians all over the country who have responded with much warmth to seeing it. It may be of interest to you to know that a large number of kinescope recordings are now being made and that the program will be seen widely during the next year both in this country and abroad where it will be seen with appropriate translations." Overnight I had become a TV personality, but the real kudo was awarded in 1956 when my wife and Fred, my six-year-old son, went to Disneyland in Anaheim, California. The first building we visited was the old-fashioned Drug Store run by Upjohn. I was immediately recognized and greeted warmly by their personnel as "Dr. Lepore of the Upjohn Grand Rounds." Son Fred's remark: "That's my Pop." What else can you ask for?

One of the fans of the Upjohn Grand Rounds was Dr. Virginia Kneeland Frantz, a talented professor of surgical pathology at P&S whose brother, Dr. Yale Kneeland, was a stellar teacher and professor of medicine at P&S; they comprised a rarity in American medicine, a brother-and-sister team. She praised the show and was a regular viewer. After one of the telecasts she sought me out and told me how much she enjoyed it. She thought the camera techniques were exceptionally good. She was especially intrigued by the appearance of one of the panelists, who looked "positively owlish." The truth of the matter, that I could not divulge at the time, was that the panelist, apprehensive over appearing on television, had arrived drunk at the television center. Steve and the moderator filled him with black coffee and walked him about. The moderator was cautioned not to call upon the panelist for the first half hour of the show by which time he had sobered up. No wonder he "looked owlish." What a hangover! After the first Grand Rounds telecast, I was appointed to the advisory committee for Grand Rounds and served on it until the series was terminated.

One of the most interesting evenings I have ever spent was in preparation for the Grand Rounds of December 1961 on "Lesions of the Brain." The participants included Macdonald Critchley of London, Wilder Penfield of Montreal, Michael DeBakey of Houston, Irving Cooper of New York, and Eugene Pendergrass of Philadelphia. While the Upjohn Grand Rounds were noted for their spontaneity and liveliness, they were the culmination of a great deal of intensive preparation by the producer, Stephen Schwartz, and his staff. The day before the telecast was spent in getting the panelists to know each other and to let them have access to some information about the patients being presented without giving away their diagnoses or outcomes. The day ended with dinner served in the private dining room of our hotel suite. Following a leisurely and delicious meal, there was time for conversation. With this fascinating group of people the conversation, off the record or "under the rose," could be stimulating and exhilarating or it might be stilted and boring. Should this be left to chance or should some plans be made to encourage a dialogue involving all of the panelists? Knowing that we would be sitting around the dining table for several hours, I thought I would prepare myself for it by reading a recently published book, *The Torch*—a historical novel on the life of Hippocrates, written by none other than Dr. Wilder Penfield, a panelist, the director of the Montreal Neurological Center. If the after-dinner conversation was going well, my plan was to listen and learn. If it faltered, I was prepared to engage Dr. Penfield in a discussion of his new book, which had received an excellent review in the *New York Times* that week. As luck would have it, after the sumptuous meal and the wine, the conversation lagged and I decided to initiate a conversation with Dr. Penfield about his book. My first question was how he had come to write this fascinating historical novel. I struck a real geyser. Dr. Penfield, a Greek scholar, regaled us with tales of his yearly field trips to the Greek Islands, seeking to pursue his hobby of Greek lore and Hippocrates and Grecian medicine. Soon everyone at the table had a question for Dr. Penfield and the dialogue sparkled. The answer to my first question was in the Prologue to *The Torch*, presented so beautifully that I will quote it verbatim for my readers' enjoyment:

> This is a story from the life of Hippocrates the physician—a story of what may have happened one spring twenty-four hundred years ago. Many things have not changed since Hippocrates was young and Daphne (his wife) came to the island of Cos. The sky and the wind and the bird songs, and the sound of the sea, are just as they were. Man's brain was as swift then as it is now, and the physicians found problems in the practice of medicine

not unlike those of today. Hippocrates lived in the golden age of ancient Greece. When he began to study the secrets of nature critically, it was as though he had lighted a torch in the darkness, holding it high so that those who were trying to help the sick could see at last, and examine cause and effect. The first clear statement of the scientific method—the method that has created modern medicine and natural science—is to be found in the Hippocratic writings. Copied and recopied century after century, they served the world for more than two thousand years as a textbook of medicine.

Today men call him the father of modern medicine, and the Hippocratic Oath is still the practicing physician's moral code. But in spite of all this, history provides scanty reference to the man himself—and how it was that the torch was lit has been forgotten. —Now, since history has brought us new and relevant facts, it may be hoped that the picture painted here in this historic novel is clear and true. If so—the man so nearly lost in the darkening mists of time will live again and we shall see and understand, at last, the lighting of the torch.[2]

On Wednesday evening, 20 April 1960, I participated in the Upjohn Grand Rounds Number Nine on closed-circuit television from the Ohio State University College of Medicine, Columbus, Ohio. The topic was "Gastrointestinal Problems, Medicine or Surgery?" The panel was made up of the following clinicians and educators: Dr. Richard B. Cattell, director and surgeon-in-chief, Lahey Clinic; Dr. Philip J. Hodes (moderator), professor and chairman, department of radiology, Jefferson Medical College; Dr. Franz J. Ingelfinger, professor of medicine, Boston University School of Medicine; Dr. Michael J. Lepore, assistant clinical professor of medicine, Columbia University College of Physicians and Surgeons; Dr. Rodney Maingot, surgeon, Royal Free Hospital, London, England; Dr. Richard Schatzki, clinical associate in radiology, Harvard Medical School; Dr. Owen H. Wangensteen, professor and head, department of surgery, University of Minnesota Medical School; and Dr. Robert M. Zollinger, professor and chairman, department of surgery, Ohio State University College of Medicine. This proved to be a very interesting evening for me for it pitted me as the only other medical attending against the formidable Franz Ingelfinger, who in addition to his superb qualifications, was also the editor of the *New England*

---

2. Wilder Penfield, *The Torch* (Boston & Toronto: Little, Brown and Company, 1960), pp. 3–4.

Journal of Medicine. I was also asked by Steve Schwartz to keep an eye on Dr. Richard Cattell of the Lahey Clinic, regarded by many as the greatest biliary-tract surgeon of this century. Dr. Cattell had never before appeared on television and he was subject to unpredictable momentary lapses of memory, a forerunner of the disease that shortened his life.

My instructions were to step in, if anything untoward occurred, and improvise for a minute or two. With this in mind, I was seated next to the great surgeon. The moderator, Phil Hodes, performed very well, fomenting pros and cons and using his panel with consummate skill. Dr. Zollinger, always keen and knowledgeable, and at times acerbic, fanned the discussion in his inimitable fashion, pitting surgeon against physician. The program lasted for ninety minutes, during which a great deal of ground was covered. Dr. Ingelfinger and I differed on the management of three of the four patients that were presented. I later found out that the viewers voted with me. Dr. Cattell handled himself with the wisdom, skill, and judgment for which he was famous and, fortunately, there were no memory lapses. At the end of the program he turned to me and said, "Thanks for holding my coat"—a welcome tribute from a great surgeon. The next one to congratulate me was Steve Schwartz, a rabbi's son and a good friend, who threw his arms about me and yelled, "Michael, tonight you were the Cardinal of American Medicine!" In the limousine on the way back to our hotel, Dr. Franz Ingelfinger, seated next to me, said, "Mike, you were marvelous tonight. I could see that you were very experienced in clinical decision-making and it paid off. I saw in consultation perhaps 100 patients with ulcerative colitis last year but treated none of them on a one-on-one basis."

Years later, in 1972, I received the following letter from R. P. Trubey, manager, professional communications, The Upjohn Company:

> Dear Dr. Lepore:
>   We of Upjohn experience a vicarious lift each time one of our eminent film "alumni" is honored; and we extend our congratulations on your appointment as Professor of Clinical Medicine at New York University School of Medicine. As a matter of interest only, Kinescopes of the two Grand Rounds telecasts in which you participated (Diagnosis and Management of Acute Abdominal Problems and Gastrointestinal Problems—edicine or Surgery?) had, as of March 1, 1972, been shown 8,466 and 4,417 times, respectively, to cumulative audiences of 164,079 and 95,010 doctors, nurses and students.

It was clear that the vision I had of teaching in a medical school without walls via television was being magnificently brought to reality through the efforts of Steve Schwartz and his team. By 1962, seven years after their initiation by Steve Schwartz, I heard the Upjohn Grand Rounds were going to be discontinued. I sent the following letter to Mr. W. Fred Allen, vice president, The Upjohn Company, Kalamazoo, Michigan:

Dear Mr. Allen:

I have recently learned, to my disappointment, that the Upjohn Grand Rounds have not been continued. As a member of the Advisory Committee to the Grand Rounds, and as a moderator of the first presentation and as one whose interest in the program has never flagged, I would like to ask you to initiate, if you will, a review of the considerations having to do with the future of its superb and already famous teaching program. Since I understand that you were responsible for introducing this important program which has added so much lustre to the Upjohn reputation, it seems all the more fitting that your advice be sought concerning the continuation of this service to the physicians of this country and abroad.

It is hardly necessary that I indicate to you how highly I have regarded this educational section of the Upjohn Company, as a vehicle for transmitting vividly and authoritatively to audiences around the world the newest and most important trends in a variety of fields. Witness the impact of the latest clinic which brought before the world of medicine superb audiovisual Rounds of Dr. Irving Cooper's operation for Parkinson's disease. With this presentation, Upjohn anticipated the American Medical Association, LIFE magazine and other agencies in presenting the facts to the physicians of America. To mention another, Dr. Owen Wangensteen's discussion of gastric hypothermia appeared in the Upjohn Grand Rounds long before the recent upsurge of medical and public interest in this form of therapy. You have had then, in the Upjohn Grand Rounds, the essence of truly Hippocratic bedside and operating room medicine and surgery presented by some of the greatest people known in world medicine. As a result, these films are, as you know, still circulating and they still attract large audiences and, perhaps most interestingly, are being referred to as one might to a definitive written article on the subject discussed. It has been my pleasure not infrequently to hear a doctor say, "I heard Doctor So-and-So say this on the Grand Rounds telecast."

The contribution has therefore been a very important one and one that I feel should be continued even if one may find it difficult to judge its contributions to the Upjohn Company in dollars and cents. In this day, when all of the pharmaceutical manufacturers are the recipients of so much ill-advised and unfair criticism from people with curious and at times questionable motivation, it seems to me vital that every effort should be made to support the unselfish, constructive and educational ideals represented to date by the Upjohn Grand Rounds.

The phenomenal success of the Grand Rounds is almost entirely due to its producer, Mr. Stephen W. Schwartz of New York, whom I have been privileged to know since the very inception of this program,. Mr. Schwartz has brought to this field a brilliant, imaginative mind with a flair for communicating the advances of modern medicine to physicians and lay persons. He has the educational background and the dynamic and vigorous personality needed to attract the national and international figures in medicine and to enlist their participation and active collaboration. This is no mean feat when you consider the caliber of the persons involved. I have no hesitation to tell you that there is not enough money in the world to attract men of this caliber to a program sponsored by any pharmaceutical manufacturer. The appeal to these men has had to be on the basis of the value of the program as a teaching exercise. It has been in this spirit that they have participated and without this spirit the program would die.

The future development of the program lies in ensurance that the skills and brilliance of Mr. Stephen Schwartz and his contacts with the leaders in medicine be permitted to flourish and be utilized by Upjohn.

I would hope that serious consideration be given to re-instituting the Upjohn Grand Rounds as a service not only to American medicine, but also to world medicine.

I shall look forward to hearing from you regarding these constructive suggestions.

With best wishes, I remain

Sincerely yours,
Michael J. Lepore, M.D.

cc: S. W. Schwartz

Mr. Allen's reply was cordial and conveyed the impression that the Grand Rounds would be curtailed but not abandoned:

October 25, 1962

Michael J. Lepore, M.D.
The Roosevelt Hospital
The Upjohn Gastrointestinal Service
428 West 58th Street
New York, New York

Dear Dr. Lepore:

Thank you for your letter of October 17. You have certainly described Upjohn Grand Rounds most eloquently and I find it easy to agree with your conclusion.

We have not said that we were discontinuing Grand Rounds. It did seem wise for us to curtail our expenses in 1962 to this extent, but at no time have we intended to leave the impression with any one that Grand Rounds has been completely abandoned.

Whether not we are able to renew this activity in 1963 has not been decided yet, but you may be sure that it is being given careful consideration.

I would like to take this opportunity to express my appreciation to you as a member of the committee on Grand Rounds and also for your thoughtfulness in having written.

Best wishes.

Sincerely yours,
W. F. Allen

November 13, 1962

Mr. W. Fred Allen
Vice President
The Upjohn Company
Kalamazoo, Michigan

Dear Mr. Allen:

I would like to thank you for your letter of October concerning the Upjohn Grand Rounds and am pleased to know that you found my comments to be appropriate.

I am glad to hear that the Grand Rounds have not been abandoned and hope I shall have the pleasure of seeing you when the next one is produced.

Sincerely yours,
Michael J. Lepore, M.D.

But, alas, other matters were influencing the decision on continuing the Grand Rounds. I do not know all of the facts, but I learned later that Steve Schwartz was not too happy with his relationship with the McAdams Agency. In January 1962 he left that agency to start his own company, Medical Television Productions, Inc., in the business of selling, packaging, and producing, for pharmaceutical companies and other clients, "telecasts, radio programs and motion pictures addressed to professional medical audiences." Since he would now be competing with the McAdams Agency for clients, including Upjohn, the road ahead would be far from smooth. Steve chose never to discuss this matter with me and I respected his privacy by not asking any questions. For all practical purposes, the Grand Rounds were over but they had been great fun while they lasted.

Steve did some very interesting things after starting his own firm, but they were never of the magnitude or scope of the original Grand Rounds. Finally, illness came to this brilliant young man causing his death from carcinoma in 1979 at the age of fifty-five.

In his short paper of 1957 titled "Medical Education and Television,"[3] Steve Schwartz said:

> Postgraduate medical education, like undergraduate medical education, to be fully successful must be interestingly and dynamically presented. The television technic can succeed only when it provides a contribution that cannot be met by the traditional methods, such as books journals, lectures, etc. To employ television for a review of facts will therefore not suffice. The merit of the new medium lies in its ability to bring before the medical profession critical intelligences at work. Since the days of Hippocrates this has always been the stuff of which good medical education has consisted. Osler once pointed out that medicine is learned on the wards and not in the classrooms. The new electronic medium can take us all into the wards, operating rooms, the pathology laboratories and more important, into the minds of our great teachers. We are happy to note that this project (Grand Rounds) stemmed from the vision of one of our pharmaceutical manufacturers.
>
> The Upjohn Company—has supported this project, thus making the series available without cost to every physician. The response to the project has been gratifying. One midwestern physician who traveled 200 miles to attend a telecast stated subsequently that "I would go a thousand miles to see and hear these men again."

Since the first Grand Rounds closed-circuit telecast of 18 January 1956, pioneered by Stephen Schwartz, many changes and some advances have occurred in the field. The public has accepted and welcomed more and more explicit discussion and viewing of medical and surgical events on open circuits. Topics that Steve and I and organized medicine feared to present before the general public are now daily occurrences on open circuits. There seems to be no end to the craving of the general public for more and more information about its health. Excellent teaching programs sponsored by organized medicine and its specialty groups are regularly seen each Sunday on cable television, supported by various pharmaceutical companies, foundations,

---

3. Stephen W. Schwartz, "Medical Education and Television," Medical Annals of the District of Columbia 26, No. 1 (Aug. 3, 1957), pp. 29-31.

and medical societies. They are of very high quality and serve to keep many physicians and surgeons on the cutting edge of new developments in diagnosis, therapy, and management.

As I compare these sometimes elegant productions, I discern a trend that I think is not in keeping with the Oslerian teaching concepts that Steve and I fought for and preserved in the original Grand Rounds. The trend in the newer programs is to deviate from the case-presentation format that was the hallmark of the original Upjohn Grand Rounds. Patients seldom appear on these new programs and I believe this detracts from their teaching and learning impact. The sessions each Sunday consist mainly of questions and answers posed to the invited panelists, and they appear to be well rehearsed. This is indeed a valid method for teaching medicine, but it could be done on radio without the expense of television and it lacks the excitement, drama, and dynamism of case presentation, whicht take us to the patient's bedside, the wards, the emergency room, the operating room, the laboratories, and the front line scene of the action.

Grand Rounds in the Oslerian tradition have virtually disappeared from major teaching hospitals, their place taken by lectures by visiting peripatetic professors subsidized by pharmaceutical firms or a tax on the attending staff. Patients are almost never presented. Slide presentations packed with data are the norm. I take this to be a step backward in medical education and believe measures should be taken to replace or supplement these lecture sessions with the case presentations that were the hallmark of the Oslerian "natural" method of teaching that revolutionized American medical education at the turn of this century. If the major hospitals did this and arranged for their conferences to be videotaped, the best ones could be made available to affiliated and smaller institutions across the country. To set the standard, I believe we need a renewal of the Upjohn-type Grand Rounds of forty years ago, sparked perhaps by a modern-era communications wizard and teacher, another Stephen W. Schwartz.

Like Abraham Flexner who revolutionized American medical education at the turn of the century, Steve was not an M.D. He was an educator, professor of English at CCNY. He had the brilliant knack of grasping concepts of clinical medicine and scientific research with ease and could communicate their essence to lay persons as well as professionals with consummate skill and ingenuity.

Steve Schwartz was the son of a rabbi and had a brilliant brother, Dr. William B. Schwartz, who is renowned as a medical scholar and teacher. Their mother was a talented poet who brightened my day as my sixty-fifth birthday approached, sending me the following poem:

Able-gentle and brilliant, Dr. Michael Lepore
  whom thru the years we've loved more and more
not alone for his selfless untiring devotion
  but for the great faith and courage he instills without question!
Would there were more like him in this manacle age
  to help bring peace and love rather than guns and rage
watch over him father—for years untold
  so he may help and heal both young and old.
May god guide your path—Michael—to the mountain peak
  as Moses with his Commandments the summit did seek

Lovingly
Molly V. Schwartz
Feb.1975

In a recent issue of *JAMA*,[4] Dr. George D. Lundberg, the editor, published a concise editorial on "The Demise of National Medical Television." He pointed out that:

> . . . in the summer of 1993, three National Medical Television Networks existed: Lifetime Medical Television, Medical News Network and American Medical Television. In August 1993, Lifetime Medical Television ceased operations after nearly 10 years of significant educational service. And then there were two. In August 1994, Medical News Network was canceled, after having never really gotten off the ground except in elaborate program development and national market testing. And then there was one. In December 1994, after 5 years of successful programming for physicians, other health professionals, and patients, first on the Discovery Channel and then on CNBC, the owners of American Medical Television (NBC Cable, The American Medical Association, the Orbis Broadcast Group, and Dr. Art Ulene) voted to dissolve the partnership, ceasing operations before February 1995. And then there were none.
>
> As with any complex venture, the reasons for these failures were complex. But the common reason was the bottom line. Television is a powerful communication medium. Americans get most of their scientific and medical information from television. Arguably, there has never been a time of greater need for wide distribution of accurate and reliable new medical information to medical scientists, clinicians, economists, policy makers, and, of course, the public. I cannot personally believe that a $1-trillion-a-year industry that runs on information flow cannot support at least one properly managed medical television network.

---

4. *Journal of the American Medical Association* 273 (March 15, 1995), p. 891.

Something will surface to fill this obvious vacuum. The closing paragraph of this editorial is a plea for help:

> As ideas occur to you about how we can re-create national medical television and retain ethical, professional control of its content (i.e., like the high quality, peer reviewed biomedical literature) please call or write. Think about it. It's serious!

I believe the AMA should spearhead a drive to support Medical Television as a very important key element in continuing medical education (CME). Since there is no free lunch, I suggest that the AMA ask its members to contribute a significant sum annually to a fund to support CME, with especial emphasis on teaching by television. We should organize a national commission on television CME consisting of experienced practicing clinicians as well as academicians, who will determine the scope of the program and its goals. It ought to be lean and mean and relevant to the problems faced by practicing clinicians in every category. It should also include a small number of laymen picked with great care. The pharmaceutical houses will, I am certain, participate and support this effort. I believe CNN, CSPAN, etc. should pitch in with their facilities and support. I am really amazed that the big three caved in and wonder what we can learn from their failure.

Chapter 21

⌒⌒

The Iceman Cometh to Park Avenue

I N 1948, ONLY TWO YEARS AFTER RETURNING from military service, I took Dr. Walter Palmer's advice and leased a small office in a nice building at 944 Park Avenue at a rent I could afford. In those days, to avoid garage fees, it was still possible to turn the car keys over to the doorman who would see that the car was not ticketed by the cop on patrol. I asked my sister, Lucille Lepore Russo, R.N. to manage the office and perform R.N. duties as well. Lucille, a Bellevue Nursing School graduate, was the head nurse and ward instructor on Ward B6 of the A&B Building of Bellevue on the Third Medical Division (the NYU Division). She also was the night supervisor of the entire A&B building, for three months, an enormous responsibility for a young nurse. She was highly regarded by her superiors and a valued member of their nursing staff. When Dr. William Tillet, the NYU professor and chairman of the department of medicine, learned that she was planning to leave Bellevue to work with me, he called me and tried to persuade me to let her remain at Bellevue. We had a friendly chat and he pleasantly agreed that the move to my office was in my sister's best interest and wished her well. As I look back, this was one of the best decisions I have ever made. Her loyalty, intelligence, skill, and common sense were major assets to my practice of medicine. With her help, my private practice flourished. I continued to use a few hours each week in Harkness Pavilion, but I soon realized that the downtown office had many advantages. The patients who came to me did so because they sought my personal care and not primarily because I was a staff member of a vast medical center. Their telephone calls were handled by me or my nurse, not by strangers who knew them only as numbers on a list. This personal approach to the practice of medicine quickly paid off in major dividends. With the rapid growth of my practice, it soon became evident that we needed more space and we began looking around for it. One day, while I was driving down Park Avenue, my sister saw an empty doctors' office. It was at 550 Park Avenue on the southwest corner of 62nd Street with a desirable street-level entrance on Park Avenue and a lobby entrance on the side street. We made an appointment with the renting agent to inspect this spacious and well-located office. The suite consisted of three enormous rooms with high ceilings plus a foyer and reception area. It had been occupied by only one physician since the construction of the building in 1917. The physician was the famous Evan Evans, renowned consultant, internist, and eminent diagnostician of the Roosevelt Hospital staff and professor of medicine at the Columbia University College of Physicians and Surgeons in the days when it was located on 58th Street near Tenth Avenue in Manhattan. Dr. Evans himself drew up the plans for the office and no major changes had ever been made. The office still had antique wall fixtures and, I was to learn later, was still on direct electric current that would require a major electrical conversion out of my pocket. Dr. Evans, then in his eighties, owned the ten-room, three-bathroom apartment above the office. An accomplished pianist, he practiced regularly on his grand piano and his music would waft into the medical office, for our enjoyment. Periodically he would drop into the office, visiting with me and querying me about my research and teaching. He would shake his head and remark that medicine had become so complicated, and I in turn would comment that it must have been even more difficult in his heyday to deal with sick people and their diseases without the aid of the laboratory and the radiologists. After my initial visit, I brought my beloved wife to see the office that had caught my eye. She, too, was enchanted by the suite and challenged by the prospect of decorating it. The office had been empty for nearly two years because it would have required major construction alterations for multiple occupancy, and single occupancy required the payment of a substantial rental for those days. The reconstruction costs would have been prohibitive and I knew I could not afford them. I decided to make no structural changes and planned to use the office in much the same manner that Dr. Evans had employed for many years. I signed the lease and turned the furnishing of the office over to my wife and a close friend, Miss Kay Comiskey, who was a skilled interior decorator working pro bono. The two of them had a wonderful time and, through their efforts, the office was quietly but not frighteningly elegant and much admired for its ambiance by people from all walks of life who came to seek my advice. The entrance foyer was nicely arranged, the waiting room was capacious measuring 20 x 20 feet. Special mahogany doors donated to me by Mr. Joseph Pirozzi, my friend and patient, sealed off the consultation room, which measured 20 x 24 feet, so that utter privacy was maintained for all patients. The next area was the toilet and a small laboratory space. Next was a large (18 x 28 feet), immaculate, well-equipped examining room. There were no gimmicks, no fluoroscope, no x-ray, no diathermy, merely a sturdy examining table, an instrument cabinet containing proctosigmoidoscopes, vaginal specula, several chairs, a clothes tree, a beam balance and sphygmomanometers, ophthalmoscope, and otoscope, and several stethoscopes. What the patient got when he visited me was the doctor himself, no gimmicks but intense concentration on the patient with no interruption by beepers or telephone calls. The examining room was large enough to break down into multiple little examining cubicles. Since I never saw more than one patient at a time, I had no need for multiple examining rooms or mass production of any sort. I have always felt with Francis W. Peabody that "The treatment of a disease may be entirely impersonal; the care of the patient must be completely personal."[1] For the next thirty years this marvelous office would be the focal point of my career in the personal practice of medicine. In those days a Park Avenue office was the goal of many doctors. Park Avenue was the Harley Street of America. The avenue was lined with offices of most of the leading teaching clinicians in New York. This was before hospital-based office became commonplace and before the takeover of hospital teaching and practice by the full-time system. Nowadays the large offices have been replaced by rabbit-warren cubicles, the denizens no longer the key professors controlling medical and surgical services. Abortionists abound and chiropractors, podiatrists, and cosmetic surgeons are in abundant supply as are rectal specialists, endodontists, cataract specialists, and laser operators. Advertising by doctors, forbidden in my early days, is now rampant, filling pages of the tabloid newspapers. Is it any wonder that our profession is now viewed as a business or trade?

When I announced my move in 1948 to the office at 944 Park Avenue, I received several nice letters, one of them from Dr. Walter Palmer, wishing me well and adding that he was sure I would do well.

One rather disturbing remark was made to me in 1953 when I moved to 550 Park Avenue by Dr. Franklin Hanger, one of the full-time professors at P&S, who said, "I see you have taken over Evan Evans' large office on Park Avenue. I hope you can keep it full." My reply to this unsolicited carp was, "My aim is to keep my patients moving on schedule so that the office will never be full." I thought it was a cheap shot to take at a young man striving to excel. First the full-timers tell me to get a downtown office, then they envy my success. "Catch 22"!

---

1. Francis Weld Peabody, "The Care of the Patient," *Journal of the American Medical Association* 88 (March 19, 1928), pp. 877–82.

My private practice grew rapidly with some referrals from my colleagues at Columbia-Presbyterian and many self-referrals from satisfied patients from all walks of life. The downtown office was much more convenient to reach than the Medical Center and preferred by most of my patients. Referrals from doctors on the staff of other major hospitals were numerous and interesting. The referring doctors, fearing the loss of the patient, preferred to send them to a consultant with a downtown office not physically connected with a medical center. Over the years I have found that word of mouth from satisfied patients was the best source of referrals to my practice. Furthermore, many of the doctors who referred patients to me were prodded by their patients who had heard of me through their friends or relatives. This is why to this day I am a firm believer in freedom of choice in selecting a doctor. I can quote many instances of lives that were saved because a patient or the family decided to change doctors when things were not going well. Those politicians who claim that freedom of choice is unnecessary are absolutely wrong and my advice to the public is that they fight like tigers to preserve their right to choose a personal doctor.

Over the years, through my practice, I encountered many interesting people from all walks of life and I enjoyed knowing them and helping them. Early in my days at 550 I was consulted by Major Henry Hooker, President F. D. Roosevelt's friend and law partner, who had served as our ambassador to England. There was nothing seriously wrong with Major Hooker but he had been a patient of Evan Evans and he seemed to enjoy coming in to see me for a checkup in the relatively unchanged sumptuous office previously occupied by Dr. Evan Evans. One day, Major Hooker told me an interesting story. It was during WW II that the queen of the Netherlands was being entertained at dinner in the Roosevelt town house nearby with the president as host. Major Hooker received an invitation to attend. This led him to telephone Dr. Evans, asking if he had some medicine that he could take to keep alert during the dinner. Dr. Evans said, "There is a new medicine on the market that will help you. I will call the pharmacist and have him deliver it to you. Take a tablet before dinner." The major had a great time and managed to monopolize the conversation with the queen, no mean feat with President Roosevelt at the table. After the dinner, Roosevelt called him aside and said, "Henry, what the hell did you have to drink before you came to dinner? I couldn't get a word in edgewise at dinner." The major replied that he had not had anything to drink before coming to dinner. "But," he said, "I did take a new pill that my doctor prescribed." "Let's call him up and find out what it was," said the president. The medicine was

Benzedrine. No wonder he monopolized the conversation! Years later I would remember this story when I was consulted by Mr. Malcolm Muir, the dynamic publisher of *Newsweek* magazine, who told me he was meeting with General Eisenhower the next day to persuade him to run for the presidency. Mr. Muir told me he wanted to be on his toes, alert, and keen, and asked me to prescribe some medication to assure this. I remembered the Major Hooker story and told him about it. I recall saying, "Mr. Muir I've known you for some years and I don't believe you need any stimulant. Just be your usual dynamic self." Mr. Muir returned from his visit with Eisenhower's acceptance. Mr. Muir had been referred to me by Dr. Byron Stookey, the famous neurosurgeon who was also one of my patients. Mr. Muir's number-one man at *Newsweek* was Theodore (Ted) Mueller, who became my patient and friend. He was a most unusual person who had a great deal to do with *Newsweek*'s success. I learned from him that an outstanding newsman has high professional standards equivalent to those of any dedicated physician. During one of his visits, Mr. Mueller asked me to name the teacher who meant the most to me. My answer was Dean George Hoyt Whipple of Rochester. I forgot about this conversation for several years until one day, after Mr. Mueller's death, I was visited by his attorney, Mr. John M. Keating, and Gibson McCabe of *Newsweek* carrying a large well-wrapped parcel. Mr. Keating read the following letter to me.

November 13, 1962

Dr. Michael J. Lepore
550 Park Avenue
New York 21, New York

Dear Dr. Lepore:
    As executor and trustee of the estate and long-time friend of Theodore F. Mueller, I would like to record how the gift by Ted to you of the picture of Dean George Hoyt Whipple came about.
    As you know, Ted was extremely fond of you. He very highly respected you as a Doctor and I think loved you as a friend. From anecdotes he told me you apparently had taken him in the evenings on different occasions from his hospital room to visit Association meetings with you and to learn of some of the professional activities of the various medical associations. I knew him intimately and knew that partly because of his somewhat lonely life he was very deeply appreciative to you for this camaraderie.
    He was a truly great man. As you know he was Publisher of Newsweek Magazine. He had come up the hard way and he made a great contribution to Newsweek and the publishing field.

In his visits with you, you had told him about the great esteem and high regard in which you held Dean George Hoyt Whipple of the Medical School at the University of Rochester. You apparently had told Ted how you felt that your training under Dean Whipple and your association with him had contributed to and molded your career in medicine and had left such an important imprint on your whole life.

When he was in the hospital in his last illness, he felt you had devoted so much of your all to him that he wanted to give you something to show his appreciation. He told his secretary that you had spoken of a portrait of Dean George Hoyt Whipple which was in a place of honor at the University of Rochester. He told her that she should get some of the Newsweek staff in the Rochester area to go see the picture and see what the best and most effective way of reproducing it would be.

The Newsweek employee found the picture, examined it and reported that an excellent reproduction could be made by an artistic photographic process. Ted authorized and directed him to employ an outstanding photographer-artist to make the best possible reproduction of the painting. The work had practically been completed at the time of Ted's death. The artist who had made the reproduction arranged for the framing and shipment to us, after which it was presented to you.

The picture is an artistic reproduction of a portrait of a great man, George Hoyt Whipple, Dean of Rochester Medical School which was given by a great man, Theodore F. Mueller, Publisher of Newsweek Magazine to you to show his appreciation to a great man who had expended his all for him.

Cordially yours,
John M. Keating

JMK:B

This handsome 28 x 24 inch colored oil portrait of my beloved Dean has been hanging on the north wall of my home library since its arrival in 1962, serving to inspire me to live up to the promise this great man saw in the eighteen-year-old student he interviewed and accepted for medical school in 1929. There is a little more to add to this story. Ted Mueller had originally wished to have a bust made of Dean Whipple for presentation to me. The Dean felt that, at age 83, he lacked the patience to sit for a bust and the decision was made to substitute a copy of a portrait that I had seen and admired.

Chapter 22

~~~~

Songs My Patients Taught Me

It is a safe rule to have no teaching
without a patient for a text, and the
best teaching is that taught by the
patient himself.

—Sir William Osler, 1904[1]

THE EDUCATION OF THE PHYSICIAN begins in his childhood and
his home, continues in college and medical school, and persists
for the rest of his life. For the physician as well as his patient,
survival and success depends upon constant renewal and assimilation
of new facts and concepts. It is an old saw that fifty percent of what
is taught in medical school will be obsolete in five years, the faculty
uncertain which half it will be. A phase of the education of the doctor that is seldom addressed in medical school is the role of the
patient in his training and development. Again I quote Sir William
Osler: "To study the phenomena of disease without books is to sail
an uncharted sea, while to study books without patients is not to go
to sea at all."[2] "Medicine is learned by the bedside and not in the classroom."[3]

The tools of my professional specialty of internal medicine are
not surgical instruments, endoscopes, x-ray machines, lasers, and
ultrasound, they are the five senses that God has blessed us with, a
pair of strong hands, a plain stethoscope, a retentive memory, good
health, a wholesome lifestyle, integrity, tenacity, and humility combined with confidence, the courage of my convictions, and something
called judgment, wisdom, and common sense. Above all, I have been

---

1. Sir William Osler, "On the Need of a Radical Reform in our Methods of
Teaching Medical Students," *Medical News* 82 (1904), pp. 49–53.

2. William Osler, "Books and Men," *Medical and Surgical Journal* 144 (1901),
pp. 60–1.

3. Robert Bennett Bean, ed., *Sir William Osler: Aphorisms Collected by Robert
Bennett Bean* (Springfield, Ill.: Charles C. Thomas, 1901).

the advocate for my patients, ready to make any sacrifice to cure some, relieve others, and comfort all. My purpose is to improve or save lives and never to destroy them.

In the sixty-four years since I entered medical school, I have had the great pleasure and privilege of learning much from my illustrious teachers, many of them famous men and women. To them I owe a great debt that I can never repay.

This narrative provides some of the details of their impact upon my life and career. But there is another group of people who have affected my life to a major degree and taught me many wonderful things. They are my patients, some famous, a few infamous, and most somewhere in-between.

One afternoon in March 1956 I received a telephone call from my friend and colleague Dr. Carmine T. Vicale, a brilliant neurologist, asking me to see Miss Greta Garbo, who was having abdominal problems. I arranged an early appointment at my 550 Park Avenue office on a Monday morning. In spite of a raging blizzard with no traffic moving, Miss Garbo arrived promptly for her appointment having walked the distance from her apartment on East 52nd Street to my office on 62nd Street wearing her galoshes and her floppy felt hat. As luck would have it, because of the blizzard I was unable to leave my home in Englewood, New Jersey, and remained there like a caged lion. My staff had managed to get to the office and the telephones were working. The situation was explained to Miss Garbo, who was very gracious and understanding, and she was given another appointment.

On March 20, 1956, Miss Garbo arrived for her consultation. She was then fifty-one years old, appeared ill and slightly wan, but clearly just as beautiful as her movies had shown her to be. She was charming, had a throaty voice with no trace of an accent, and she was a good historian. I learned from her that she had been admitted to Harkness Pavilion earlier that year by her physician, Dr. Dana Atchley, one of our senior professors. During her stay, she underwent many studies and was told they were negative for any organic disease. She continued to experience right-lower-quadrant pain and nausea and sought advice from other consultants. One of them, a gynecologist on the Memorial Hospital staff, examined her and said she had an ovarian tumor and recommended admission to Memorial Hospital for an operation. She sought another opinion, that of Dr. Anthony D'Esopo, professor of obstetrics and gynecology at P&S, who found no evidence of an ovarian tumor. He recommended that she see me in consultation, asking Dr. Vicale to arrange the appointment. I took a complete and thorough history and examined the patient from head to toes. The only significant findings were definite tenderness in the right lower quadrant and suspicion of a mass in the region of the cecum. Miss Garbo was a world traveler and had ample opportunity to acquire intestinal infections. My diagnosis was that she had an amebic granuloma of the cecum. This was quickly confirmed by obtaining a warm purged stool for ova and protozoa in Dr. Howard Shookhoff's laboratory. The stool contained cysts and trophozoites of Entamoeba histolytica, the causative agent of amebiasis of the cecum and amebic dysentery. At this point I would ordinarily have admitted her to Harkness Pavilion for treatment.

She was reluctant to do this because she did not wish to embarrass Dr. Atchley. She said she would be willing to take any medicine I prescribed. She lived nearby and would keep in daily touch with me and come to my office as often as necessary. I too, was not anxious to upset Dr. Atchley, who had told one of our surgeons, "I do my own gastroenterology," after it was suggested that he ask me to consult on a V.I.P. of his with recurrent major GI bleeding. I kept my fingers crossed, followed Miss Garbo closely, and cured her of the amebiasis with several courses of amebicidal agents. I had occasion to review her Harkness admission hospital record and the GI x-rays done during that admission. Sure enough, Dr. Ross Golden, the famous radiologist, had seen a contracted, conical, irritable cecum consistent with amebiasis and called it to the attending's attention. The attending told Dr. Golden that he felt he was overdiagnosing amebiasis, but he requested two stools for ova and protozoa. They were negative, but I knew that in an economy move, Mrs. Hulse, our expert parasitologist whose laboratory had for years been on the eighth floor of the Presbyterian Hospital, had been moved to the Board of Health building on 168th Street and Broadway, a long city block from Harkness Pavilion. The powers that be had never figured out how on a freezing day in March, trophozoites in the stool could survive the trip and the long wait in the laboratory necessitated by the relocation of the laboratory outside of the main hospital building. For Garbo fans, I am pleased to report that her feet were not, as rumored, too large. She wore shoe size 8AA, in keeping with her general physique. She weighed 130 pounds and her height was 5 feet 7 inches. I found Miss Garbo to be an excellent, intelligent, and cooperative patient. She was very considerate and never in a hurry. On one occasion she was accompanied by her good friend of many years, Mr. George Schlee. The latter was an urbane and debonair gentleman who, viewing a photograph of my beautiful wife and my young son, asked "Is this your production?" Both Greta Garbo and I laughed as I said, "He sure is."

I have often wondered what might have happened to Miss Garbo if she had been operated upon by the gynecologist who thought she had an ovarian tumor.

I recall that many years ago, Texas Guinan, the night-club hostess, was operated upon for what unexpectedly turned out to be amebiasis of the colon and did not survive. The lesson in the Greta Garbo story is that even the high and mighty should call for consultation in a puzzling case. The consultant in tropical diseases (now called geographic medicine), must have a high index of suspicion triggered by a good knowledge of the travel habits and lifestyle of his patients. Equally important is access to a reliable laboratory with first-rate technicians familiar and experienced in recognizing protozoan pathogens. We teach our students, over and over again, the importance of obtaining warm purged stools for immediate examination, but this advice is frequently disregarded. All too often, in our major hospitals, stool specimens languish on shelves for prolonged periods before they are examined by sometimes inexperienced technicians.

A good tropical-disease specialist must be a fearless coprologist. My internship and residency at Duke University Hospital and my military experience in WW II with soldiers returned from service in North Africa, the CBI theater, the Mediterranean, and the Pacific, and my stay on Tinian and Saipan taught me a great deal and was worth its weight in gold for me and my patients in the years that have followed.

In closing the Greta Garbo episode, I must record that I complained to the powers that be at Columbia-Presbyterian that a diagnosis of amebiasis of the cecum had been missed in a famous patient because of inadequate laboratory facilities and false economy in moving the tropical-disease laboratory to an outside site. My recommendation was that the laboratory and its highly skilled technician be returned to its former base within the medical center proper, a suggestion that fell upon deaf ears. To my knowledge nothing was done about this. This was a factor, when the opportunity arose, in my decision to establish the Upjohn Gastroenterology Service at another major teaching hospital.

C.C., a Patient with Cystic Fibrosis

When I returned to Columbia-Presbyterian in 1946 from military service in WW II most of my time was spent rebuilding my practice and resuming my teaching activities in the Vanderbilt Clinic and Presbyterian Hospital. I quickly renewed my association with Ross Golden, professor and director of radiology, and sought to continue with my clinical investigation of malabsorptive disorders, including sprue, celiac disease, and small-bowel and pancreatic disease.

In those days there were no NIH funds for research and little or no support existed for GI research or laboratory space within the department of medicine. The emphasis in the department of medicine was on general internal medicine. A small research unit focused its attention on diabetes, Addison's disease, metabolic disorders, hypertension, and electrolyte imbalance. It is hard to believe, but in those days a serum amylase determination at Columbia-Presbyterian had to be arranged by appointment two or three days ahead. There was no provision for an emergency amylase test. The reason for this was that a senior professor at the Medical Center, who was a well trained biochemist, did not approve of the rather crude tests for amylase then in vogue in several other hospitals in New York and he refused to use them, preferring a more complex and time-consuming procedure that was less available to us. I looked into the matter and was able to persuade the powers that be to permit us to use the less-complicated and easily performed tests in use at Bellevue Hospital. We were then able to get an emergency serum amylase in the same way we did a blood sugar at any hour of the day or night.

Since I had a very pleasant experience in 1931 doing research at the Babies' Hospital, I renewed my friendship with that staff and came to know and admire Dr. Dorothy Andersen, a talented pathologist and research scientist who was the first to describe the entity of fibrocystic disease of the pancreas. In addition to that disease, she was also greatly interested in childhood celiac disease. She had a laboratory and a technician for studies of malabsorption, including stools for fat and starches and serum carotene and Vitamin A levels, as well as pancreatic enzyme assays. Later I was able to persuade her to add D-xylose absorption studies to these.

With time, in an informal manner, I became the chief gastroenterology consultant for the Babies' Hospital and saw many of the patients with inflammatory-bowel disease, celiac disease, and fibrocystic disease of the pancreas, and I followed those who survived to childhood and adolescence in the Vanderbilt Clinic. Dr. Andersen made her laboratory facilities available for some of my patients.

Cystic fibrosis of the pancreas, named by Fanconi in 1936, and clearly and comprehensively described as a disease entity by Dorothy Andersen in 1938, is a generalized, serious, hereditary disease of children, adolescents, and young adults due to dysfunction of exocrine glands. "It is the most common lethal genetic disease of the white race. In the United States it affects 2 in 2500 white, 1 in 17000 blacks and 1 in 90,000 full-blooded Asians. It is transmitted as an autosomal recessive trait, so that 4 percent of the white population carry the lethal gene."[4]

The disease is characterized by the combination of symptoms of pancreatic exocrine insufficiency with those of chronic pulmonary disease, with the latter usually dominating the clinical picture, accounting for most of the deaths and much of the morbidity. In the past, most of the early experience had come from the autopsy rooms of large medical centers. As therapy and diagnosis improved with the advent of potent antibiotics, the life span of many of the children was prolonged to the point that significant numbers outgrew their pediatric age limit and survived to adolescence and young adulthood. When they reached this point in their lives, they were assigned to my Cystic Fibrosis Clinic in the Vanderbilt Clinic, where they were followed by me and by members of the pediatric staff. Dr. Andersen had been joined during the war years by a very able and well-trained pediatrician who shared her research interests. He was Dr. Paul A. di Sant'Agnese, an M.D. graduate of the University of Rome, 1938, whose training included residencies at the Post Graduate Hospital, Willard Parker Hospital, and the Koplik Fellowship in Pediatrics at the Babies' Hospital. He was awarded a doctor of science degree in medicine by Columbia University in 1948. Dr. di Sant'Agnese and I became close friends and collaborators for a number of years before he accepted an important position at the NIH in pediatric research. With the discovery by di Sant'Agnese, et al., in 1953 of high levels of sodium and chloride in the sweat of patients with cystic fibrosis, a simple non-invasive test made it possible to diagnose and screen patients with the disease. For many years it has been the gold standard for the diagnosis of cystic fibrosis, a position from which it may be dislodged by more sophisticated and more specific tests. As with many discoveries, serendipity and keen clinical observation led Dr. Andersen and her group, including Dr. di Sant'Agnese, to make this important contribution. They had noted that children with cystic fibrosis were prone to dehydration, collapse, and serious illness during a severe heat wave in New York in 1951. The children's parents also reported that when they kissed the children, their sweat was very salty. Dr. di Sant'Agnese pounced on these leads and, encouraged by

---

4. W.N. Kelley, Ed. in Chief, *Textbook of Internal Medicine* (Philadelphia: J.B. Lippincott, 1992), pp. 1732-35.

Dr. Andersen, organized a team effort to test sweat levels of sodium and chloride in these children.

Dr. di Sant'Agnese had the knack of bringing people together in cooperative and team efforts. He enlisted the assistance of Dr. Robert Darling, newly appointed professor of physical medicine and rehabilitation, and Dr. George A. Perera, associate professor of medicine, an authority on adrenal and renal function and hypertension. Their efforts culminated in a short and well-designed experiment reported in the *American Journal of the Medical Sciences* in January 1953, vol. 225, pp. 67–70, followed by a more complete report entitled "Sweat Electrolyte Disturbances Associated with Childhood Pancreatic Disease," published in the *American Journal of Medicine*, vol. 15, December 1953, pp. 777–84, a classic in its field. In passing, it should be mentioned that this was before the era of enormous NIH grants, the support coming in part from a gift for celiac research of the United Fruit Company and in part by the Robert Bacon Whitney Fund for Cystic Fibrosis of the Pancreas. In those days a little bit of money went a long way. I do not recall that there was any money for gastroenterology at Columbia-Presbyterian at that time. Only by scrounging from other departments, such as pediatrics and radiology, and later from surgery, was it possible to pursue my research interests in gastroenterology. The department of medicine was focused on general internal medicine and the subspecialties were struggling to develop.

Through Dr. di Sant'Agnese I met and cared for a patient with cystic fibrosis whom I shall never forget. C.C. was a pretty, dark-haired, lively teenager of fourteen who had been referred to Dr. di Sant'Agnese in the Vanderbilt Clinic for diagnosis and treatment of cystic fibrosis, undiagnosed for years by a multitude of physicians. She had classical cystic fibrosis of the lungs, pansinusitis, and steatorrhea. A strongly positive sweat test clinched the diagnosis.

What set C.C. apart from our other patients with cystic fibrosis were bouts of very severe abdominal pain relieved only by Demerol in heavy dosage. These attacks had been occurring three to four times a year and had eluded diagnosis. Shortly after the Cystic Fibrosis group at Columbia-Presbyterian assumed the care of C.C., I was asked to see her because of one of these attacks of pain. The pain seemed very real, dull and constant, starting in the epigastrium and radiating across the left upper quadrant through to the back and causing the patient to assume the fetal position. I was certain on clinical grounds that the pain was of pancreatic origin and I ordered STAT serum amylase tests that were elevated, a rare finding in cystic fibrosis and probably caused by inspissated pancreatic juice blocking the pancreatic ducts.

Other possibilities had been ruled out by radiologic techniques then in vogue, including cholecystograms, intravenous pyelogram, and meticulously performed roentgen studies of the stomach, duodenum and small bowel. Between the attacks she was free of abdominal pain and was able to function. During 1959 her attacks became more frequent and more prolonged. Soon she was habituated to Demerol and posed a serious problem in management. In May 1959, after thorough discussion and consultation with Dr. Milton Porter, our chief pancreas surgeon, Dr. di Sant'Agnese and I decided with Dr. Porter that something more should be done and agreed on a right thoracolumbar sympathectomy and splanchnicectomy with celiac ganglionectomy which was done on 12 May 1959. It failed to relieve the pain and the patient continued to have severe bouts of pancreatitis requiring Demerol. We theorized that with each bout of pancreatitis her exocrine pancreas would atrophy sparing the endocrine function of the islets of Langerhans so that she would not become a diabetic. The frequency of the attacks and escalating requirements for Demerol led us to consider removing a substantial portion of the pancreas. Dr. Porter at that time was performing partial and subtotal pancreatectomy for severe relapsing pancreatitis in adult patients and had achieved some promising results. The situation was discussed at length with the patient's father and mother, who agreed and granted permission for the operation. On 10 May 1960, the patient underwent exploratory laparotomy, splenectomy, left hemi-pancreatectomy, and a prophylactic appendectomy. The pathologists' diagnosis on the submitted tissue was, "Chronic pancreatitis, Cystic fibrosis of the pancreas, clinical, chronic peripancreatic lymph-adenitis. Normal spleen and appendix." Additional notes were, "On section the normal architecture of the pancreas is lost, instead is seen a white fibrotic surface with areas of yellow coloration which may represent adipose tissue. Microscopic sections demonstrate the pancreatic parenchyma is scanty. There is extensive fibrosis and marked fatty infiltration. The stroma shows minimal lymphocytic infiltration. Many ductules contain inspissated eosinophilic material. The islets of Langerhans appear relatively unaffected."

Mirabile dictu, the operation was successful and for a time C.C. gained weight (30 pounds), had no need for Demerol, and was able to attend school on a regular basis. *This remission lasted for two and one-half years.* In early 1963, she had a recurrence of abdominal pain requiring Demerol and her pulmonary disease worsened, failing to respond to antibiotics.

At her wish and her family's, this wonderful and brave young lady, only nineteen, died at home in 1963 of bilateral bronchopneumonia due to hemolytic Staphylococcus aureus, coagulase positive. But this is not the end of the saga of C.C. Her father was a talented lawyer who, spurred by his child's illness, decided to do everything he could to help other children with cystic fibrosis. He was especially struck as I was by the inability of the afflicted to afford medications, especially antibiotics, and the expense of frequent and long hospital admissions. In our discussions, we agreed that children with cystic fibrosis should be eligible for state assistance and classified as physically handicapped, making them eligible for state-paid medical care, hospital care, and medications. Mr. C. fought for the passage in Albany of several bills for this purpose. These bills were passed during Governor Nelson Rockefeller's tenure, giving comfort and solace and substantial help to those afflicted with this disease. Paul di Sant'Agnese left the Babies' Hospital in New York in 1960 to become chief of the Pediatric Metabolism Branch of the National Institute of Arthritis, Metabolism and Digestive Disease of the NIH, where he has remained and flourished, continuing his work with cystic fibrosis and developing a group of distinguished and outstanding disciples who revere him as their mentor. To all of us interested in cystic fibrosis, the recent (1989) identification of the gene that carries cystic fibrosis is one of the major discoveries of this century, bringing hope for a revolution in the treatment and prevention of this disease. The two teams credited with this discovery, led by Lap-Chee Tsui and John Riordan of the Toronto Hospital for Sick Children, the other by Francis Collins of the Howard Hughes Medical Institute of the University of Michigan at Ann Arbor, almost certainly deserve a Nobel Prize. In the 1940s, when our team at Columbia-Presbyterian was struggling to keep our patients with CF alive, who would ever have dared to believe that its cause would be found, paving the road to improved therapy, prevention, and ultimately a cure? This was a marvelous song my patients taught me and I shall never forget it.

Anatole Broyard: *Intoxicated by My Illness*[5]

Another patient who taught me a great deal was one I never met in person. He was Anatole Broyard, a noted essayist, critic, and

---

5. Anatole Broyard, *Intoxicated by My Illness* (New York: Clarkson Potter, 1992), pp. 33–58.

columnist of the *New York Times* whose prose and Gallic comments I have enjoyed for years.

I suppose he might be included among my "patients" because he was once admitted to one of my hospitals, St. Vincent's Medical Center in New York City, with a high fever of undetermined origin. This was his only illness prior to that of 1989 that proved to be very serious, ending with his death from prostate cancer on 11 October 1990. It was during his terminal illness that he published a sprightly essay in the *New York Times*, republished in *Hippocrates*[6] and again in a book of essays posthumously in 1992, describing his difficulties in finding a physician in Cambridge who could satisfy him as a patient. The title was "The Patient Examines the Doctor." Broyard said: "When in the summer of 1989 I moved from Connecticut to Cambridge, Massachusetts, I found that I couldn't urinate. I was like Alex Portnoy, in *Portnoy's Complaint*, who couldn't fornicate in Israel. I had always wanted to live in Cambridge and I was almost persuaded that I couldn't urinate because I was surprised by joy, in C. S. Lewis' phrase. When my inhibition persisted, I began to think about a doctor, and I set about finding one in the superstitious manner most people fall back on in this situation. I asked a couple I knew for a recommendation." They recommended their internist who, in turn, recommended a urologist. The latter proved to be an able and competent individual who examined him thoroughly and, after complete studies, informed him that he had cancer of the prostate that had already spread to his lymph nodes and bones. Broyard did not feel that he wished to put his life in the hands of this urologist. By his own admission, Broyard's expectations were of a very high order, leading to the editorial comment in *Hippocrates* that "All he wants is a physician who treats body and soul, appreciates the tragedy of illness, looks good in scrubs and thinks like Oliver Sacks." That is a large order in this era of narrow subspecialization, high technology, procedure-oriented medicine, and doctors in a hurry.

These considerations led Broyard to select another urologist to take over his care. This one was regarded as the best in Cambridge and the most respected in the field of prostate cancer. Broyard's initial impression was positive but it did not take long before the patient realized that, despite his reputation and medical knowledge, this urologist failed to communicate and relate well to this patient. He was so

---

6. Anatole Broyard, "The Patient Examines the Doctor," *Hippocrates: The Magazine of Health and Medicine*, April 1992, pp. 74–78.

admired by Broyard's friends and others that Broyard stayed the course with him, albeit with some reservations. These were clearly expressed by Broyard in his essay:

> "—What do I want in a doctor? asks Broyard. I want one who is a close reader of illness and a good critic of medicine. —Also I would like a doctor who is not only a talented physician, but a bit of a metaphysician, too, someone who can treat body and soul. . . . To the typical physician, my illness is a routine incident in his rounds, while for me it's the crisis of my life. I would feel better if I had a doctor who perceived this incongruity. . . . I see no reason for my doctor to love me—nor would I expect him to suffer with me. I wouldn't demand a lot of my doctor's time: I just wish he would brood on my situation for perhaps five minutes, that he would give me his whole mind just once, be bonded with me for a brief space. I would also like to think of him as going through my character, as he goes through my flesh, to get at my illness, for each man is ill in his own way.
>
> I would also like a doctor who enjoyed me. I want to be a good story for him, to give him some of my art in exchange for his. . . . Finally, I would be happier with a witty doctor who could appreciate the comedy as well as the tragedy of my illness, its quirks and eccentricities, the final jokes of a personality that has nothing further to lose."

Broyard continues:

> "Physicians have been taught in medical school that they must keep the patient at a distance because there isn't time to accommodate his personality, or because if the doctor becomes involved in the patient's predicament, the emotional burden will be too great. As I've suggested it doesn't take much time to make good contact, but beyond that, the emotional burden of avoiding the patient may be much harder on the doctor than he imagines. . . . It may be this that sometimes makes him complain of feeling harassed. A doctor's job would be so much more interesting and satisfying if he simply let himself plunge into the patient, if he could lose his own fear of falling.
>
> This doctor is the most famous authority on the prostate in Cambridge, Massachusetts, which is crowded with doctors. He knows all there is to know about the prostate, but I cannot sit down and talk with him about it, which I find a great deprivation.
>
> There's a paradox here at the heart of medicine, because the doctor, like a writer, must have a voice of his own, something that conveys the timbre, the rhythm, the diction and the music of his humanity that compensates us for all the speechless machines.

When a doctor makes a difficult diagnosis, it is not his medical knowledge only that determines it, but a voice in his head. Such a diagnosis depends as much on inspiration as art does. Whether he wants to be or not, the doctor is a storyteller, and he can turn our lives into good or bad stories, regardless of the diagnosis."

Speaking of his highly respected urologist, Broyard made these perceptive remarks:

"We are what the French call *un couple malade*, a marriage of doctor and patient. Perhaps later, when he is older, he'll have learned how to converse. Astute as he is, he doesn't understand that all cures are partly "talking cures" in Freud's phrase. Every patient needs mouth-to-mouth resuscitation, for talk is the kiss of life. Besides talking himself, the doctor ought to bleed the patient of talk, of the consciousness of his illness, as earlier physicians used to bleed their patients to let out heat or dangerous humors.

Every patient invites the doctor to combine the role of the priest, the philosopher, the poet, the lover. He expects the doctor to evaluate his entire life, like a biographer. The sick man asks far too much, he is impatient in everything, and his doctor may be afraid of making a fool of himself in trying to reply. . . . Of course a physician may reasonably ask, 'But what am I supposed to say? All I can tell the patient is the facts, if there are any facts.' . . . But this is not quite true. The doctor's answer to his patients will come naturally, or at first unnaturally, from the intersecting of the patient's needs with the doctors' experience and his as-yet-untried imagination. He doesn't have to lie to the sick man or give him false assurances. He himself, his presence and his will to reach the patient, is the assurance the sick man needs."

(Shades of Walsh McDermott who said "There is a time in illness when the doctor *himself* must be the treatment.")

"Just as a mother ushers her child into the world, so the doctor must usher the patient out of the world of the healthy and into whatever physical and mental purgatory awaits him. The doctor is the *patient's only familiar in a foreign country*.

To help the doctor reach the patient, and to help the patient reach the doctor, the hospital ought to be less like a laboratory and more like a theater, which would be only fitting, since no place contains more drama. Originally the patient was protected by the sterility of the hospital. Only the sterility went too far; it sterilized the doctor's thinking, the patient's entire experience in the hospital. But the sick man needs the contagion of life. Death is the ultimate sterility."

Broyard concludes his essay with these inspirational comments and advice:

> "Not every patient can be saved, but his illness may be eased by the way the doctor responds to him—*and in responding to him the doctor may save himself*. But first he must become a student again; he has to dissect the cadaver of his professional persona; he must see that his silence and neutrality are unnatural. . . . It may be necessary to give up some of his authority in exchange for his humanity, but as the old family doctor knew, this is not a bad bargain. *In learning to talk to his patients, the doctor may talk himself back into loving his work*. He has little to lose and everything to gain by letting the sick man into his heart. If he does, they can share, as few others can, the wonder, terror, and exaltation of being on the edge of being, between the natural and supernatural."

There is much wisdom in this essay written on his deathbed by a talented and perceptive layman. Broyard, the dying patient, expressed with exquisite skill and feeling what our patients are asking of us in medicine. Yet how few there are in medicine who follow his precepts. This must change if medicine is to remain the great profession passed on to us by Sir William Osler and the other great clinicians of our glorious past. I firmly believe as did Broyard that "In learning to talk to his patients, the doctor may talk himself back into loving his work." Even more so if he learns to listen to the patient and becomes skilled in non-verbal communication as well.

Written with the Gallic eloquence of a talented writer, it is the *cri de coeur* of a human being facing the end of his life with courage and the determination to express his views on patient care as it prevails in this era of modern medicine even in the best of hands. Procedures and technology have taken over. The psychiatrists and lawyers in our society are among the few that are rewarded for speaking with people. The art of medicine is neglected and seldom taught because of the lack of role models, inadequate compensation, and the lack of time and commitment to better communication with patients. The press and television emphasize what appears to be wrong with health care and its "providers." The arbiters and critics are largely laypersons, politicians, lawyers, anthropologists, sociologists, and economists with very little knowledge of what it takes to practice good medicine.

Anatole Broyard's message is one of the best statements I have ever read from a layman giving the reasons or lack of reason for selecting a doctor. Would that this essay be reprinted and presented to every medical student in America, accompanied by Dr. Francis W. Peabody's great classic, also written during the author's terminal illness in 1926–27, "The Care of the Patient," which concludes with these immortal words:

> "Disease in man is never exactly the same as disease in an experimental animal, for in man the disease at once affects and is affected by what we call the emotional life. Thus, the physician who attempts to take care of a patient while he neglects this factor is as unscientific as the investigator who neglects to control all the conditions that may affect his experiment. The good physician knows his patients through and through, and his knowledge is bought dearly. Time, sympathy and understanding must be lavishly dispensed, but the reward is to be found in that personal bond which forms the greatest satisfaction of the practice of medicine. One of the essential qualities of the clinician is interest in humanity, for the secret of the care of the patient is in caring for the patient."[7]

---

7. Francis Weld Peabody, "The Care of the Patient," *Journal of the American Medical Association* 88 (March 19, 1927), pp. 877–82.

Chapter 23

~~~

Mr. J. Peter Grace, Chairman of W. R. Grace and Company

Grace is courage under pressure—
the best ones die moving forward.

—Ernest Hemingway

FOR THE FINAL CASE PRESENTATION of patients who have taught me so much and given me great pleasure in the personal practice of internal medicine, I present the saga of the illness of Mr. J. Peter Grace, the grandson of the founder of W. R. Grace and Company who became its chairman in 1945 and built the firm from a $5 million concern to a $5 billion corporation during his unprecedented forty-seven years of tenure as its chairman. "Sir Peter," as I dubbed him in deference to his position as head of the Knights of Malta, admired the Archangel Michael, "who loved heights,"[1] as did Sir Peter who spent much of his adult life soaring above 30,000 feet in his private jet plane pursuing international and national business ventures that at latest count employed 50,000 employees. A great believer in and defender of capitalism and an enemy of waste in government, he somehow found and made the time for many philanthropies and above all for his beloved Roman Catholic Church as well as a host of non-sectarian causes. Like his grandfather, he was a personal friend and advisor to four American presidents and several cardinals and monarchs. A devoted family man with nine children and twenty grandchildren, he was blessed with a loyal, charming, and intelligent wife, Margaret, who gave stability to his sometimes roller-coaster lifestyle.

Sir Peter greatly admired the Archangel Michael and in jest, he would twit me that I inherited his name through the accident of my

---

1. Henry Adams, *Mont-Saint-Michel and Chartres* (Garden City, N.Y.: Doubleday & Company, Inc., 1959), p. 1.

birth on St. Michael's Day, 8 May 1910, and reminded me of the archangel's enormous accomplishments. On several occasions during his serious illness, which had its ups and downs, Sir Peter reminded me of Saint Michael and often called me his "security blanket," always available and accessible and in control of his case even when he was 30,000 feet above the earth or thousands of miles away from home. For those who may like to know more about the archangel, I quote from the opening paragraph of Henry Adams's famous classic.

> The ARCHANGEL loved heights. Standing on the summit of the tower that crowned his church, wings up spread, sword uplifted, the devil crawling beneath, and the cock, symbol of eternal vigilance, perched on his mailed foot, Saint Michael held a place of his own in heaven and on earth which seems, in the eleventh century, to leave hardly room for the Virgin of the Crypt at Chartres, still less for the Beau Christ of the thirteenth century at Amiens. The Archangel stands for Church and State, and both militant. He is the conqueror of Satan, the mightiest of all created spirits, the nearest to God. His place was where the danger was greatest; therefore you find him here. For the same reason he was, while the pagan danger lasted, the patron Saint of France. So the Normans, when they were converted to Christianity, put themselves under his powerful protection. So he stood for centuries on his Mount in Peril of the Sea, watching across the tremor of the immense ocean,—immensi tremor oceani,—as Louis XI, inspired for once to poetry, inscribed on the collar of the Order of Saint Michael which he created. So soldiers, nobles and monarchs went on pilgrimage to his shrine; so the common people followed, and still follow like ourselves.[2]

For the past twenty-five years I have been a medical consultant to this wonderful Grace family and nicknamed by them "Dr. Mike." This relationship was cemented when a talented son of Sir Peter, Dr. William R. Grace, served his medical internship and residency in 1969–1971 at St. Vincent's Hospital and Medical Center in New York with a rotation through my gastrointestinal service. Dr. Grace went on to become an outstanding oncologist and chief of oncology at St. Vincent's.

In 1970 the Sisters of Charity of St. Vincent's Hospital and Medical Center in New York, the organizers and owners of the hospital, decided to appoint a lay board to advise them in the management

---

2. Ibid.

of the Medical Center. The first chairman of the board of trustees was Mr. J. Peter Grace who, true to form, sought to make some administrative and financial changes. In 1972 my first occasion to witness this aspect of Sir Peter in action was at a dinner meeting of the directors of departments of St. Vincent's Hospital with the trustees and key Sisters of Charity. I recall that one of the directors of a major department complained that the trustees were not raising enough money for St. Vincent's Hospital and rather bluntly stated that trustees should be primarily money raisers. Sir Peter stood up and conceded that financial matters were important, but, playing the doctor, his diagnosis of what was sorely needed at St. Vincent's Hospital was more than mere money. He then, in his striking approach to problem-solving, asked the audience whether any were readers of *Town and Country* magazine. Several in the audience said yes. Sir Peter then said, "This month's issue has an article on the best doctors and medical services in America and there is only one doctor named from St. Vincent's Hospital. He is sitting at this table. His name is Michael Lepore. What St. Vincent's Hospital needs is two more doctors like Mike Lepore to attract new patents and to improve the quality of teaching research and patient care." I knew then that I had a real friend on the board.

In the fall of 1989, Sir Peter developed right-hip pain while playing tennis; x-ray films revealed a tumor of the right hip and proximal femur. The question was whether this was a primary bone tumor or metastatic. In 1978 he had undergone a radical resection of a subcutaneous mass measuring 4 x 3 x 2 cm from his left loin at the Columbia-Presbyterian Medical Center by an excellent plastic surgeon. The diagnosis was leiomyosarcoma. Finding the slides of the original tumor at this late date was not easy, but with the help of Dr. Rafaele Lattes, professor of surgical pathology, and Dr. George Hyman of P&S they were located and reviewed by Dr. Lattes, who agreed with the diagnosis of leiomyosarcoma. The slides were also reviewed by Dr. Andrew G. Huvos of Memorial Hospital, a renowned specialist in the pathology of bone tumors, who agreed with Dr. Lattes.

Dr. Joseph Lane, head of the Memorial Hospital Bone Tumor Section, saw the patient in consultation at Memorial Hospital on 3 January 1990. He felt that the diagnosis of leiomyosarcoma was unlikely and favored malignant fibrohistiocytoma or chondrosarcoma, primary bone tumors both of which were potentially curable without sacrificing the extremity. He recommended that the first thing to do was to establish a tissue diagnosis, and he recommended doing this with an intratrochanteric approach to avoid injury to the cortex of the femur at the site of the tumor. Mr. Grace decided that he wished to have his operation in St. Vincent's Hospital by Dr. Patrick Boland, an outstanding orthopedic surgeon who is on the Memorial Staff as well as St. Vincent's and trained by Dr. Lane. The biopsy was done on 5 January 1990 at St. Vincent's Hospital by Dr. Boland. Slides were reviewed by Dr. Huvos as well as the St. Vincent's Hospital pathology staff, and the unequivocal diagnosis of leiomyosarcoma identical with that of 1978 was made. On 10 January 1990, Mr. Grace underwent enbloc resection of the right hip and proximal femur and insertion of a custom proximal femoral prosthesis for leiomyosarcoma by Dr. Patrick Boland at St Vincent's Hospital. His postoperative recovery was smooth except for a large hematoma at the operative site requiring needle aspiration. The patient cooperated marvelously with his rehabilitation at St. Vincent's Hospital. Muscle mass, strength, and motion all improved remarkably with only a slight limp. He made an early return to his corporate responsibilities and was soon traveling all over the world via his private jet on corporation business.

At this point I must say that I have never seen a patient who was as uncomplaining as Sir Peter. He had been a great athlete, a three varsity letter man at Yale, class of 1936. He was an Olympic-caliber polo player as well and played professional hockey for a time. He had no vices except for a pipe that he loved to smoke for relaxation. He was a teetotaler and enjoyed good food and good company.

He knew his central office and key employees by their first names and was easily accessible to them for help with personal or family problems. He was a hands-on manager who remembered faces and names. He had a fantastic memory and could handle millions of dollars the way most of us manage one-hundred-dollar bills. He had great curiosity and would ask question after question when faced with a new development and God help you if you failed to pass his interrogation. I have been the personal physician to many brilliant persons but this man was, to my way of thinking, the one at the top of the heap. He did, of course, make his share of mistakes given the world in which he lived and, like Mayor Fiorello LaGuardia, when he did err "it was a Lulu." Nevertheless, the phrase from *Hamlet* is most appropriate for this great man. "He was a man, take him for all in all, I shall not look upon his like again."[3]

To our dismay, on a routine checkup (24 July 1992) a chest x-ray revealed multiple metastases in both lungs. He was without symptoms

---

3. *Hamlet, Prince of Denmark*, Act I, scene ii, in *The Complete Works of William Shakespeare* (New York: Crown Publishers, Random House, 1975), p. 1075.

or adverse clinical signs and we were all startled by these findings, especially since his chest x-ray six months before had been perfectly clear. A needle biopsy confirmed that these were indeed metastases from the original leiomyosarcoma. It was decided to seek the advice of Dr. James Holland, renowned oncologist and head of that division at Mt. Sinai Hospital, on 27 July 1992. I accompanied Mr. Grace to Dr. Holland's office in Manhattan, as did Dr. William R. Grace and his mother, Margaret. The choice of Jim Holland was a marvelous one. He was just the right person to join our team and he warmly recalled me as one of his "esteemed" teachers at P&S many years ago. Dr. Holland's recommendation was to start chemotherapy. He was optimistic because "the slow growth of his tumor from the primary to the first metastasis in the femur is advantageous." It was thirty months since the femoral surgery.

A chest x-ray in 1991 was normal—"We will plan to treat him with dactinomycin and dacarbazine in combination, beginning on or about August 10. He may require G.C.S.F.—additional chemotherapeutic options for later include Ifosfamide with mesna and Doxorubicin." Intravenous chemotherapy was given by Dr. Holland to Mr. Grace as an outpatient while he continued to fulfill his business obligations and the demands of his many board meetings that necessitated his flying by private jet to national and international meetings and conferences. In order to make this feasible, he had private-duty nurses who accompanied him whenever he traveled. They were able to telephone me from the plane at any hour of the day or night. I remained on twenty-four-hour call for Mr. Grace from the day of the first metastases to his femur in 1989 until his death in April 1995. I was able with the assistance of excellent nurses to cover many ailments early on by ordering antibiotics, anti-emetics, or sedatives wherever they might be. One itinerary I remember well was to the following countries and cities (17 September – 1 October 1993) Bangkok, Hawaii, Hong Kong, Tokyo, Ireland, Guam, Belgium, Indonesia, Singapore, Malaysia, and Australia.

My attitude toward Sir Peter was that if the president of the United States has medical and nursing care on an around-the-clock-basis, an important corporate giant, ill with a serious condition, should have all the assistance he needs to ensure his safety and protection against infection on the important business trips required of him as the head of a $5 billion corporation employing 50,000 people.

In March 1993, because of progression of the pulmonary metastases, he was given more aggressive and intensive chemotherapy, including Adriamycin, Doxorubicin, and Ifosfamide, resulting in neutropenic sepsis requiring an emergency admission to St. Vincent's

Hospital (3–30–93 to 4–7–93). He responded well to supportive measures and granulocyte promoting factor. In July 1993 we were able to obtain liposome daunorubicin, and this was given with some benefit and was well tolerated. In December 1993 he was given a course of intravenous Taxol plus radiotherapy to the left lung with a favorable response. In March 1994 a subcutaneous right-deltoid mass was excised, the pathology report was again the same tumor, a leiomyosarcoma. In May 1994 he was given a course of radiotherapy to the right upper lung with a positive response. Of all of the therapy given the patient, the most effective seemed to be radiotherapy, and during his illness he received three courses of radiotherapy to the lungs with some benefit. A discouraging event toward the end of the patient's life was the appearance of a metastatic nodule in the tongue and multiple lesions of the right quadriceps muscle. Worst of all was that, despite therapeutic measures, the pulmonary metastases increased in size and location. Finally, despite selective radiotherapy to the lungs, dyspnea, wheezing, and cough increased, unresponsive to therapy, and necessitated his emergency admission to St Vincent's Hospital on 11 April 1995. He was clearly terminally ill and needed I.V. morphine drip to control dyspnea, pain, and discomfort. Despite all of this, he enjoyed seeing his family and friends who came from far and wide to say goodbye. A distinguished and loyal visitor was his great friend, His Eminence John Cardinal O'Connor, who spent several long sessions with Mr. Grace before he died.

The funeral in St Patrick's Cathedral was attended by over 1,200 participants and conducted by His Eminence, who was the celebrant as well as the homilist.[4] I was in the audience and thrilled by Cardinal O'Connor's personal and marvelous appraisal of Sir Peter.

"If you want to know Peter Grace then you have to look at his faith," the Cardinal said. "He felt very personally the obligation God had placed upon him," and believed that he was called to "use his life to carry out God's will. . . . I think he saw W. R. Grace [the family business] as an instrumentality for doing this," the Cardinal said. Power, wealth, and possessions were "toys" to Mr. Grace, he said. "His life was his faith." Though he was known for his intense commitment to his company, Cardinal O'Connor said in his homily that it is a "misreading" to believe that the company was Mr. Grace's main concern or that he tried to "buy his way into heaven" through charitable work.

---

4. Claudia McDonnell, "This was a Believer," *Catholic New York* 14, no. 31 (April 1995).

"Nothing of the sort," he said. This was a believer. He noted that Mr. Grace had "a simple faith" and was deeply devoted to Mary, especially under the title of Our Lady of Lourdes. One of his most "poignant" experiences with him was a pilgrimage to Lourdes to pray for Mr. Grace's recovery, he said.

What further comment can this writer, the personal physician to this great man, make to describe what it means to have been in this position? First of all, I am humble that God gave me this opportunity to know this person intimately and I am proud of the medical school and universities and hospitals that made it possible for me to cope with the demands of this trust and ability to cope with them. You may rest assured that the team I brought together—which included his wife and family; the nurses, especially Miss Martha Kelly; Dr. Patrick Boland, superb orthopedist and friend; Dr. Anthony Gagliardi, topflight pulmonologist; Dr. James Holland, the great oncologist and excellent clinician and humanist; Mr. Grace's physician-son, Dr. William R. Grace, the distinguished oncologist; and Dr. George Schwarz, eminent radiotherapist—all played important roles not only in prolonging Sir Peter's life but maintaining the quality of his life and making possible the many wonderful deeds he was able to accomplish during his last years.

Despite all we could do for him. Sir Peter died on 19 April 1995 in the very same Room 1601 of the John Coleman Pavilion of the St. Vincent's Hospital where my beloved wife Ardean died in 1987. The closing weeks of his life had been marred by inaccurate and poorly informed statements concerning the W. R. Grace Company and its board of directors.

I personally felt that the criticism was ill-timed, unfair, and most of it untrue, and took pleasure in arranging to have the following obituary published n the *New York Times* of 20 April 1995:

> GRACE-J.PETER, BELOVED FRIEND VALIANT IN ILL-NESS, LOYAL DEFENDER OF HIS FAITH. A TRULY GREAT AND GOOD AMERICAN, OUTSTANDING BUSINESS LEADER, GENEROUS PHILANTHROPIST, SILENT BENEFACTOR TO MANY. "HE WAS A MAN, TAKE HIM FOR ALL AND ALL, WE SHALL NOT LOOK UPON HIS LIKE AGAIN." WE MOURN HIS DEMISE AND CELEBRATE HIS LIFE. TO HIS BELOVED WIFE, MARGARET, HIS NINE CHILDREN AND OTHER MEMBERS OF HIS DEVOTED FAMILY WE EXTEND OUR CONDOLENCES AND PRAYER.
>
> THE LEPORE FAMILY

In my four years of military service in WW II, I saw and participated in the care of many soldiers and marines with combat injuries
and witnessed extraordinary examples of guts and courage under fire.
To my mind, Sir Peter, when ill, exemplified Ernest Hemingway's definition of Guts as "Grace under pressure." This trait Sir Peter exhibited to the utmost degree. He never complained to me about his plight
and serious illness. He inspired all of those entrusted with his care to
look ahead and to keep trying no matter what the odds. He loved
fighters and did not have much use for quitters.

The story of W. R. Grace and Company has been beautifully written by Marquis James, the outstanding biographer of his day and
twice Pulitzer Prize-winner who would probably have won another
Pulitzer if the book entitled *Merchant Adventurer—The Story of W. R.
Grace*[5] had been published when James completed it in 1948. For rea-
sons not completely known the book was suppressed by the Grace
Corporation, probably for fear of antagonizing Peruvian and Chilean
governments. Galley proofs were stored in the basement of the lower
Manhattan Grace warehouse until they were rediscovered by
Professor Lawrence Clayton, a historian and professor at the
University of Alabama, whose father had been a trusted Grace
employee and executive in the early days of the firm. Through
Professor Clayton's efforts the book was finally published in 1993.
The book jacket vividly and accurately describes its contents:[6]

> This fast-paced, beautifully written biography tells the story of
> one of American's most successful immigrants. First arriving
> here as a teenager in 1846, Irish-born William R. Grace worked
> his way up from ordinary seaman to become master of a vast
> commercial empire, reformer of the Democratic party, and New
> York City's first Catholic mayor.
>
> Grace's fortunes started to rise when he began supplying
> ships in the Peruvian guano trade. By the late 1860's he was a rich
> man; his New York firm operated vessels around the world,
> helped build railroads in Latin America, and ran guns to Peru for
> its disastrous war against Chile. Yet he still had time to battle
> Tammany Hall during his two terms as mayor and to pursue such

---

5. Marquis, James, *Merchant Adventurer: The Story of W. R. Grace*, with an
Introduction by Lawrence A. Clayton. Scholarly Resources Inc.: Wilmington, Del.
6. Ibid.

new business opportunities as the growing rubber market and the building of what is now the Panama Canal.

Marquis James's expert telling of this true-life Horatio Alger story—which some say could have won him his third Pulitzer—was suppressed by the Grace Corporation when James finished it in 1948. Rediscovered in the firm's archives thirty years later by Professor Lawrence Clayton, it is now being published for the first time.

For the reader interested in the colorful world of sailing ships and Yankee captains, in the exploitation of Latin American resources and North American know-how, in the ruthless tactics of Gilded Age politics, or in any of the many other arenas that William Grace entered—and frequently dominated—*Merchant Adventurer* will prove compelling as literature and tremendously informative as history.

In 1945 J. Peter Grace (1913–1995) was elected President of W. R. Grace and a new era began, lasting nearly a half century. That story needs to be told by someone of the caliber of Marquis James, and I hope this will soon happen. In the meantime I will treasure the autographed copy of *Merchant Adventurer—The Story of W. R. Grace* given to me by Sir Peter with his handwritten inscription, "To Dr. Michael Lepore, who is the very best in any field that he chooses and who is a gentleman and a scholar and a super friend. With warmest regards, Peter."

In closing this chapter dear friend, I bid you adieu until we meet again!

Doctor Mike

Chapter 24

~~~

Birth of the Upjohn Gastrointestinal Service

O NE AFTERNOON IN OCTOBER 1961, I received a very pleasant surprise. Out of the blue, without any previous discussion, one of my patients, Mrs. Janet Upjohn Stearns, made an appointment to come to my office at 550 Park Avenue to discuss an important matter. She was a member of the Upjohn family, her grandfather, Dr. W. O. Upjohn, had founded the pharmaceutical house in Kalamazoo, Michigan. Her husband was Dr. William Stearns, a highly regarded chest specialist on our staff. Mrs. Stearns was referred to me in 1958 because of a mysterious ailment that had begun in her childhood and had eluded diagnosis despite much effort by many consultants. Her symptoms were chiefly abdominal, consisting of recurrent severe abdominal distention, flatulence, recurrent foul diarrhea, cramps, fatty-food intolerance, weight loss, weakness, and episodes suggestive of hypoglycemia. She was known to be allergic to a wide variety of foods and medications. I examined her carefully and did a workup for malabsorption that led me to diagnose her ailment as non-tropical sprue. Assisting me to make this diagnosis was the fact that one of her children had severe celiac disease. I prescribed a strict low-gluten diet, vitamin therapy, and elimination of offending foods. She cooperated to the letter and soon was feeling better than she had in years. She had just returned from a visit to her mother in Kalamazoo, where she learned that she was being given a large gift of Upjohn corporate stock to use as she saw fit. Her mother was aware that her daughter had suffered a rather turbulent life, complicated in part by her previously undiagnosed ailments. Now that she was physically much improved due to her new therapeutic program, her mother advised her daughter to use her inheritance to help others and to do this during her lifetime so that she might witness in person and enjoy the happiness that comes from helping others. Mrs. Stearns said she had hurried home with her mind made up to do something major to help me to develop gastroenterology at Columbia-Presbyterian. As a patient of mine, she had been admitted to Harkness Pavilion and was pleased with her treatment. She also observed how difficult it was to perform an adequate malabsorption workup in a setting lacking a formal commitment to the specialty of gastroenterology. She said she was preparing a letter of gift and a proposal for establishing an endowed chair in gastroenterology and a gastrointestinal section for diagnosis, treatment, and research. She was also interested in advancing the care of ambulatory patients with digestive ailments.

When I arrived home after my interview with Mrs. Stearns, I shared the good news with my beloved wife. Her immediate reaction was that of joy and pride that this opportunity had arisen. I cautioned her that this was far from being a *fait accompli*. In fact, I was certain that the concept of a part-time salaried professor who continued his personal practice of medicine while administering an important section would be strongly opposed by the full-timers. Given the Bard professor's clearly expressed hostility toward subspecialties, acceptance of the major gift and proposal seemed unlikely.

The following day, a Saturday, when I made my rounds in Harkness Pavilion, I stopped by the eighth floor of the Presbyterian Hospital where the department of medicine had its headquarters, looking for someone to share my good news. The only person in his office on that Saturday was my good friend and teacher, Dr. Dickinson W. Richards, Nobel laureate in 1956 for his work with cardiac catheterization. He listened with obvious pleasure to the news that Mrs. Janet Upjohn Stearns was making a major proposal to strengthen gastroenterology at Columbia-Presbyterian. He congratulated me and suggested that I call Dr. Stanley Bradley, the Bard professor, at his home nearby and he gave me his telephone number. He said he thought Dr. Bradley should know about the proposal before leaving for a long vacation in Europe on the following Monday. I dialed the number and Dr. Bradley answered. Rather than greeting the proposal with joy or warmth, he was obviously nettled and annoyed that I was bothering him at home for a "matter that could wait." I was almost completely turned off by this reply and I did not tell him I was calling at the behest of Dr. Richards. I also did not tell him that Mrs. Stearns had expressed the desire to proceed as quickly as possible with plans for the proposal, citing pressing tax and financial matters that needed to be settled before the end of the year.

Since the Bard professor would be away for at least one month, Mrs. Stearns and I decided to send her letter of proposal to Dean H. Houston Merritt for his review. Copies of the letters follow:

A PROPOSAL FOR THE ENDOWMENT OF A CHAIR
IN GASTROENTEROLOGY
OCTOBER 1961

For a number of years I have been greatly interested in the future of the Columbia-Presbyterian Medical Center and through my own illness I have become familiar with the Center, its facilities and its staff. The nature of my illness has been such as to acquaint me particularly with the Center's assets, deficiencies and needs in the realm of Gastroenterology, and my experiences, observations and inquiries have made it quite clear to me that there is a great need for the encouragement, support and vigorous development of the specialty of Gastroenterology in the Medical Center.

I should like to do what I can to help strengthen the teaching and training program and the research activities and to improve the care and management of patients with gastrointestinal ailments. While I am interested in physical facilities and laboratories, I am more interested in the people staffing them. I feel there has been of late too much emphasis upon physical plants and interior decoration to the exclusion and at times neglect of the real purpose of our hospitals, namely, the treatment and the healing of the sick. I should like to see within my own lifetime that my gift is resulting in the alleviation of human suffering not only in the wards and clinics of this medical center but also the private and semi-private services.

It is my belief that an important function of a university medical center is to set an example of the practice of medicine for others to emulate. Modern treatment of many patients with gastrointestinal diseases often requires special facilities, highly skilled personnel and complicated techniques of study. I know from personal experience that the care of such patients often imposes inordinate demands upon the standard facilities of the general medical or surgical services and it is often impossible for the patient to obtain and the institution to provide the necessary services.

It seems to me that much suffering might be alleviated and lives saved by better coordination of the specialized services needed for the optimal treatment of patients with gastrointestinal diseases.

I am therefore interested in the creation of a special Gastrointestinal Unit under the direction of Dr. Michael J. Lepore within the Columbia-Presbyterian Medical Center to be devoted to the so-called intensive care of patients with gastrointestinal ailments. It is suggested that the unit consist of 4–6 beds with special facilities for metabolic studies and appropriate diagnostic and therapeutic equipment and personnel skilled and specially trained for this purpose. These should be available for occupancy by patients in all economic categories, the one common denominator being their need for expert care under the direction of the Gastrointestinal Section. This unit, concentrating skilled personnel, special techniques and special apparatus should do much to advance the care of these patients and should serve as an example and inspiration to the community and to the world.

After giving this matter much thought I have decided to submit the following proposal for your consideration, hoping that my action will stimulate others to donate additional funds for this very important area of medicine.

Trustees of the College of Physician and Surgeons
Columbia University
New York

Gentlemen:

A PROPOSAL FOR THE ENDOWMENT OF A CHAIR
IN GASTROENTEROLOGY
OCTOBER 1961

I propose to endow a Chair in Gastroenterology in the Department of Medicine along the following general lines, but on the condition that it be designated the UPJOHN PROFESSORSHIP IN GASTROENTEROLOGY; and the further condition that its first Professor be Dr. Michael J. Lepore. This Chair will be in memory of my grandfather and the father who together combined qualities of great vigor and tenacity of purpose and warm human understanding with a sincere desire to help their fellow man.

It is my personal desire that every effort be made to strengthen the teaching and training program, improve research activities and improve the care and management of patients with gastrointestinal ailments in the clinics and the ward services of this medical center. Inevitably, it is hoped that the benefits accruing to the ward and clinic patients will be transmitted to the private and semi-private patients so that people in all economic categories will benefit from the proposed program. This Chair should carry with it a substantial part-time salary and the incumbent should be encouraged (let alone permitted) to conduct a private practice without restrictions. I say this because, based on my experience as a patient, I know that over and above a good knowledge of medicine, skill in the care of the sick patient, coupled with compassion, sympathetic understanding and an emphasis on human values, are qualities which are a great asset to a physician; particularly is this important to one who is responsible for setting an example to student, house staff and the community. The qualities are to a great degree evoked by the doctor-patient relationship which comes from caring for private patients. For any unduly concerned about this emphasis I quote from an illustrious source: "If the University has secured the right type of man and if it has provided him with **** facilities and opportunities commensurate with his needs and desires, he will neither want to do too much private practice nor will he have to. His tastes lie in other directions. There is no need for special prohibitions. One has only to recall the names of Delafield, of Osler, of Halsted and others to confirm this statement."

Having found in Dr. Michael J. Lepore the individual who, I am convinced, has the vigor, energy, vision and qualities of leadership necessary to promote the objective of a sound program in Gastroenterology, and who also possesses the finest qualities of the true physician, scientist and healer, I am prepared to give impetus to the program by providing some or all of the necessary initial funds. I have at my sole disposal certain charitable funds which presently produce between $10,000 to $15,000 per annum which would provide for the part-time salary for this Chair and perhaps for some expenses. There is a possibility that the fund may be considerably increased in the near future, and if so, greater benefits for the program might be provided. Beyond this, however, I am prepared to currently provide additional substantial support for such phases of the program as are specified by Dr. Lepore. My feeling is that this program deserves the support of others as well as myself and it is hoped that it will stimulate others to donate additional funds for this important area of medicine.

I wish to emphasize that it is my desire that Dr. Michael J. Lepore be in charge of this program and that my offer is directly and absolutely contingent upon this stipulation.

Because of certain important tax and legal aspects, it is essential that some decisions regarding this proposal be reached in the near future. To that end I shall be glad to commence at once the discussion of the various problems involved.

Very truly yours,
Janet Upjohn Stearns

Pending the return of the Bard professor, I discussed the Upjohn proposal with a number of close friends and colleagues at Columbia-Presbyterian. They were uniformly delighted with the proposal and felt it was high time that this sort of recognition and opportunity had come to me. Dr. Charles Flood's comment was that there was room for two professors of gastroenterology at P&S. I continued to feel uneasy about the Bard professor's hostile attitude and knew I had my work cut out for me. I knew also that if he did not approve and lend his support, it would be virtually impossible for me to do the job.

When the Bard professor returned from his vacation, I met with him and discussed the project. I could see that he had reservations about my plans. I then submitted a plan in writing for the development of a GI unit at P&S. At a subsequent meeting with him, we went down a checklist I had prepared as conditions for the gift prepared by me with Mrs. Stearns. Dr. Bradley had discussed this with the executive committee of the department of medicine. Of the list of a dozen or so conditions, a number, I believe it was four, failed to get his approval and that of the executive committee. At this juncture, I must say that during the weeks that preceded my meeting with Dr. Bradley, anticipating a negative response from him, I had been thinking of other options. First and foremost, I had made up my mind that I really wanted to pursue this opportunity even if it would involve leaving the Medical Center for another hospital. Fueling this decision was the tremendous difficulty in gaining hospital admission for my busy practice due to the shortage of beds. Secondly, the great abdominal surgeons who had dominated the scene at Columbia-Presbyterian for the past thirty years were either retired or on their way, their replacements chiefly vascular and cardiothoracic surgeons with limited interests in the fields of gastroenterology. I had discussed this with Mrs. Stearns, who wondered whether we should consider Roosevelt Hospital, an affiliate of P&S, which had two major attractions: a new building, the Winston, under construction, and a very well-regarded surgical staff that was especially strong in the field of gastroenterology.

When Dr. Bradley told me that he could not accept a significant number of the conditions we had placed on the Upjohn gift, my answer was ready. I said, in that event, the gift will not be made to Columbia-Presbyterian. He asked whether I alone could make that decision. My answer was that with Mrs. Stearns prior approval, I was empowered to do this. He expressed his disbelief that after twenty-five years at P&S and my fine record that I would leave. I assured him that I certainly might go elsewhere. He then wondered whether Mrs. Stearns could be persuaded to contribute to the construction of the Black Laboratory building. I said she had clearly indicated that she and her family were not interested in bricks and mortar. Their major interest was in people. In retrospect, perhaps I might have tried to work out some sort of acceptable compromise, but I guessed, instinctively, that the Bard professor and I would not get along harmoniously. Following this meeting, negotiations were initiated with Roosevelt Hospital. There we were greeted with open arms and offered space in the new Winston Building. I was promised that I would never have any problem with admission of my private patients. This promise was kept. The hospital enjoyed an excellent reputation, was affiliated with P&S, and was geographically near my office at 550 Park Avenue. Our medical students at P&S thought it was their best affiliate. Most of the house staff was from P&S. I had a meeting with Dean Merritt regarding the shift to Roosevelt. He assured me that my appointment at P&S would continue when I transferred to Roosevelt. Roosevelt made certain that I had office space and some facilities to get the Upjohn Gastrointestinal Service underway. It was also agreed that I be a member of its Executive Committee.

Chapter 25

Roosevelt Hospital, 1962–1965

Establishment of the Upjohn Gastrointestinal Service, Clinic and Foundation

ROOSEVELT HOSPITAL IN 1962 was largely dominated by its excellent surgical service. There were three chiefs of surgery, Drs. Frederick Amendola, Howard Patterson, and James Thompson, all of them good abdominal surgeons. They served without salary and seemed always to be at the hospital. Their assistants were also first-rate. The medical service had two chiefs, Dr. Julian M. Freston and Dr. Arthur J. Antenucci, also non-salaried. All of these men had substantial and remunerative private practices. The trustees, led by an outstanding chairperson, Mrs. Donald Bush, were prominent in the business and social world of New York. Some were wealthy. A member since 1931 was Dean Willard Rappleye, now retired from his post at P&S and becoming more active on the Roosevelt board, where I believe he was aggressively promoting the inauguration of Flexnerian full time starting with the department of medicine. I was not aware of these activities when I first joined the Roosevelt staff.

In my verbal agreement with Roosevelt Hospital, the Upjohn Gastrointestinal Service controlled up to twenty beds scattered among the several medical floors. It was assigned interns in rotation as well as two residents paid for by hospital funds. Upjohn funds paid for two to three fellows in a day when fellowships paid $5,000 per annum. In my discussion with Mrs. Stearns I stipulated that I needed a topflight administrator to take care of the many non-medical details inherent in running a first-rate academic and teaching service in gastroenterology. The person I was able to persuade to accept this position, Miss Martha Swensson, had worked with me before WW II as the administrator of the personnel medical department of the Columbia-Presbyterian Medical Center. This was without doubt the best appointment I have ever made. She was able to spare me the burden of many administrative duties. Above all, she knew what I was trying to do and set the highest standards for the service. The talented attending physicians, residents, and fellows that flocked to our doors appreciated, as I did, the skill, dedication, tact, innovation, and loyalty of this marvelous person. She was an excellent money manager who made dollars go a long way.

When I arrived at Roosevelt Hospital I found, in keeping with the situation in most community hospitals, their outpatient department was a second-class operation, poorly housed, understaffed, and ill-equipped. The status of the outpatient clinic may be gauged by the fact that full attendings were no longer obligated to work in the out-patient service. This was a far cry from the Vanderbilt Clinic where, in those days, everybody served, even the senior professors. I had already made up my mind that the Upjohn Clinic would be attended by every physician on my staff including full attendings. The real problem in achieving this goal was to find the space and to create the facilities to house this innovative unit that was to reflect the philoso-phy and wishes of its donor and its designated leader and director. I located an area of Roosevelt Hospital that had at one time functioned as an observation ward and was no longer being used for that pur-pose. The area needed to be rebuilt to serve its new purpose. I was advised that new construction at Roosevelt Hospital was in gridlock at the New York City Building Department and there were many proj-ects that had been stalled there for years. I discussed this matter at some length with a devoted patient and close friend, Mr. Joseph Pirozzi, a building contractor and a former Commissioner of Internal Revenue who said he would look into it. He had friends in high places and was on a first-name basis with Mayor Robert Wagner. Within a few weeks of his intercession, Roosevelt Hospital was granted per-mission to proceed with construction of the Upjohn Clinic. Mrs. Stearns provided the funds for this and the project proceeded at a brisk pace. The clinic consisted of a waiting room and four private examining rooms, an endoscopy unit and a conference room and library equipped with state-of-the-art audiovisual equipment. The Endoscopy Suite was I believe, the first of its kind in the city. To staff it, I knew I had to have a nurse-educator selected by me and under my administrative control. This would not be easy to accomplish through the customary routes but I was learning the secret of how to get "unorthodox" things done to initiate innovations. The secret was to discuss the innovation and enlist the chief administrator's interest. The decisive stroke was to offer to have the Upjohn Foundation pay for the salaries and other expenses involved. This was how I obtained administrative approval to recruit a cracker-jack nurse supervisor from the Vanderbilt Clinic, Miss Margaret Reid, to become one of the key members of my team at Roosevelt. A graduate of the Presbyterian Hospital's School of Nursing and the holder of a B.S. degree in nursing and a Master's degree in public health from

Columbia University, Miss Reid had worked with me for years in the Vanderbilt Clinic and was excited by the challenge of the new service and was very happy to join our team. She would be the chief nursing supervisor of the Upjohn Clinic in charge of the Endoscopy Unit and the care and instruction of patients with ileostomies or colostomies, the forerunner of an enterostomal service. Unfortunately, Miss Reid became ill with a malignant primary brain tumor during her second year with us. Despite valiant efforts at the Neurological Institute, Miss Reid died after a prolonged battle to overcome the disease. Our loss at the Upjohn was grievous and we never really got over it. She was everything we had sought for in her position and left a heritage we have never forgotten.

The Upjohn Clinic and Service flourished and our conferences were well attended by surgical as well as medical attendings, pathologists and radiologists, house staff and medical students. I knew I must be doing something right when, one day, several new members of our house staff rushed by saying they had to get to the Upjohn GI Conference on time so that they did not miss a minute of it. They said "This Dr. Lepore is better than Ben Casey," a popular young "movie" doctor of that day.

Interesting new patients were referred and I was frequently asked to consult on complicated problems. One of the most interesting patients I was asked to see was a seventy-year-old man with a history of recurrent massive upper GI tract bleeding with melena and anemia requiring multiple transfusions. I was asked to see the patient in Hackensack Hospital in February 1964. When I arrived at the hospital, I was met by his family physician and his surgeon and soon the patient's bed was surrounded by an attentive young house staff. The history of his illness was that he had enjoyed good health until February 1963 when he had his first episode of painless GI bleeding manifested by the passage of tarry stools, weakness, and anemia. He was transfused two units of blood. There was no hematemesis. Investigations, including a GI series and barium enema, failed to identify the cause of the bleeding. A second episode of melena necessitated hospital admission on 12/29/63 when his hemoglobin had fallen to 10.2 gm per 100 cc. Exploratory laparotomy was performed. The stomach and duodenum were examined and found to be grossly normal. Several small bluish areas were seen in the small bowel. The colon was examined and found to be grossly negative. The postoperative diagnosis was Weber-Rendu-Osler disease. The patient was given two units of blood and discharged with a hemoglobin of 13.3 gm percent and a hematocrit of 45 percent. On 1/2/64 he was readmitted with "massive" tarry stools and a hemoglobin of 10.2 gm percent and hematocrit of 31 percent. He required six units of blood preoperatively. He was again explored and it was apparent that he was bleeding from the "lower portion" of the duodenum without any evidence of peptic ulcer disease. A pyloroplasty was performed. Complete hematological study failed to reveal any evidence of a coagulopathy or hematological disorder other than an iron-deficiency anemia. Six days after, he bled again and was re-admitted to Hackensack Hospital on 1/28/64 and given three units of blood. The surgeon spoke of exploring the patient once again. It was at this juncture that I was asked to see the patient at the family's request. I reviewed the patient's history quickly at the bedside and confirmed the details. I then proceeded with a methodical and careful physical examination starting at the top and proceeding to the bottom. I called for a tongue blade and after the usual struggle, a flashlight was located as well as a tongue blade. His tongue was normal without any telangiectases or macroglossia. On the left buccal mucosa there was a 2.5 cm blue bleb nevus that no one else had noticed. I asked whether there were any more of these. The answer was no but I persisted, looking at the sole of the feet and sure enough there was a similar lesion on the sole of the right foot. I quickly completed my examination, including a rectal examination. I then asked for the GI x-ray films. When I reviewed these, previously called "normal," I saw in the transverse duodenum several lesions that might well be blue bleb nevi. Putting together the pieces of this puzzle, I felt certain that the bleeding was coming from one or more blue bleb rubber nevi of the transverse duodenum. The transverse duodenum is retroperitoneal and difficult to palpate and examine for bleeding. I also knew that it would take a very seasoned and experienced surgeon to attempt to resect this area of the duodenum without causing injury to pancreatic and biliary ducts. I told the group and the family what I thought was wrong and what was needed. I recommended that he be transferred to my service at Roosevelt Hospital where we were equipped to perform fiberoptic gastroscopy and other tests to localize the site of hemorrhage. This was done at gastroscopy by Dr. James Gabriel. No bleeding site was found in the stomach or proximal duodenum. By using an instrument called a diagnostotube we were able to establish that the bleeding was coming from the transverse duodenum. Operation was advised but the patient demurred and wished to go home on medical therapy. Inevitably, he re-bled and on 1/19/64 had to return to Roosevelt Hospital, where he underwent extensive surgery by Dr. Frederick Amendola, a superb abdominal surgeon, the best of a very talented group of abdominal surgeons at Roosevelt Hospital. The diagnosis of bleeding from blue bleb nevi of the duodenum was confirmed. The operation consisted of a partial distal duodenectomy and partial jejunectomy with primary end-to-end duodeno-jejunostomy. His postoperative course was complicated by further bleeding requiring re-operation on February 29, 1964, when another blue bleb nevus in the descending limb of the duodenum 4 cm distal to the ampulla of Vater, bled furiously. Dr. Amendola was able to stem the bleeding by transfixing the bleeding vascular malformation. The patient was discharged on 4/7/64 to the care of his local physician. The saga continued. I last saw the patient in July 1969 when he was admitted to my service at St. Vincent's Hospital because of melena, anemia with a hemoglobin of 7.7 gm per 100 cc and hematocrit of 27 percent. Stools converted from guaiac positive to negative. He responded well to two units of whole blood. Selective visceral angiography failed to reveal a bleeding site. He was discharged, improved, to the care of his family doctor.

In his excellent monograph, "Vascular Spiders and Related Lesions of the Skin," Dr. William Bennett Bean had this to say:

> There is a characteristic variety of bluish nevus of the skin found in association with angiomas of the gastrointestinal tract which cause serious bleeding. The larger angiomas have some of the feel and look of rubber nipples, are compressible and refill fairly promptly from their rumpled compressed state. I have called them rubber-bleb nevi though they vary in size, shape and numbers. This lesion has been described by surgeons but has not been emphasized in writings of internists and gastroenterologists—While much less common than hereditary hemorrhagic telangiectasia, the syndrome of erectile bluish nevi of the skin and angiomatoses of the gut associated with enteric bleeding is definite. It should be known better.[1]

One of the most popular and best-attended teaching conferences at Roosevelt Hospital was the Clinico-Pathology Conference, or CPC, held once monthly. The cases selected for discussion were patients who had died, usually from an ailment that had not been detected prior to the autopsy. The attending physician selected to discuss the problem had never seen the patient in question and knew nothing about the autopsy findings. This added spontaneity to the session and placed the discussant under considerable strain, usually quite evident to the audience of peers, house staff, and medical students. These

---

1. William B. Bennett, *Vascular Spiders and Related Lesions of the Skin* (Springfield, Illinois: Charles C. Thomas, 1958), pp. 178–179.

CPCs focusing upon case presentations were successfully promoted at the Massachusetts General Hospital by Dr. Richard Cabot. The purpose was to indicate how a seasoned clinician goes about problem solving when faced with a patient he has never seen. When performed by an expert, nothing can match the clinical case presentation for its teaching value and contribution to the art of diagnosis. At every medical school where I have studied or taught—Rochester, Duke, Yale and Columbia University College of Physicians and Surgeons—the CPC has been a key part of the teaching and learning program. Yet, in recent years, the material for these sessions has been limited by the low autopsy percentages in all teaching hospitals. Rates as low as twenty percent and even less are now acceptable whereas in the past, a hospital would lose its accreditation if its autopsy rate dropped below fifty percent. Various explanations have been offered for this sharp decline, one being that the hospitals are not being reimbursed for performing autopsies. Another is that with the advent of newer diagnostic technology such as CT scanning MRI, ultrasonography, fine needle biopsy, and interventional radiology, plus elegant batteries of all sorts of biochemical data, the clinician no longer needs the autopsy to confirm or deny the accuracy of his diagnosis. The truth of the matter is that the autopsy still reveals that a substantial number of clinical diagnoses are missed. Some believe that clinicians are not as aggressive in seeking autopsy permission because of the fear of uncovering a missed diagnosis or an error in management. Some families deny permission for an autopsy on a family member because "he or she has suffered enough." Others fear that finding something at autopsy might uncover a pre-existing ailment that might void an insurance policy recently issued. In this climate, it is no wonder that house staff and their attending physicians are not as aggressive as they used to be in pursuit of postmortem examinations. When I interned in medicine at Duke in 1935–36 I set a record for autopsies that I do not believe has been equaled—100 percent. I attribute this in part to the Johns Hopkins system then in vogue at Duke of being on call around the clock, seven days a week, unless another intern would exchange calls with me. We did not have intensive-care units in those days. We took care of the very sick on our wards as well as those with diagnostic problems. As a result, I knew my patients well and to this day I can still recall some of them by name and ailment. Needless to say, to achieve a 100 percent autopsy rate there also had to be an element of plain luck. My patients knew me well and knew that I worked very hard to save their lives and so did their families. No money was changing hands. The families felt that they wanted to do anything in their power to help their "doctor" save other lives.

With this introduction, let me tell you about the one and only time in my three years at Roosevelt Hospital that I was asked to discuss a difficult case problem at a CPC. Two weeks before the conference I was asked by the chief of medicine to discuss that month's case and given a summary of the patient's complaints, hospital course, and the usual laboratory and x-ray findings. When I read the protocol, I realized that the patient's symptoms were chiefly of cardiac origin, with intractable congestive heart failure, in a seventy-one-year-old black woman who had been treated for over fifty years at Roosevelt Hospital. During the last three years of her life she was troubled with diarrhea with as many as twelve loose or semi-solid stools per day. She also had polyarthritis, albuminuria, renal insufficiency, and hepatomegaly. I wondered why this case had been assigned to me, given my special interest in gastroenterology. One of my staff warned me that the chief of medicine had said he was assigning this case to me because he knew I would miss the diagnosis because it had been missed by all of the senior attendings, including himself. This was like waving a red flag in front of me, and so I approached the CPC with every intention to succeed in making the diagnosis. When I stepped to the podium, I prefaced my approach to the CPC with these remarks:

> On several occasions I have been asked by members of the resident staff to explain how one should conduct a clinico-pathologic conference. Expertise at clinico-pathologic conferences is a great art to which I lay no claim. (Quite frankly I prefer to make the diagnosis in the living patient.) I look on it not as an opportunity to exhibit great knowledge that I do not possess, but rather as an important teaching and learning experience for both the speaker and the listeners. When I am an observer in the audience, my interest is not so much in the final diagnosis as in witnessing how a colleague goes about solving a complex problem on the basis of a protocol and a word picture of the preceding events presented in the form of an abstract. In some ways it has the fascination of watching a detective at work. My approach to our diagnostic problem of today will be to try, by careful scrutiny of the protocol, to arrive at a single diagnosis that will fit the clinical picture. The history is one of progressive and intractable congestive heart failure in a seventy-one-year-old black woman without known hypertension or previously documented rheumatic or vascular disease.

I then discussed briefly, a number of conditions that I felt were not responsible for her illness. My final conclusion was: "I believe that this unfortunate old friend of the Roosevelt Hospital cared for by us for nearly fifty years of her life, died of a rare and unusual disease affecting multiple systems and focusing its major effects on the heart. I believe that this patient had primary systemic amyloidosis."[2]

Having made this statement, I sat down and waited for the pathologists's report. Dr. Richard Fredericks, the pathologist who had performed the autopsy, came quickly to the point, showing a photograph of the markedly enlarged heart and microscopic slides of heart and muscle stained with Congo Red and Crystal Violet that clearly documented my diagnosis of amyloidosis. The facial expression of the chief of medicine was something I would have liked to have seen preserved in a photograph. Dismay and frustration were visibly portrayed. My staff was exuberant and delighted that their chief had triumphed once again in another showdown at Roosevelt. I received a rare ovation for my presentation and was further rewarded by its selection for publication in the *New York State Journal of Medicine* as an outstanding teaching contribution.

----

2. Michael J. Lepore, "Cardiac Failure in Elderly Female," Clinico-Pathologic Conference, *NY State Journal of Medicine* 2 (May 1966), pp. 1222–1229.

Chapter 26

~~~

Consultant and Physician
to President Herbert C. Hoover

"I outlived the bastards."

O N 7 JANUARY 1964, I WAS ASKED by Dr. Ralph Boots to see, in consultation, former President Herbert C. Hoover, who was suffering with gastrointestinal complaints. President Hoover had requested the consultation in writing. The request is in my possession. It is written in pencil on plain white stationery in Mr. Hoover's own hand. It reads as follows:

> Dear Dr. Boots & Bowman [sic: Bauman]: It seems to me we have reached a point where our treatment for digestive gasses must be reviewed. I have asked Allan to take up the subject as to what can be done.
>
> I go for hours—sometimes a whole night awaking every few minutes endeavoring to expel stomach gases. It seems everything turns to gas in a few minutes irrespective of medication of pills and drugs.

The reasons for my selection as the consultant were not entirely clear to me, for all of the previous consultants had been chosen from the staff of the Columbia-Presbyterian Medical Center. I had left that institution after completing twenty-five years of service in 1962 to found and direct the Upjohn Gastrointestinal Service at the Roosevelt Hospital. I was well known to Dr. Boots, Dr. Schullinger, Dr. St. John, and Dr. John Lattimer, the doctors involved in President Hoover's care. Dr. Boots, the physician in charge, was rather skeptical that anyone could help Mr. Hoover and was quite blunt in telling me this while we were riding in the elevator to the Waldorf Towers, Apartment 31A, occupied by Mr. Hoover.

The consultation was quite formal and was held in the living room of the spacious apartment occupied by President Hoover as a residence and office for many years. We were surrounded by items recalling some of Mr. Hoover's great contributions to public life and also much personal memorabilia. A lovely oil portrait of his deceased wife graced one wall adding elegance and charm to the room. Two cupboards housing her priceless collection of Chinese porcelain occupied key corners. In the southeast corner of the room was Mr. Hoover's desk where much of his writing was done. There was a fireplace in the wall that contained artificial logs and coals. Over the mantlepiece were numerous testimonials of honors rendered and tributes paid to this great man. They were quite diversified, ranging from The Humanitarian Award of the Jewish Theological Seminary of America to a memorandum dated 5 July 1962 from Secretary of Defense Robert McNamara congratulating President Hoover on having saved the American people 750 million dollars during the fiscal year 1963 by virtue of the implementation of economy measures in the Federal government recommended by the first Hoover Commission (1947–49). There were other unusual items in this beautiful room that I was later privileged to learn more about from Mr. Hoover. Among them was the cast-iron gnome standing at the doorway of the living room. It was a "Tommy Knocker" a memento of days in the mines where these little gnomes were regarded as good luck omens and served to warn the miners of impending danger or disaster. In 1963 Mr. Hoover wrote to a friend:

> The Tommy-Knockers were the gnomes who for centuries had given benevolent aid to the hard rock miners mostly by warning of rock falls and water breaks. They were associated with fairies, generally, and we all believe in fairies. —They had a long record with the happiness of the miners. I had occasion to meet the mining gnomes in person in a Russian mine. The Russian miners so believed in them that they cast life-size figures of them in the machine shops and placed them in needed spots around and in the mines. . . . To prove my belief in their efficacy, I brought one of them home, although he weighs many pounds. He still guards the entrance to my apartment in the Waldorf-Astoria.[1]

There was also a sword in its scabbard hanging on the north wall. I was to learn that it had been presented with great ceremony to President Hoover in Helsinki before an enthusiastic audience of Finns.

I was introduced to Mr. Allan Hoover, the younger son of the President who acted as his father's spokesman. Herbert Hoover, Jr., was in California but kept in touch by telephone. Dr. Ralph Boots, Mr.

---

1. Herbert Hoover to Joseph Milliken, 23 May 1963. In *Herbert Hoover: The Uncommon Man* (Hoover Presidential Library Association Inc. , 1974), p 8.

Hoover's physician of nearly thirty years, briefed me on the details of the history. We were joined later by Dr. Rudolph Schullinger, who had operated upon Mr. Hoover on two occasions.

President Hoover's medical history was essentially as follows. In 1937 he was found to have a macrocytic anemia (HgB 14 gm, RBC 3 million) for which he was given liver-extract injections until Vitamin B-12 became available for general use. In 1956 he experienced his first bout of biliary colic. In the spring of 1958 he underwent cholecys- tectomy by Dr. Rudolph Schullinger at Harkness Pavilion. The patient's liver was described as normal by Dr. Schullinger. In the fall of 1958 hepatomegaly was first noted, as well as ankle edema. These were attributed at first to congestive heart failure, but the liver did not recede after digitalization. Hepatomegaly progressively increased until his liver edge reached the "pelvic brim." Mr. Hoover was seen in con- sultation by Dr. Franklin Hanger, a renowned liver specialist, who felt that he had non-icteric viral hepatitis and expressed the opinion that the patient had only six months to live. The patient was not jaundiced and his liver chemistries were surprisingly normal, with a negative cephalin flocculation test and normal serum bilirubin and alkaline phosphatase. Needle biopsy was discussed but vetoed by both Dr. Hanger and Dr. Arthur Blakemore, who also saw the patient. In ret- rospect, I believe that his hepatitis may well have been due to Hepatitis C acquired from his transfusions. At the time none of the hepatitis viruses had been identified.

In August 1962, despite pallor and failing general health, the patient went to West Branch, Iowa, to dedicate his Presidential Library. Upon returning he was immediately hospitalized in Harkness Pavilion with profound anemia (HgB 4.0 gm) and positive stool gua- iacs. Barium enema revealed a carcinoma of the transverse colon. He was operated upon by Dr. Schullinger, who found a bulky carcinoma of the transverse colon as well as several polyps. The tumor had invaded the serosa. A wide resection was done with an end to side ileotransverse colostomy. No gross liver metastases were seen but biopsy of the enlarged liver was not performed. The regional nodes were negative for carcinoma.

The next major episode of illness occurred in May 1963, the patient allegedly having been well in the interim. The illness consisted of one GI hemorrhage after another, manifested by tarry stools. This ailment was attributed to bleeding from "stress ulcer," although this was not documented. Melena and anemia were the chief manifesta- tions. Fiberoptic gastroscopy was in its infancy and was never done. The patient refused to go to the hospital. He was transfused with packed red cells repeatedly and finally stopped bleeding. During this

illness he developed acute urinary retention. Dr. John Lattimer inserted a Foley catheter and it was still present in January 1964, when I first
saw the patient.

Since the episode of bleeding in May 1963, the patient had continued to have positive stool guaiacs and anemia, and he required
repeated transfusions of packed red cells. In December 1963 the
patient developed diabetes and he was started on insulin. It was at
about this time or perhaps a little before that a major disagreement
had arisen between President Hoover's sons and Drs. Boots,
Schullinger, and St. John. The latter, a distinguished abdominal surgeon then retired, was a friend and advisor of many years standing.
Both Allan Hoover and Herbert Hoover, Jr., told me that the three
doctors, through Dr. St. John who acted as their spokesman, stated
that in their opinion President Hoover had lived his life and they recommended abandoning supportive and therapeutic measures, letting
nature take its course. This horrified both sons and their wives and led
to several acrimonious discussions, during which it was clearly stated
by both sons that so long as their father was not in great pain and so
long as he retained control of his mental faculties, they felt that every
effort should be made to prolong his life and to keep him comfortable no matter what expense or effort it might entail. Mr. Allan
Hoover was quite certain that despite their reluctant acquiescence, the
doctors failed to treat his father aggressively and did not perform the
tests and studies needed to accurately monitor his progress or decline.

President Hoover also had made it abundantly clear to his doctors
that he was tired of hospitals and refused to enter any hospital preferring, no hurry about it, to die in the comfort of his Waldorf-Towers
apartment among his familiar faces and surroundings. Really what he
desired was home care in modern dress with the trimmings of state-
of-the-art technology. This, then, was the background of the illness
for which I was called to see President Hoover on 7 January 1964.

When I examined President Hoover that day, I was impressed by
his history, which was clearly that of gastroesophageal reflux and
severe heartburn consistent with an esophageal hiatal hernia. The hernia had been missed on a gastrointestinal series done in Harkness
Pavilion. I spotted it in some x-ray films during the course of this
consultation. On physical examination he was an elderly, alert man
wearing a hearing aid. He was belching frequently and in moderate
distress. His mucous membranes and conjunctivae were slightly pale.
There was no icterus and no spider angiomata or other vascular
lesions seen. The tongue was rather large but there was no papillary
atrophy. He was nearly edentulous. There was the excisional scar of a
small epithelioma of the lower lip in this longtime pipe smoker. No

enlarged nodes could be felt in the neck. The neck veins were not distended. There were no carotid bruits. The thyroid gland felt normal. The chest was sightly increased in its AP diameter. The heart was not enlarged. There was a grade 2 systolic murmur audible over the entire precordium. The sounds were of good quality and regular in rate and rhythm. The lungs were emphysematous. No basal rales were heard. The abdomen was protuberant and thin-walled. The liver was remarkably enlarged, relatively smooth, non-tender, extending 13 cm below the xiphoid and 15 cm below the right costal margin in the midclavicular line. The enlargement of the left lobe was really quite striking. The spleen was easily felt, 2FB below the left costal margin. There was no ascites. The scars of previous operations were well healed. No other masses could be felt. There were no bruits. There was much peristaltic activity. A Foley catheter was in place. Rectal examination revealed mild prostatic enlargement and some tenderness. The extremities were free of edema. The peripheral pulses were normal. There was rather severe onychomycosis of the toenails and the fingernails of the left hand. Laboratory studies at this time revealed moderate anemia, positive stool guaiacs, glycosuria, hyperglycemia, albuminuria, and moderate elevation of B.U.N.

When I had completed my examination, the President asked me, "Doctor, what do you think is wrong?" I replied, "I would like to discuss this with Drs. Boots and Schullinger, and then we will come back to discuss it further with you." Then we left the room and reviewed the problem. I stated flatly that his GI troubles were coming from reflux esophagitis, related to his hiatal hernia, which could be managed medically with a strict medical program. Dr. Boots's reaction was that the patient would never follow a medical program. As tactfully as I could, I disagreed. My appraisal was that President Hoover, with his brilliant engineer's mind, could not fail to comply with my therapeutic plan if he were thoroughly informed about it in clear and unequivocal terms, with an explanation as to its rationale. With the approval of his doctors, I returned to President Hoover's bedroom and used one of his pads of white paper on which I drew a rough sketch of the esophagus and the stomach and the hiatal hernia. The patient listened to me carefully and when I had finished, he said, "You're the doctor. I'll do as you say." I had stressed that the head of the bed should be elevated six inches on blocks to reduce the reflux of acid gastric juice into the esophagus. Every two hours an ounce of Gelusil antacid was to be swallowed. The diet was to be bland and in small feedings. What I did not mention to him was replacing his bed with an electronically operated hospital bed. I knew there would be reluctance to give up the bed that he and his wife had slept in for many years. I did discuss this with Miss Marshall, his head nurse. She said "Give me some time and I think I shall be able to arrange it. It would not only help the patient but will make nursing care much simpler when he is acutely ill." Within forty-eight hours, the symptoms of heartburn and eructation that had plagued the president for so many nights and days were markedly improved and he asked Miss Marshall to thank me and to request that I see him again. When I returned a few days later his improvement had persisted and after a pleasant chat, I started for the door when he called to me and handed me a large, beautifully designed antique-looking book resembling the original *De Re Metallica* of Agricola, which had been translated by President and Mrs. Hoover into English from its original Latin, a classic mining text of the sixteenth century that is still in use as a standard reference work. It took the Hoovers five years, from 1907–1912, to complete while they were living in London. This book, autographed by President Hoover, is among the most treasured items in my personal library.

You may well imagine how busy I was when I was called to see President Hoover. The new Upjohn Clinic and Service had been established at Roosevelt Hospital and occupied a great deal of my energy and time. My personal practice continued to thrive and, all in all, I was having the time of my life enjoying every minute of it. After seeing President Hoover, I arrived home quite late and was having a snack in our kitchen when our son, Fred, joined me and asked me what sort of day I'd had. My reply was: "I want to tell you about it. I know you want to study medicine. You've told me this since you were ten years old. I know you don't want to study it just because it's easy, because I think you can see that I work hard at it. This morning when I left here at six o'clock to get down on time for my teaching rounds at Roosevelt Hospital, I saw a miserable old Italian man who was dirty and smelly, hostile, spoke no English, and nobody wanted to take care of him. I spoke to him in Italian and found out that he was complaining that there was a cockroach in his cup of coffee, a legitimate complaint. I made a quick Army-style inspection of the Ward kitchen, found it to be dirty and the source of roaches. My complaint to administration created a bit of a stir but it provided some results. Then I saw other people on my teaching rounds and later in the day I was asked to see one of the greatest Americans that ever lived." Fred asked, "Who was he?" I said President Herbert Hoover and continued, "I have a note here, written by him that I want you to treasure. In it, he tells his doctors that he would like to have a consultant called for his stomach complaints, and this is why your Daddy was called to see him. I want you to cherish this because I think this is an experience we will be very proud of. Later today I saw and examined this wonderful man and I am sure I'm going to help him. I immediately liked him and I think he liked me." Then I said to Fred, "Now I'm tired. It's been a long day. Let's go to bed."

"But this is what medicine is about. You're going to meet some of the least-wanted and some of the most-respected people in the world, and there's just no finer way to live, because there is a common denominator, the doctor who brings hope, help, and sympathy to those seeking his advice. They are sick or think they are and that is why you're here. This is what medicine is all about. At its best it is a very personal one-on-one way of life."

From time to time, the President would ask me to visit him and to advise him. Then one day Allan Hoover told me that his father wished me to become his personal physician. I was honored by this request and told Allan that I certainly wanted to help his father but recognized that this might create a problem, because I had originally been called as a consultant. He said he would get in touch with several leaders in American medicine as well as the American Medical Association. I believe one of the persons consulted was Dr. Dwight Wilbur of San Francisco. I was told that there should be no ethical objection to my serving as President Hoover's doctor if he so wished and if I were willing to do so.

The patient's next major episode of illness was an acute right kidney colic that occurred on 22 February 1964. He became gravely ill with gross hematuria, chills, and high fever, and sepsis. His NPN rose to 67 mg percent and a drop in hemoglobin to 7.1 percent occurred. He again refused hospitalization. An intravenous pyelogram was done in his bedroom but it was unsatisfactory. It was assumed that he had passed a kidney stone. The patient then developed bronchopneumonia and needed antibiotic therapy. Ampicillin was used with a good response. An oxygen tent was brought in and used. Diabetes was controlled with insulin. Transfusions of packed red cells were administered. After some anxious days, he recovered and slowly regained his strength. The transfusion requirement became less heavy and his stool guaiacs became negative or only faintly positive. Constipation was controlled by milk of magnesia and mineral oil by mouth and nightly oil-retention enemas, the latter preventing fecal impaction, which had been quite a problem. The Foley catheter dropped out in March 1964 and was never reinserted.

When a person as prominent as President Hoover is seriously ill, the press and the public are eager for news and will spare nothing to get information. Fortunately, President Hoover had on his staff of volunteers two dedicated newsmen who had served pro bono to restore his public image following the defeat for re-election in 1932.

The men were very experienced and devoted to Mr. Hoover. They were Neil MacNeil, a former managing editor of the *New York Times* and Frank Mason, president of I.N.S. Mr. MacNeil told me that after he retired from the *New York Times* he decided to volunteer to help President Hoover to overcome the adverse publicity that he was receiving from the general press. He felt that Mr. Hoover had been badly treated by F.D.R. and the Democrats and that his great accomplishments as a humanitarian had been ignored. He was the political scapegoat of the press and blamed for a depression he had never caused or abetted. Hoover welcomed the assistance of these two seasoned newspapermen and cooperated with them until the very end. So when I was faced with questions from the press, I was able to refer the reporters to the two experts. Whenever Mr. Hoover was seriously ill, I would issue a daily bulletin and at times a twice-daily report. I was amazed by the mail these bulletins generated from across the country from my former teachers, Deans, patients, students, and residents, as well as some total strangers. Dr. McCann, my revered first professor of medicine, wrote that my bulletins were first-rate, concise, and informative. Dean Wilburt C. Davison of Duke wrote to tell me how proud he was that one of his boys was taking care of the former president and great humanitarian. He also confided that he had worked under Hoover's auspices in food relief in Belgium after WW I but that he had never had occasion to meet him in person.

Once I was appointed President Hoover's personal physician, I went on twenty-four-hour call for him. This was not as difficult as it sounds because there were nurses around the clock, with double teams on each eight-hour shift when serious complications rose. The nurses were free to call me at any time. When the President was seriously ill, I slept in one of the bedrooms adjoining his. It gave him great comfort to know that I was physically present when he needed me. During periods of very serious illness, I would be assisted by one of my Upjohn fellows or a resident from Roosevelt Hospital. Blood for transfusion was obtained from carefully selected donors, usually house staff at Roosevelt Hospital. The Upjohn fellows and residents who served with pride by caring for this great man were Dr. Jesus E. Noyola from Mexico, Dr. Sheldon V. Smith, Dr. H. Keith Johnson, Dr. Harry M. Friedland, Dr. Frederick A. London, and Dr. Moishe L. Schmidt, the Lubin Fellow.

President Hoover had in the past experienced an acute reaction from a blood transfusion and he feared recurrences. I made it my practice to start every transfusion myself and remained with the patient until the transfusion was completed. At least forty transfusions were given during my watch, all of them without an adverse reaction. I pay tribute to the chief blood-bank technician at Roosevelt Hospital, the late Mrs. Lisji Bielukas, who expended considerable effort to find suitable donors, stimulated to do so because Mr. Hoover had saved her life when she was just a child in Europe and needed the food the Hoover-directed ARA supplied to keep her from starving to death. Dr. Rudolph Garrett, the chief of pathology at Roosevelt, also told me on several occasions that it was Mr. Hoover's food relief that saved his life when he was growing up in Europe.

Some time later I learned that Frank Mason had commented that President Hoover's recovery from his episode of renal colic, sepsis, and bronchopneumonia was almost miraculous and perhaps metaphysical. When I was queried about this in an interview with Ray Henle, the radio commentator, I replied that I was not a metaphysician, but I know that on a number of occasions I have witnessed the turn of the tide of illness toward recovery by just being present at my patients' bedside, inspiring them to fight to get well despite overwhelming odds. As Walsh McDermott had said, there are times in serious illness when the physician himself must be the treatment.

Following his acute illness in the spring of 1964, President Hoover resumed his usual activities, reading, writing, receiving visitors, and keeping in touch with the world outside. One of my duties was to screen the list of visitors and to place some limit on the length of visits. I left this largely to Miss Marshall, the head nurse who knew a good deal about the visitors. She knew those who seemed to cheer up the president and those that might upset him. President Hoover very much enjoyed President Truman's visits. In fact, he was the first to tell me that Harry Truman would go down in history as a great president. When I asked him why, he said he was very courageous, made good decisions, could communicate very well with the public, and was an outstanding leader. At the time Mr. Hoover told me this, Truman was not so highly regarded by others. Since then, most people would agree that Truman was one of the great presidents who adorned the office. Having served on Tinian in WW II, preparing for the planned invasion of Japan, I strongly agreed with President Truman's decision to drop the atom bomb, sparing both sides enormous combat casualties. President Hoover took great pleasure in telling me the story of Truman's quickly and without fanfare ordering the changing back of the name of Boulder Dam to the Hoover Dam, righting a serious wrong perpetrated by Franklin D. Roosevelt in one of the petty and partisan actions of his presidency.

President Hoover's general condition gradually improved, but his anemia recurred and on 20 March he was given 2 units of packed red cells. He received another 2 units on 15 April, 2 units on 10 June, and

2 units on 29 August. He was kept on Ampicillin 250 mg four times daily to clear up a urinary-tract infection. In addition, it was felt that he was mentally clearer while on the antibiotic, suggesting that there might be some degree of hepatic encephalopathy accounting for periodic drowsiness. It was also found that chlorothiazide, a diuretic, had a similar effect upon his alertness, so this was stopped.

Slowly but surely, the tenth of August was approaching, the ninetieth birthday of the thirty-first president of the United States. Only one other president of the United States had lived to 90—John Adams, the second president, who served from 1797 to 1801, was born 19 October 1735 and died 4 July 1826.Preparations were being made for this occasion. Mr. Hoover's favorite sport, second only to fishing, was baseball, and the New York Yankees was his favorite team. He was especially proud of Joe DiMaggio and his two major-league brothers, Vincent and Domenic, all products of the Boy's Club of San Francisco, the sons of a fisherman. President Hoover knew all the Yankee ballplayers by the numbers on the back of their shirts. President Hoover was asked to be present at the Yankee Stadium to throw out the ball on his ninetieth birthday. Because of his precarious health, I advised him not to go. Arrangements were made for the Boy's Club of New York City to pick a member to toss out the first ball. Mr. Hoover would be watching the game on his television set in the living room of his apartment. Bob Considine, the sports reporter and a good friend, would join the president. I was also asked to be present. Before the game started, President Hoover asked me to pose with him for a photograph by Ivan Dimitri, the well-known photographer. I shall always treasure that picture. While it was being taken, Mr. Dimitri was on his knees on the hardwood floor. It was President Hoover who noticed the photographer's position, called out to his head nurse, Miss Marshall, and asked her to get a pillow for Ivan Dimitri so that he could kneel on it with less discomfort. That afternoon Mr. Hoover also presented me with a beautiful Bulova wristwatch as memento of the occasion. We watched the baseball ceremonies on television with Bob Considine. The young Puerto Rican boy from the Boys' Club, who had been selected to throw out the first ball in place of the president, stood up and threw the ball to Elston Howard, the Yankee catcher, and missed him by a few yards. Mr. Hoover sent the message to the boy not to worry; he himself was not too great a ballplayer at Stanford and was glad to serve as the team manager.

One of the highlights of this year was having dinner with President Hoover in his dining room with my beloved wife and our son who was then fifteen years old and a six footer. When I introduced my son to the president, he remarked "Doctor, they feed them better nowadays."

Following the President's birthday there was no essential change in his condition except for a slowly progressive weakness and drowsiness, which seemed quite marked on Friday, October 16th, when his hemoglobin had fallen to 9.8 gm percent with hematocrit of 28. His prothrombin time, which had fallen to 20 seconds (control of 13 seconds) on 1 October 1964 had risen with Vitamin K therapy to 14 seconds on 15 October 1964.

At this time the nonfasting blood sugar was 210 mg percent, Na 128 mEq/l, K 5.2 in mEq/l, chloride 101 mEq/l. Serum urea nitrogen was 32 mg percent. The decision to transfuse him was made and the blood was obtained for Saturday, 17 October. While we were searching for a vein for transfusion at 3:55 P.M., the patient suddenly vomited 500 cc of clotted red blood and shortly thereafter vomited a similar amount. Hematocrit taken at this time had dropped to 26 percent. He complained of great thirst. B.P. had dropped to 100/70. Pulse 84. Transfusions of packed cells were started. Despite replacement of two units, that evening his hematocrit had not risen. Blood replacement was continued and by the next day his hemoglobin was 12.0 gm, hematocrit 35, and the vital signs were stable. However, he had become very drowsy, and an ominous sign was the rise in serum urea nitrogen to 89 mg percent. He was passing tarry stools and regurgitated bright red blood on several occasions and on others dark blood. Enemas were given to clean out the large bowel. The question of passing a tube into the stomach to empty it was considered. We also discussed the possibility of gastric cooling or even a Sengstaken-Blakemore balloon. These matters were discussed with Dr. Howard A. Patterson, a renowned abdominal surgeon and president of the American College of Surgeons, and Dr. J. Beall Rodgers, who saw the patient in consultation. It was our opinion that gastric cooling was contraindicated at this time. A venous cutdown was performed in the left forearm under local anesthesia by Dr. J. B. Rodgers. This facilitated intravenous therapy. Fortunately, the scalp needle introduced into a vein of the left ankle did yeoman service and provided us with an additional route for administration of blood and fluids. Blood replacement amounted to a total of 17 units from 17 October through 19 October 1964, the BUN had risen to 150 mg percent, taken while glucose was being infused steadily. Total serum bilirubin was 12.9 mg percent, direct was 0.9 mg percent. Ceph. flocc. was trace positive. Blood ammonia was 454 mg percent and the patient was unresponsive. A nasogastric tube was passed, 19 October 1964 through the right nostril and 2700 cc of old clotted blood and secretions were aspirated while irrigation with ice water was performed. After some time the gastric returns were clear and there was no evidence of fresh bleeding. Intravenous therapy was continued and Modumate and calcium gluconate were added to the infusions. Urinary output was good. With hemorrhage arrested, efforts were instituted to clear the GI tract of blood. Milk of magnesia was instilled via the nasogastric tube. Neomycin was instilled into the stomach to reduce the bacterial flora of the gut in an attempt to control ammonia production. Gentle colonic lavage removed old blood and tarry material from the large bowel. Later that day the BUN had begun to fall to 128 mg percent and the vital signs were stable. That night at 10 P.M. auricular fibrillation occurred at a relative slow rate. At 3:20 A.M. he was resting comfortably. At 6 A.M. a change occurred manifested by clamminess, profuse sweating, hypotension, and weakness of his pulse, which was grossly irregular. Irrigation with the nasogastric tube revealed evidence of a fresh hemorrhage of considerable magnitude. Gastric lavage with ice water was administered. The patient's general condition was steadily deteriorating. His respirations were labored, stertorous, and bubbling. Following this renewed hemorrhage for a time, his respirations were less labored. Then Cheyne-Stokes respirations ensued. The patient was now in deep coma and never regained consciousness. He subsequently experienced generalized clonic convulsions, which was followed by a lesser one soon after. His blood pressure gradually became unobtainable and then his respirations stopped. The heart continued to beat irregularly but slowly and then stopped at 11:34 A.M. on 20 October 1964.

My final diagnosis on the Certificate of Death was as follows:

> Part I. Death was caused by:
> (a.) Immediate cause:
> gastrointestinal hemorrhage due to
> (b.) Peptic ulceration of esophagus and possible esophageal varices due to
> (c.) Esophageal hiatus hernia and postnecrotic cirrhosis of liver.
>
> Part II. Other significant condition:
> Diabetes mellitus.

It was my impression that the massive loss of blood into the GI tract had precipitated hepatic coma and that this in turn had been complicated by pre-existing chronic renal disease with azotemia and hyperkalemia. The announcement of the death of a former president of the United States, especially one as famous as Herbert Hoover, is headline news. A protocol for simultaneously notifying the major news services had been prepared by Neil MacNeil and Frank E.

Mason. The *New York Herald Tribune* erroneously reported that morning that I personally had given the announcement to two wire-service reporters who had been allowed into the Hoover suite. Of course, I had been so busy that I had not seen the newspaper report. Frank Mason had and he was quite upset because the report was inaccurate and could be regarded as a breach of professional etiquette on the part of the doctor as well as the press. Frank Mason was one of the breed of journalists who treasured professionalism and accuracy in reporting and would not tolerate any deviation from this normal code. He fired off a letter to the editor of the *New York Herald Tribune* that elicited an apology and correction. Mr. Mason's letter is reproduced here in its entirety to emphasize that the best of journalists also have high standards of integrity and regard for the truth.

The Waldorf-Astoria Tower
New York, New York 10022
October 21, 1964

Mr. James G. Bellows, Editor
New York Herald Tribune
230 West 41 Street
New York, New York 10036

Dear Mr. Bellows:

As a volunteer staff aide to President Herbert Hoover for over 25 years, and as a former President of the International News Service and newspaper and radio station owner, interested in accurate newspaper reporting, I am sending you this memorandum to correct, for your files, misstatements which appeared in the New York Herald-Tribune this morning about the announcement of the death of Mr. Hoover.

Myths and legends inevitably proliferate in history about any great leader. But it is probably rare to have them published as a matter of record within a few hours after his death.

The New York Herald Tribune on page one this morning (October 21, 1964) states:

"Then, three hours later, his physician, Dr. Michael J. Lepore, stepped before the two wire-service reporters who had been allowed into the Hoover suite and read a statement he had penned in black ink on Waldorf stationery."

This is not true. The facts are that the President's physician, Dr. Lepore, at no time during this illness has appeared before any newspapermen or has spoken to any newspaper or radio reporter, either directly or by telephone about Mr. Hoover. Nor were any newspaper men "allowed into the Hoover suite."

Dr. Lepore handed the Bulletin announcing Mr. Hoover's death at 11:35 A.M. to me in Mr. Hoover's suite, 31-A of the Waldorf Towers. I carried the bulletin from Apartment 31-A by elevator to the press suite, 2200, of the Waldorf Towers. As we had previously arranged, I handed it to Mr. Neil MacNeil, who for many years as a volunteer, has served as Mr. Hoover's editor and press representative.

In accordance with our arrangement, Mr. MacNeil immediately instructed each of the two wire service men to call his news desk. When each had his editor on the wire, Mr. MacNeil dictated the death announcement to them so that both wire services could carry the flash simultaneously. Mr. MacNeil followed the flash by dictating to the two wire service reporters a statement which Mr. MacNeil and I had previously written to be held by Mr. MacNeil until Mr. Hoover's death had been announced.

When Mr. MacNeil finished dictating the one-page release, he was taken by Mr. Ray Henle to a combination television, radio, still picture and press room, on the fourth floor of the Waldorf-Astoria. This room had been arranged through the initiative of Mr. Henle of the National Broadcasting company as a joint enterprise with other broadcasters.

When Mr. MacNeil reached the crowded room, he repeated the same announcement in the same words which he had made to the wire service men a few minutes before in the press suite. Mr. MacNeil then returned to his press suite on the 22nd floor.

There are the exact facts—and I have checked and rechecked them for accuracy.

Very truly yours,
Frank E. Mason

"What is it like to witness the death of a great man?" I was asked by Ray Henle in an interview. "Oh, yes, I was there. In fact I was in residence in his apartment occupying the spare bedroom. He had on his ninetieth birthday given me a wristwatch and I couldn't help, as I counted his pulse and listened to his heart and looked at this watch— I couldn't help associate the friendship and to realize that this watch was the instrument by which I was monitoring the last seconds of his life. When death occurs to a dear friend and great man, it's always a lonesome and heartrending experience. Death is a personal one-on-one relationship of physician and patient, whether he is the greatest man in the world or the most common, sharing the same doctor. For me this is the essence of the personal practice of medicine. It means that we are privileged, because of our honorable profession, to usher people into the world and to usher them out. There is a little bit of us that goes each time one of our patients goes. It's not easy. I've done this for my own father and mother and it's not easy because it is a lonesome, solitary experience when you are alone standing there tolling off the counts, and then making the pronouncement of death. And I knew I had witnessed the death of just about the finest human being I had ever known."

President Hoover had made arrangements before his death to have a postmortem examination done at Columbia-Presbyterian Medical Center. This was done and I attended it. There were no surprises. The clinical diagnoses were confirmed. There was no evidence or recurrence of the carcinoma of the colon. The bleeding was attributed to two tiny benign gastric ulcers of the cardia of the stomach suggesting to some observers the diagnosis of a rare entity, Dieulafoy's erosion.

When a president or former president of the United States dies, since each has served as commander-in-chief of the armed forces, the funeral arrangements are taken over by the army. President Hoover had three funerals, the first at the cathedral-like St. Bartholomew's Church across the street from the Waldorf Towers, the second in the impressive and historic Capitol Rotunda in Washington, D.C., and the last in a grassy field in the little village of West Branch, Iowa, where he was born in humble Quaker surroundings, son of a blacksmith, orphaned at eight, and, despite much adversity, by dint of his brilliant mind, tenacity, and courage, rising to become the greatest mining engineer of all time, then the thirty-first president of the United States and finally the highest accolade, a great humanitarian.

Attendance at the funeral was by invitation. Large crowds attended each one. My beloved wife Ardean and I were invited to attend all three funerals. Each guest was given a typewritten set of instructions.

"PRESIDENT HOOVER—CORTEGE"

N.B. Retain small green ticket (St. Bartholomew's Church 8:30 A.M.) until after the service at Rotunda of Capitol

Friday, October 23

1. Deliver luggage to Waldorf Towers lobby between 6:00–8:00 A.M. It will be tagged and delivered to you on arrival at Madison Hotel, Washington, D.C.

2. Present your admission card at St. Bartholomew's Church, 50th Street entrance, no later than 8:15 A.M.

3. After the service, take any limousine, after the 5th car, for transportation to railroad station.

4. Hotel reservations at Hotel Madison, Tel. No. Code 202–483–6400.

Saturday, October 24

You will be briefed regarding other details on arrival in Washington.

Sunday, October 25

Be at Rotunda no later than 9:15 A.M. for service and removal motor escort to Military Air Transport Field (National Airport)

Ar 1:55 P.M., West Branch, Iowa
3:00 P.M. Services at Hoover Memorial Library
Return by plane to New York City

Thousands of New Yorkers walked by the bier that night paying their respects. The simple and short funeral service at St. Bartholomew's was well attended by a veritable Who's Who in America. My wife and I were pleased that our favorite psalm, the twenty-first, was included. It is impossible for me to name all of the mourners, but I do remember these: President Lyndon B. Johnson, Hubert Humphrey, Barry Goldwater, Jim Farley, John Connolly, Bernard Baruch, Eddie Rickenbacher, Senator Keating, Admiral and Mrs. Lewis L. Strauss, the widow of General MacArthur, and the Milbank family, and many strangers. At the end of the service, friends greeted each other over the pews. As we left St. Bartholomew's, Ardean and I made certain that we stepped into our designated limousine and the cortege headed downtown toward the Pennsylvania Railroad Station where we boarded the train for Washington, D.C. We were met in Washington, D.C., by President Lyndon B. Johnson and Lady Bird. I was pleased to see how warmly they greeted the Hoover family and invited them to stay at the White House. We and some other guests were taken to the Madison Hotel, across the road from the White House, where we would stay. On Saturday, Ardean and I were treated to a guided tour of the White House, the first for both of us. Ardean was especially delighted to see, closeup, the furnishings and the decor of the beautiful mansion.

That evening we were invited to a cocktail reception hosted by Mr. Ray Henle, the radio news commentator, a favorite of President

Hoover. There we met a bewildering assortment of men and women prominent in the world of politics, congress, the senate, and numerous friends and relatives. Everyone appeared to be enjoying the occasion until one of the guests, Mr. Arthur A. Curtice from California and a close friend of the Hoovers, suddenly collapsed and the call went out for a doctor. I responded quickly with my ever-present stethoscope in my rear trouser pocket. When I arrived at Mr. Curtice' side, a gray-haired distinguished appearing man was bending over him. I identified myself to him and he in turn informed me that he was Admiral Joel T. Boone who had been the White House physician for President Hoover. Since I had the stethoscope I proceeded to examine our patient and quickly decided that he was suffering with an acute cardiac arrhythmia, atrial fibrillation. Admiral Boone knew that the nearest hospital was the George Washington University Medical Center. He felt the best way to get the patient there was to put him into one of the taxicabs waiting at the hotel door. This we did and arrived very quickly at the emergency room. Here we were quickly met by an alert and keen young medical resident who just happened to be a graduate of my medical school, Rochester. An electrocardiogram confirmed the diagnosis of atrial fibrillation and it was recommended that the patient be admitted for treatment and observation. By this time Mr. Curtice was very alert and was extremely reluctant to enter the hospital since this would mean that he would miss the flight with us the next morning to Cedar Rapids and to West Branch. I told the patient that it was unwise to take the flight and urged him not to do so. Finally I called the hospital's chief of cardiology and explained what was happening. After some arm-twisting by me the doctor agreed to come to the hospital despite the late hour to review the situation and to persuade the patient to remain. This he did, although he did admit that he was miffed with me at first, because he felt his resident could have handled the situation. Later, after he had seen the patient and met with me, he graciously admitted that I was absolutely right and that he was glad he had come in to see the patient.

Fortunately, Ardean had returned to the Madison Hotel when she saw that I was busy with an emergency. Not the first and not the last time!

On Sunday, the 25th of October, we were driven to the Capitol Rotunda (our first visit there) arriving well before the 9:15 A.M. service was to begin. On the way, we saw the casket on wheels of the caisson, with Blackjack, the handsome black horse without a rider, slowly following the casket, the symbol of a presidential funeral. In the Capitol Rotunda we were asked to line up in a formation supervised by the army. Mrs. Lepore and I were in the second row, directly behind President Lyndon B. Johnson and Lady Bird. The chaplain dated back to President Hoover's occupancy of the White House and had known him quite well. His words were well chosen and to the point. I especially remember that he said that only a few months before they had buried the youngest martyred President (JFK) and now they were burying the oldest former president. He mentioned the abuse that Mr. Hoover had suffered when he left the White House and said he had outlived these bad moments and emerged as a great humanitarian. At this point in his eulogy, I had a good look at LBJ who shed tears in visible evidence of the emotion he was feeling. I decided then that LBJ had some real points in his favor. I also remembered that during his eighties, a reporter asked Mr. Hoover how he felt toward his enemies and detractors; he replied, "I outlived the bastards."[2]

From the Capitol Rotunda we were driven to the Military Air Transport Field (National Airport) where we boarded the Columbine, the presidential airplane, heading for Cedar Rapids, Iowa. The plane was full of interesting people, including the Hoover family as well as their friends. An Army Lt. Colonel was in charge. Among those on the Columbine were Admiral and Mrs. Lewis Strauss, Mrs. MacArthur, the Milbank family, and other prominent persons. The flight was smooth and uneventful for the first hour, but then another medical emergency occurred. I was made aware of it by the Lt. Colonel in charge. He said he was sorry to disturb me but he was concerned about one of the passengers, Barry Goldwater's brother-in-law, who was slumped over in his seat up front. Armed with my trusty stethoscope I hurried down the aisle wondering, What next? He was sitting upright in his chair, sweating profusely and having difficulty in responding to questions. I quickly found out that he was a diabetic, had taken his insulin before coming to the Capitol Rotunda, but had skipped breakfast. I asked the Lt. Colonel to get me the emergency bag. He nearly choked when he realized that he had locked the bag in the cargo bay of the airplane and to get at it would necessitate breaking formation and landing at the nearest airport. The army officer was quite embarrassed, for until now his arrangements had been flawless. Having been in the army myself in WW II, I could understand his

---

2. Richard Norton Smith, "'Outliving the Bastards': Herbert Hoover as a Former President," in *Farwell to the Chief* (Worland, Wyoming: High Plains Publishing Company, 1990), p. 25.

dilemma. Breaking formation would lead to an investigation and the discovery of the oversight that the medical emergency bag that should have been up front with the pilots was sealed below. I said, "Hold on, I think he is in insulin shock and if we can stuff him with coffee and sugar and orange juice, it might just work to bring his blood sugar up. But be quick about it." Fortunately, these items were available. With the patient gradually losing consciousness, I was able to get him to swallow the coffee and sugar and orange juice. Luck was with us, for he began to respond and soon he was his normal self. I kept close watch on him throughout the trip and also at the graveside for the interment.

When we reached Cedar Rapids, a funeral cortege was formed, and I shall always remember that at every hamlet and town on the road to West Branch the people had come out waving flags, many of them with tears streaming down their faces, as they paid homage to the blacksmith's son from West Branch who had achieved fame and enormous success in almost every field of endeavor.

The sight of the tiny cottage where the thirty-first president was born is something I shall never forget. Only in America is it possible to soar so high from the humblest of origins. America was blessed in many ways by the life of Herbert Hoover. He lies buried forever in a hillside near his Memorial Library, joined by his beloved wife, who died in 1944. Tears well from my eyes as I write this. They are not those of sadness, they are those of joy that our great country that can and has produced a Herbert Hoover will always overcome its problems and conflicts and produce more people like Hoover to lead us to the summit of our expectations. TO EACH HIS FARTHEST STAR!!

To have been his personal physician and friend is one of the greatest joys of my professional life. There is a lesson in this story for all of those who aspire to be and those who are members of our glorious profession of medicine. We must have excellent, dedicated physicians for all of our people. We must provide access for all sick persons to the best of medical care. A few men and women will rise above the average by dint of greater ability, better opportunity, and innate wisdom and experience. When these gifted persons have in their care the leaders of our country, there is the opportunity to influence attitudes and support by these leaders for medical education, health care delivery, research and primary care, and the preservation of the personal practice of the best of medicine.

I close this chapter on President Hoover with a letter from his son, Allan, which I shall cherish forever.

The Towers

October 31, 1964

The WALDORF-ASTORIA
New York 10022

Dear Dr. Lepore:

It is not possible to convey to you in mere words the gratitude in our hearts for all you did for our father.

You gave him so much more than your medical genius: stimulating encouragement, a feeling of security and complete confidence.

Dad trusted you, and our entire family shared his opinion that you are a truly good man, Dr. Lepore and a great and dedicated doctor.

Sincerely and gratefully,
Alan Hoover

Dr. Michael J. Lepore
550 Park Avenue
New York, New York

Chapter 27

~ひ~

Problems at Roosevelt Hospital:
The Bête Noir of Full Time

THE UPJOHN GASTROINTESTINAL SERVICE had come to Roosevelt Hospital in early 1962 like a breath of fresh air in a torpid climate. One of the reasons for selecting Roosevelt Hospital for launching this innovative service was the new eleven-story Winston Building for private and semiprivate patients then well underway. It would serve as an excellent base for delivering health care in an up-to-date, state-of-the-art facility, replacing or supplementing the older Roosevelt facilities. The location of the hospital was in a relatively safe area of Manhattan easily reached by bus or subway. The story of the genesis of the Winston Building is worth repeating. The attending staff had been urging for years that Roosevelt must build new facilities to compete for patients as well as for staff. A fund-raising drive was started but, despite valiant efforts, the momentum stalled at a level that would provide for only a four- or five-story building. Dr. Frederick Amendola, one of their finest surgeons, told me that at a meeting of the executive committee he strongly objected to settling for a small building that they would soon outgrow and urged that they plan for at least a ten-story building, borrowing money if necessary to pay for it. He said he was sick and tired of seeing Roosevelt settle for chicken coop-like structures like the Russell Memorial Building when it should aspire to higher goals. Dr. Amendola's impassioned plea to "go for the gold" seemed to have frightened many of his colleagues, who thought it was too ambitious. Little did they know that sitting at the head of the table was an individual, Mr. Garrard Winston, a trustee, who would soon pledge ten million dollars for the construction of a modern eleven-story building for patients. At that time, the sixties, this was more than adequate funding for this project. The building would be named for him. This building was well underway when Mrs. Stearns and I initiated discussions with the Roosevelt Hospital trustees. I remember how exciting it was when we climbed up the steel skeleton of the new building while administrative officers described the scope of the construction and the new facilities envisioned, including what was most unusual in those days, central air conditioning. We were told that if we wished, we might have the top floor of the building for the Upjohn Service. Since Mrs. Stearns had made it very clear in her letters that she was not interested at that time in bricks and mortar but very committed to supporting new ideas and people with original concepts, this offer was reviewed and then rejected because of the large sum of money needed to finance it. Within one year of our entry to Roosevelt Hospital, we had built a modern, functional outpatient clinic that was functioning marvelously, lifting outpatient care and teaching to a level never before seen at Roosevelt Hospital. On 1 April 1963, the Upjohn Gastrointestinal Clinic was formally dedicated in a reception attended by its donor, Mrs. Janet Upjohn Stearns, and many distinguished guests including Mr. Peter Terenzio, chief administrator of Roosevelt Hospital; Dr. Charles Flood of P&S; Drs. Frederick Amendola, James Thompson and Howard Patterson, chiefs of surgery; and Dr. Arthur J. Antenucci, chief of medicine. Mr. Joseph Pirozzi, without whose help the clinic might never have been built, was present. My beloved wife Ardean was the hostess and poured high tea.

Roosevelt never had a gastroscope until the Upjohn Service purchased several. Gastroscopy with fiberoptic instruments equipped for biopsying as well as photography was revolutionizing the field of gastroenterology. I had assembled an excellent group of attending physicians, fellows, and residents, including Dr. James B. Gabriel, a seasoned and able gastroenterologist and endoscopist who was my second in command. The administrative staff, headed by Miss Martha Swensson, was dedicated and enthusiastic in promoting our goals. The clinic was well attended and actively engaged in the personal care of patients and the teaching of medical students, house staff, and fellows. The nursing staff under Miss Margaret Reid was a stellar element of our division. All in all, everything was moving along very smoothly, perhaps too much so, for before long we began to notice some areas of concern. First Mrs. Stearns obtained a major six- or seven-figure gift from her mother, Mrs. Grace B. Upjohn of Kalamazoo, Michigan, for the construction and installation of the latest state-of-the-art x-ray facilities for gastrointestinal imaging. I requested that this magnificent gift be acknowledged by placing a plaque on the wall with an inscription of gratitude to Mrs. Upjohn. You may imagine my surprise when I was told by Mr. Peter Terenzio, the chief administrator, that one of the two chiefs of medicine had objected to this, saying that nothing like that had been done for previous donors of gifts to the radiology department. I pursued the matter further and won my point, but the chief of medicine was not happy, because in the past he had always prevailed when a policy dispute arose. At about the same time, even though I was on the executive committee of the Roosevelt Hospital, I was not privy to important discussions that were taking place involving major changes in the professional staffing of the hospital. The hospital had decided that the era of voluntary heads of departments was ending and the future development would be to turn to full-time salaried directors and chiefs of service. At the time we came to Roosevelt, almost no department heads were on full-time salary. The three chiefs of surgery and the two chiefs of medicine received no salary and relied almost entirely on their substantial private practices. They had almost no office space worthy of the name at the hospital and very little administrative staff. The failure to provide salaries, space, and adequate staff for these heads of service was in the hallowed tradition of Roosevelt Hospital over its many years of existence. It was not entirely a matter of idealism that motivated the men (there were no women) to compete for these unsalaried positions. There was a substantial financial advantage in being a chief of service in a prestigious modern hospital with the chief exerting considerable control over admissions, operating time, and bed occupancy. The attending staff at Roosevelt was carefully limited in number and there was a flexible arrangement whereby, when beds were in high demand, certain staff members would be shut out while others could admit their patients. In periods of low occupancy, the gates could be opened at the admitting office for patients whose doctors had limited admitting privileges. I am not privy to knowing the income of the various chiefs of surgery and medicine at Roosevelt, but I am certain that it was substantial. For the surgeons, the emergency room was a significant source of revenue. The Room 100 Workmen's Compensation Clinic was, if not a gold mine, a coal mine. Since surgeons had less need for an outside office than the medical men, it was understandable that they could spend most of their time in their hospital, preferably in the operating room. By comparison, the medical chiefs spent much more time than the surgeons in their outside offices and were less visible to the house staff and medical students.

This system had worked very well for nearly one hundred years but it was beginning to wear thin. The most vulnerable area was in the department of medicine, and it was here that the opening wedge of full time would soon appear.

In my book, *Death of the Clinician: Requiem or Reveille?*, I listed in detail my objections to the Flexnerian full-time system, which has never worked satisfactorily. Yet, to this day, seventy or more years after Flexner's original proposal, whenever lay persons decide to reform medical education and training, full time is promoted as the panacea for all ills. So it was at Roosevelt Hospital that the trustees decided to go to full time in the department of medicine. Were there any other options? Of course there were. The first and foremost could have been geographic full time with faculty serving patients on fee-for-service or in a faculty group practice setting. The doctors would earn their salary the old-fashioned way, by seeing private patients. The board of trustees—egged on I believe by Mrs. Donald Bush, the president, who almost certainly was influenced by Dean Rappleye—had decided to replace the two chiefs of medical service with a full-time salaried chairman of medicine. The chiefs of surgery, who were very highly regarded by P&S and its medical students, would continue, for the time being, to be on a voluntary part-time basis. A number of factors played a role in reaching this decision, not the least of which was that one of the chiefs of medicine had antagonized the new Bard professor at P&S, Dr. Stanley Bradley, to the degree that P&S would no longer send its students to Roosevelt for their medical clerkships. I also learned that my own re-appointment as assistant clinical professor at P&S had not been renewed. When I questioned Dean Houston Merritt about this, he told me that the chief of medicine at Roosevelt had failed to send in the recommendation. Clearly I was caught in a cross fire between the chief of medicine at Roosevelt and the Bard professor. To make matters worse, Dean Merritt, who had promised me that my appointment would be renewed and even advanced to a higher grade, and despite his good will toward me, was not taking any remedial action, considering it an intramural problem. He wanted to avoid the criticism that he was trying to micromanage an affiliate hospital.

My own feeling was that instead of micromanaging he was letting the foxes guard the henhouse. Being without assigned medical students from P&S, I was deprived of one of my major interests and opportunities to advance the teaching of gastroenterology that had inspired me to start the Upjohn Gastrointestinal Service. This was the beginning of my disaffection with the situation at Roosevelt Hospital. The *bête noir* of full time, a concept I have never believed in, was intruding into my life and my career in the least-expected place. Another problem concerned the Upjohn Outpatient Clinic, which we had built and paid for and shared with a group made up chiefly of surgeons. A Workmen's Compensation Clinic ("Room 100"), perhaps illegally lodged in Roosevelt Hospital, was to take over the entire clinic when the Upjohn Gastrointestinal Service moved into new quarters on the eighth floor of the Tower Building. The new quarters were designed to house the *inpatient* activities of the Upjohn including research in gastroenterology. If we were to lose the outpatient clinic that we had built at considerable effort and expense, the care of ambulatory patients in gastroenterology would suffer, and we *and* they would suffer a serious setback. Having seen how successfully the outpatient clinic was functioning for treatment, diagnosis, teaching, and patient care, I was unwilling to give up this area in a hospital with very primitive and unsatisfactory outpatient facilities. This was an issue that might have been resolved in an equitable fashion, but the income from Room 100 was significant and the surgeons profiting from it were looking to expand this lucrative enterprise rather than to continue to share the space with the Upjohn.

It soon became apparent that the trustees, persuaded that full time was inevitable, would start with the medical service. The decision, without any discussion with the rank and file of the voluntary staff that had served Roosevelt Hospital so well for many years, was reached by the chief of medicine and the trustees to replace the voluntary unsalaried chief by a full-time salaried chairman. The choice was, I believe, an unfortunate one and I was not pleased with it. The occupant was promised a substantial salary plus permission to add six new attendings on full-time salary. If you add to this secretarial and administrative staff, technicians, office and laboratory space, malpractice insurance and vacations, health insurance, pensions and other perks, you may well imagine how expensive this policy could be. In fact, it could bankrupt the hospital, and indeed it did within three years. I had two sessions with the new chairman of medicine whom I had known when he was a resident at Presbyterian. I learned that he had decided before his arrival at Roosevelt to discharge our two vitamin investigators because they did not fit in with his plans for the department. These two men, Drs. Herman Baker and Oscar Frank, had been studying vitamin nutrition at Roosevelt and participating with me in research into the malabsorption syndromes. They were measuring blood vitamin levels with the ingenious use of a "zoo" of parasites with known growth requirements controlled by the various vitamins. They had already published a number of excellent papers in good journals and represented one of the few real research efforts being pursued at Roosevelt. I thought their dismissal was highhanded and without consideration of the needs of the Upjohn Service.

Later, I learned that my plan to build the Upjohn inpatient unit on one of the Tower building floors was going to be allowed to proceed to the tune of spending $250,000 of Upjohn funds, only to have the space taken over as a general research area by the new chairman of the department of medicine. When I learned of this from a reliable leak, I questioned the new chairman of medicine, and got him to acknowledge that this is what he was prepared to do. I then told him that I would not put up with this brazen attempt to take us for a buggy ride. I warned him that I did not believe that the full-time system was needed or could work out at Roosevelt Hospital and told him that I would give him five years to push Roosevelt Hospital into bank-ruptcy. He beat that record, Roosevelt went through thirty million dollars in endowment and went bankrupt, not in five years, but in three. It was called the most mismanaged hospital in New York by well-informed observers. In my opinion the full-time system and its advocates and representatives ruined a successful community hospital and led to its enforced rescue by St. Luke's Hospital.

Before all of this happened, lacking confidence in this hospital, I made arrangements to take the Upjohn elsewhere, to a place where the climate would be more encouraging. When I told this story to my friend, Dr. Ross Golden, he complimented me on having the guts to make a change when I became aware of the adverse developments at Roosevelt and encouraged me to keep the fight for gastroenterology on the front burner.

Chapter 28
Internal Medicine as a Vocation (1897)

> At the onset, I would like to empha-
> size the fact that the student of inter-
> nal medicine cannot be a specialist.
> The manifestation of almost any one
> of the important diseases in the
> course of a few years will "box the
> compass of the specialties."
>
> —Sir William Osler, 1897

IN 1897, OVER ONE HUNDRED YEARS AGO, Sir William Osler, the greatest physician of modern times, was invited to lecture before the section on internal medicine of the New York Academy of Medicine. The title was "Internal Medicine as a Vocation." There was, even in that early day, concern that general internal medicine was being neglected while the subspecialties were fragmenting it. Osler argued with eloquence that general internal medicine was the backbone of medical practice and every effort should be made to strengthen it and to maintain its position as the basic foundation for the education and training of physicians. Many of Osler's arguments for the importance of general internal medicine are as valid today as they were one hundred years ago. Some have lost their relevance in a period of great change in medical education, especially in the post-graduate years. Now, the general perception is that general internal medicine has become very unattractive to the current crop of medical students who are flocking to the subspecialties and the more lucrative procedure-oriented fields of practice. Whereas in the past internal medicine attracted the brightest and the best students with their Alpha Omega Alpha keys, even the best teaching hospitals are having difficulty in matching in internal medicine and find themselves accepting lower-ranking students and foreign medical graduates in order to meet their quotas. In addition, because most of those choosing a residency in internal medicine elect to become subspecialists, our country finds itself flooded with specialists who may end up examining each other and short of men and women providing primary care. The situation is so acute that it has been called a crisis in medicine and there are threats that government intervention and Draconian measures may be needed to correct the imbalance.

What went wrong and how can we fix it? Responding to Santayana's admonition that "those who cannot remember the past are condemned to repeat it," let us review Osler's defense of the generalist in internal medicine.

Let us start with the definition of a "vocation." The *American Heritage Dictionary* (1993) has two definitions of "vocation." The first is, "A regular occupation, especially one for which a person is particularly suited or qualified." The second is, "An inclination as if in response to a summons to undertake a certain kind of work, especially a religious career; a calling (Middle English *vocacioun*, Divine call to a Religious life, from old French *vocation*, from Latin *vocātiō*, vocation—Calling, from *vocatus* past participle of *vocāre* to call."I believe Osler, a minister's son, would have preferred the second definition. He went on to say: "I wish there were another term to designate the wide field of medical practice which remains after the separation of surgery, midwifery, and gynecology. Not itself a specialty (though it embraces at least half a dozen), its cultivators cannot be called specialists, but bear without reproach the good old name physician, in contradistinction to general practitioners, surgeons, obstetricians and gynecologists." Now, nearly one hundred years later, the physician is called a "provider" by our politicians and bureaucrats and is swallowed into the maw of chiropractors, general practitioners, family practitioners, nurse practitioners, and physicians' assistants. Even worse, he is treated as a tradesman and businessman and subjected to antitrust control that might be better directed to those who make the laws, especially the lawyers. Returning to Osler: "I have heard the fear expressed that in this country the sphere of the physician proper is becoming more and more restricted and perhaps this is true but I maintain (and I hope to convince you) that the opportunities are still great, that the harvest is plenteous and the laborers scarcely sufficient to meet the demand. At the outset I would like to emphasize the fact that the student of internal medicine cannot be a specialist. The manifestation of almost any one of the important diseases in the course of a few years will box the compass of the specialties—know syphilis in all its manifestations and relations and all other things clinical will be added unto you." Osler then put his finger on one of the major weaknesses of postgraduate medical education of his day. "Each generation has to grow its own consultants. Hosack, Samuel Mitchell, Swett, Alonzo Clark, Austin Flint, Fordyce Barker and Alfred Loomis, served their day in this city, and then passed on into silence. Their works remain; but enough of a great physician's experience dies with him to justify the saying 'There is no wisdom in the grave.'" To correct this weakness in the system of medical education of that day, Osler pioneered at Johns Hopkins with his residency program, ensuring that wisdom and experience would be passed on to others. He also warns, in this essay, against "the besetting sin of the young physician, chauvinism, that intolerant attitude of mind, which brooks no regard for anything outside his own circle and his own school. If he cannot go abroad let him spend part of his short vacations in seeing how it fares with the brethren in his own country. Even a New Yorker could learn something in the Massachusetts General and Boston City Hospitals— The all-important matter is to get breadth of view as early as possible, and this is difficult without travel." In the current era, I would add to Osler's advice to New York City's physicians that they visit and communicate with their peers in the many university medical centers of this city and not confine their experience and professional relationships solely to one institution, for this can lead to chauvinism at its very worst. The people of this great city and its visitors should have available to them access to the best clinicians and institutions in the world. All it takes is a knowledgeable clinician who can put his finger on these resources and harness them in the service of his patients, without regard to whether it is at his own hospital or someone else's!

Osler continues to map out the course the budding young internist should pursue following graduation. If he has shown any signs of promise during his student and hospital days, "a dispensary assistantship should be available; anything should be acceptable which brings him into contact with patients. By all means, if possible, let him be a pluralist, and—as he values his future life—let him not get early entangled in the meshes of specialism."

Later in the lecture, Osler says: "A young fellow with staying powers who avoids entanglements may look forward in twenty years to a good consulting practice in any town of 40,000 to 50,000 inhabitants. Some such man, perhaps in a town far distant, taking care of his education and not his bank book may be the Austin Flint of New York in 1930." How would the intervening time be spent? Osler advised years of work in the outpatient clinics or dispensaries of the day, spent with ambulatory patients. "Poll the successful consulting physicians of this country today, and you will find they have been evolved either from general practice or from laboratory and clinical work; many of the most prominent having risen from the ranks of general practitioners. . . . But I wish to speak here of the training of men who start with the object of becoming pure physicians. From the vantage ground of more than forty years of hard work, Sir Andrew Clark told me that he had striven ten years for bread, ten years for bread and but-ter, and twenty years for cakes and ale and this really is a very good partition of the life of the student of internal medicine, some at least, since all do not reach the last stage. . . . [A] few words in addition about this dry-bread decade. He should stick closely to the dispen-saries. A first-class reputation may be built up in them. —Many of the best-known men in London serve ten, fifteen or even twenty years in the outpatient departments before getting wards. During this period let him not lose the substance of ultimate success in grasping at the shadow of present opportunities. Time is now his money, and he must not barter away too much of it in profitless work—profitless so far as his education is concerned, though it may mean ready cash."

I was not aware of this superb essay of Osler's early in my career, but I can attest to the wisdom of his advice to young internists and regret that it has been neglected in recent times to the detriment of internal medicine as a vocation. I worked diligently and faithfully in the Vanderbilt Clinic without pay for twenty-five years. I was fussier about being on time for my clinics than I was for my private patients. Not infrequently, my clinic duties took so much of my energy and time that I was not available for private patients. I knew this was the price I had to pay for advancing my career and education. In the clin-ic, I had to see patients with common complaints and ailments as well as the "interesting cases." Long-term follow-up of people with chron-ic ailments provided me with a grasp of medical practice that could not be obtained in any other way. While Osler justly became famous as the physician who revolutionized American medical education by bringing medical students to the bedside in the wards, he should be equally revered for his emphasis on the use of ambulatory patients in the outpatient clinics and dispensaries in the education and training of the general internist. Unfortunately, the new leaders of American medical education became more and more enamored with hospital medicine than ambulatory and primary care, leading to the neglect of the latter. Medical students were exposed to rare and esoteric diseases that they would seldom see in daily practice and failed to see com-monplace problems encountered by most physicians in the outside world. Osler's methods for educating and training the general internist were superseded by excessive emphasis on the production of narrow-gauged subspecialists to the degree that teams and committees are now needed to care for patients who in earlier days were managed by one well-trained general internist.

Osler continues: "I would like to add here a few words on the question of clinical instruction as with the great prospective increase of it in our schools there will be many chances of employment for young physicians who wish to follow medicine as a vocation. Today this serious problem confronts the professors in many of our schools—how to teach practical medicine to the large classes; how to give them practical and systematic ward instruction? I know of no teacher in the country who controls enough clinical material for the instruction of classes say of 200 men during the third and fourth years. It seems to me that there are two plans open to the schools. The first is to utilize dispensaries for clinical instruction much more than is at present the rule. For this purpose a teaching room for a class of twenty-five or thirty students immediately adjoining the dispensary is essential. For instruction in physical diagnosis, for the objective teaching of disease, and for the instruction of students in the use of their senses, such an arrangement is invaluable. There are hundreds of dispensaries in which this plan is feasible, and in which the material now is not properly worked up because of the lack of this very stimulus." In a second proposal to improve teaching in internal medicine, Osler recommends that a system of "extramural" teachers be developed along the lines of the very successful one in Edinburgh that provides employment for a large number of younger men. "If we ever are to give our third- and fourth-year students practical and complete courses in physical diagnosis and clinical medicine, extending throughout the session, and not in classes of a brief period of six weeks duration, I am confident that the number of men engaged in teaching must be greatly increased."

"Ten years' hard work tells with colleagues and friends in the profession and with enlarged clinical facilities the physician enters upon the second, or bread-and-butter period. This, to most men, is the great trial, since the risks are greater, and many drop out of the race, wearied at the length of the way and drift into specialism or general practice. The physician develops more slowly than the surgeon and success comes later. There are surgeons at forty years in full practice and at the very top of the wave, a time at which the physician is only preparing to reap the harvest of years of patient toil. The surgeon must have hands, and better, young hands. He should have a head, too, but this does not seem so essential to success, and he cannot have an old head with young hands. At the end of twenty years, when about forty-five, our physician should have a first-class reputation in the profession, and a large circle of friends and students. He will probably have precious little capital in the bank, but a very large accumulation of interest-bearing funds in his brain-pan. He has gathered a stock of special knowledge which his friends in the profession appreciate, and they begin to seek his counsel in doubtful cases, and gradually learn to lean upon him in times of trial. He may awake some day, perhaps quite suddenly, to find that twenty years of quiet work, done for the love of it, has a very solid value." A final pearl from Osler: "The environment of a large city is not essential to the growth of a good clinical physician. Even in small towns a man can, if he has it in him, become well versed in methods of work and with the assistance of an occasional visit to some medical center he can become an expert diagnostician and reach a position of dignity and worth in the community in which he lives. I wish to plead particularly for the wasted opportunities in the small hospitals of our large cities, and in those of more moderate size. There are in this State a score or more of hospitals with from thirty to fifty medical beds offering splendid material for good men on which to build reputations." This was the situation in internal medicine one hundred years ago as depicted by the greatest physician of modern times. His plea was for the preservation of the general internist or physician. He did not describe it as an easy way of life. He asked for commitment and sacrifice that most of the contemporary doctors are simply unwilling to make. Many have told me that Osler was asking far too much of doctors, who are after all only human. Nevertheless, following Osler's lead a significant number of his pupils followed his example and brought distinction, honor, and high achievement to the field of internal medicine. Many of his disciples were associated with him as students, colleagues, and collaborators. They were called Oslerians and their lives have brought great honor to American medicine as well as international renown.

I was fortunate to have one of Osler's disciples as my first professor of medicine. He was William Sharp McCann of Johns Hopkins, who was selected in 1925 by founding Dean George Hoyt Whipple to become the first chairman of the department of medicine at the new medical school in Rochester, New York. Dr. McCann was graduated in 1915 from Cornell University Medical College, where he became a highly regarded protégé of Professor of Physiology Graham Lusk. Dr. McCann, interested in biochemical and physiological aspects of medicine, was planning to intern in medicine until the day that Dr. Lusk told him that Dr. Harvey Cushing had asked him to recommend one of his students for an internship on his surgical service. Lusk was honored by this tribute and McCann was thrilled. He traveled to Boston's Peter Bent Brigham Hospital, took the day-long written examination followed by an examination of a patient with a diagnostic problem.

He did well in both phases of the examinations and was accepted as an intern on Dr. Cushing's service. He was happy to work under a surgeon. Years later he would say in his memoirs that, "Had I been left to my own devices I would have sought appointment to a medical service but the opportunity to work with Dr. Cushing ensured a good experience in neurological diagnosis and an excellent introduction to the general field of endocrinology which was beginning to develop rapidly under his aegis. In many ways Dr. Cushing could be regarded as an internist who operated."[1] Cushing was an Oslerian who had been greatly influenced by Sir William during his years as a teacher at Johns Hopkins.

It was Harvey Cushing who was summoned, while on active duty in France in WW I, to the battlefront where Revere Osler, the only child of Sir William and Lady Grace Osler, lay wounded, only to find that nothing more could be done. Revere died on 30 August 1917. It gave Revere's parents solace to know that Dr. William Darrach and Dr. Brewer of the Presbyterian Hospital unit did what they could and were joined by Harvey Cushing in their efforts to help Revere. This grievous loss almost broke Sir William's heart and many, including Lady Osler, believed that he never really recovered from the blow. Osler died of bronchopneumonia and empyema with hemorrhage at 4:30 P.M. on 29 December 1919, at the age of seventy. John F. Fulton, in his excellent biography of Harvey Cushing,[2] provides us with additional information on how it happened that Harvey Cushing was asked to write the Osler biography: "Lady Osler first thought that William S. Thayer, one of Osler's successors in the Chair of medicine at the Hopkins, was the logical person to write the Life, but as soon as she received the Boston Evening Transcript (3 January 1920) and read H.C.'s 'Sir William Osler: The Man', she was convinced that he was the only one to be entrusted with it."

The appreciation began:

> In the first shock of grief at the news of Sir William Osler's death, it is difficult for anyone who felt close to him to say what is in his heart. And the strange thing about this unusually gifted and versatile man is that everyone fortunate enough to have been brought in contact with him shares in this feeling of devotion, for he gave of himself much to all. This was true of his patients as might be expected, and he was sought far and wide not only because of his wide knowledge of medicine and great wisdom,

---

1. *William S. McCann—Memoir.* (Rochester, N.Y.: University of Rochester School of Medicine Archives, 1966), p. 81.

2. John F. Fulton, *Harvey Cushing: A Biography* (Springfield, Ill.: Charles C. Thomas, 1946), pp. 457–458.

but because of his generosity, sympathy and great personal charm. It was true also—and this is more rare—of the members of his profession for whom, high or low he showed a spirit of brotherly helpfulness untinctured by those petty jealousies which sometimes mar their relationships. "Never believe what a patient may tell you to the detriment of another physician—even though you may fear it is true" was one of his sayings to students and he was preeminently the physician to physicians and their families, and would go out of his way unsolicited and unsparingly to help them when he learned they were ill or in distress of any kind— .

Cushing continued: "So Lady Osler promptly put the direct question: Sir William left no autobiography—There is one vital question—who shall write the memoir. I know of only one man worthy and able to do it and that is you and printed by the Oxford Press—I can say no more. I leave the answer to you. There is no one here who knows everything—medicine, brain, home, friends, heart, endurance, in fact all that he was—you know all" (20 February 1920). "Clearly this was a request which H.C. could not decline. Osler had meant everything to him for twenty years. He had been a spiritual father and had had a keener understanding of Cushing's own restless nature than almost anyone, and had done much to inculcate in H.C. his love of literature and history and his undying interest in Vesalius. So Cushing, who was frantically eager to get back to his clinic after nearly four years' interruption of war, committed himself to the formidable undertaking, and it proved much more so than he had surmised." The result was Cushing's monumental Pulitzer Prize-winning two-volume, 1413-page *The Life of Sir William Osler*, published in 1925 by the Oxford Press with this dedication:

> TO MEDICAL STUDENTS IN THE HOPE THAT SOME-
> THING OF OSLER'S SPIRIT MAY BE CONVEYED TO
> THOSE OF A GENERATION THAT HAS NOT KNOWN
> HIM, AND PARTICULARLY TO THOSE IN AMERICA,
> LEST IT BE FORGOTTEN WHO IT WAS THAT MADE IT
> POSSIBLE FOR THEM TO WORK AT THE BEDSIDE IN
> THE WARDS

Harvey Cushing, the father of modern neurosurgery, bibliophile, historian, and disciple of Sir William Osler became Dr. McCann's chief in 1916 at the Peter Bent Brigham Hospital where the stamp of an Oslerian was placed upon the young intern that would guide him in his exciting career as a clinician and teacher of medicine and ultimately to the chairmanship of medicine in a new medical school that would rival Johns Hopkins. Before this would happen McCann would go to war (WW I) and return to Cornell, this time under the aegis of Eugene Dubois, then selected to succeed Walter W. Palmer as head of the metabolic and chemical division in medicine at Johns Hopkins, where he would imbibe more of the Osler mystique from the medical staff. Finally at age thirty-five in 1925 he was chosen by Dean George H. Whipple to become the first chairman of medicine at the brand-new University of Rochester School of Medicine in Rochester, New York, called by many the Johns Hopkins of New York. He had learned a great deal from his three years at Hopkins. He had seen the advantages and disadvantages of the full-time system so aggressively promoted by Abraham Flexner. From what he learned at Hopkins, he was convinced that the department of medicine should be well balanced, including salaried and full-time men and outstanding clinicians with private practices and some on so-called geographic arrangements allowing for flexibility in management. He believed that instead of having the third-year medical students assigned to the outpatient clinic, they should be assigned as clinical clerks to the wards, where there was ample time to take histories, repeat physical examinations, and carefully observe sick patients. In the fourth year, the students would be better qualified to examine outpatients under the time limits imposed by the conditions of work in the clinic. At Johns Hopkins, the senior students were assigned as clinical clerks on the wards, the opposite of Dr. McCann's deployment at Rochester. Most important was Dr. McCann's Oslerian approach to the teaching of medicine at the bedside.

When Dr. McCann began his thirty-three-year tenure as the chairman of medicine at Rochester, he made another key decision. "At the onset it was decided that the head of the department of medicine could not afford to be a specialist. A rounded, well-balanced program devoted to the best interests of patients and of medical students would preclude such specialization on the part of the Professor. As the clinic got underway, an effort was made to develop semispecialists within the broad field of internal medicine among the associate and assistant professors; yet care was taken to see that each of these men was given periods of clinical responsibility of the broadest and most varied nature possible, in order to keep him from being overspecialized in practice even though his researches might follow a narrower field of activity."[3]

---

3. William S. McCann, *The Quarter Century: 1925–1950* (School of Medicine and Dentistry, The University of Rochester), p. 77.

Dr. McCann remained faithful to his commitment to general internal medicine and was an outstanding teacher at the bedside and in the amphitheater. He encouraged his most able men to explore their interests in various subspecialties but insisted that they remain firmly based in general internal medicine. He himself had a number of hobbies in internal medicine, including an interest in pulmonary disease and pneumoconiosis or silicosis. He was an excellent biochemist and enjoyed applying biochemical and physiological concepts to the understanding of clinical disease or malaise. He had a grasp of psychosomatic factors in disease unusual for that period and applied these concepts with eloquence to the understanding of diseases such as peptic ulcer. His knowledge of renal physiology and metabolic disorders was extensive. He had pioneered in the dietary treatment of diabetes and had developed a special diet that helped keep diabetics alive when supplies of potent insulin were difficult to obtain. While at Hopkins, he wrote the chapter on "Pernicious Anemia" in Cecil's *Textbook of Medicine* and might have solved the mystery of the cause of that disease if his patients had cooperated by eating the large amounts of liver needed each day to provide what was later determined to be Vitamin B-12. He took a special interest in his students and kept in touch with them in many ways as they progressed in their careers. I received letters of encouragement, patient referrals, and nice tokens of friendship from this marvelous human being. He repeatedly told me and some friends that I was the best clinician he had ever taught, and I treasure a letter in which he called me a truly great physician, the ultimate accolade from the man who taught me how to walk. I remember when I last visited him in Strong Memorial Hospital when in his eighties he was dying of carcinoma of the colon. I knew I would never see him again and I had all I could do to keep back my tears, but we had a pleasant visit.

He may have had some reservations about my emergence as a gastroenterologist, but I reassured him that I would always be a general internist with my hobby of gastroenterology. I had kept the faith instilled in me by my superb teacher and I know he was pleased with this.

In my book, *Death of the Clinician: Requiem or Reveille?*, I pay further tribute to Dr. McCann. He was the leader of the clinicians at the University of Rochester who opposed the full-time scheme that Abraham Flexner espoused so aggressively in the early days of the school. In the book, I document the bitterness of Abraham Flexner, who resisted to the very end the modification of the full-time system eventually adopted by the clinicians of the medical school. The modification that was worked out was a form used at Harvard Medical School, where the clinicians were allowed to keep the fees collected from private patients. Dr. McCann spearheaded this change, which corrected a serious flaw in the plan promoted so vigorously and unsuccessfully by Abraham Flexner.

Dr. McCann started to write his memoir in 1964 and completed it to 1966, when his terminal illness intervened. He had reached the point in his autobiography where he was appointed professor and chairman of medicine at Rochester in 1925. So, because of illness he was unable to discuss the events of the thirty-three years that followed his designation as the Dewey professor of medicine.

In his closing remarks in his memoir, Dr. McCann made this prescient comment:

> My purpose in preparing these memoirs has been to review the development of an internist and a teacher of internists, and to describe the professional background from which he grew. Thus we can see the seed, the plant, and the soil in one comprehensive glance. The problems of the patient who is ill are essentially the same throughout history. Man himself has changed but little, his illness is always a manifestation of his struggle to adapt to the changes in the world around him. The function of his physician is to understand the nature of the patient's difficulty well enough to be able to assist him wisely in making a successful adaptation. Medical education must prepare him for this task, so that he will know the internal environment of man's body and the mechanisms for maintaining successfully the life of its component cells. It must also give him understanding of the external environment in all its aspects so that he will know where and how its stresses impinge on the struggling individual who comes to him as a patient seeking help. The medical schools were reasonably close to meeting the requirements of progressive science and technology up to the period of World War II. At that point the unlocking of the secrets of atomic energy accelerated changes in the environment so rapidly that the schools have been thrown into a state of confusion. Instead of broad growth of knowledge in people who can "grasp this sorry scheme of things entire" they have proliferated specialization in ever-narrowing fields. The internist at his highest period of development was a *generalist* skilled in the perception of the overall nature of the patient's problem. His numbers are dwindling as specialists increase. Some day the schools will have to recreate him if the medical profession is to attain its ancient role of properly caring for its patients. It will then be necessary to study the successful patterns of the past in order to create them anew.

Chapter 29

❧

The Upjohn Service Moves to St. Vincent's Hospital

T HE DECISION TO LEAVE ROOSEVELT HOSPITAL was approved by
Mrs. Stearns, and she continued to be very supportive despite
the disappointment over the unpleasant experience we had
been through. The search for a new location for the Upjohn Service
considered a variety of options ranging from setting up of an independent Institute of Gastroenterology to less ambitious plans. We
were committed to placing the unit in an academic setting with excellent teaching facilities. We looked at several hospitals and several medical schools that were interested in our proposal. While going through
these negotiations, I received a call from Dr. William J. Grace, director of medicine at St. Vincent's Hospital and Medical Center, who
said he had learned I was leaving Roosevelt and would like to invite
me to come to St. Vincent's as chief of gastroenterology. He came to
see me in my office at 550 Park Avenue. We had a warm and productive session that he initiated by saying, "I'm not interested in the
Upjohn money. I have come to see you because I would like you to
take over the position of chief of gastroenterology." When I asked
him who held the position, he said he did, and went on to say that he
was leaving gastroenterology for cardiology. I liked his approach and
asked a number of relevant questions including the arrangement for
office space, clinic space, and a research laboratory. He said that start-
up space would be made available for me and the future would
depend upon my success in promoting the unit. We spoke about the
university affiliation and he said his own academic appointment was
with New York University School of Medicine, with which St.
Vincent's had been affiliated for some years. He indicated that a significant appointment at the medical school could be arranged.

I believe that Dr. Louis M. ("Pete") Rousselot, the dynamic master surgeon who was director of surgery at St. Vincent's Hospital, may
have suggested to Dr. Grace that he try to persuade me to come to St.
Vincent's. Pete and I were old friends from Columbia-Presbyterian,
where he had trained under Dr. Allen O. Whipple and was regarded
as the best surgeon of his many pupils. Dr. Rousselot had, several
years before, tried to attract me to St. Vincent's as chief of medicine
but I turned him down.

Knowing that "Peter" Rousselot was in charge of surgery at St. Vincent's was a major factor in influencing me to seriously consider Dr. Grace's offer. Dr. Grace came to me at an interesting point in our search for a new site for the Upjohn Service. I had been approached by Dr. Arthur Localio, the great abdominal surgeon at NYU who had been a schoolmate of mine at the University of Rochester School of Medicine, Class of 1936, two years behind me. Arthur remembered me warmly as a student role model that he admired and often expressed gratitude for my encouraging him to pursue research and teaching. This he did to an extraordinary degree, becoming, I believe, the finest abdominal surgeon Rochester has ever produced. Arthur wanted me to join the NYU faculty and arranged a private dinner in his Beekman Street apartment with Dr. Lewis Thomas, then Dean and professor of medicine. The main purpose of the meeting was to discuss my faculty appointment and where to house the Upjohn unit if we decided to affiliate. It was a very pleasant occasion, for I greatly admired Dr. Thomas's extraordinary achievements and appreciated his comments and suggestions. The faculty appointment was no problem. Space for the Upjohn was a serious problem. There was none available in the brand-new University Hospital. Space in old Bellevue could be had, but I turned that down as unsatisfactory for a variety of reasons. New Bellevue was suggested but at the time, it looked as if it would never be built and was at least five to ten years in the offing. My time frame made this out of the question. Welfare Island was suggested and dropped like a hot potato. I knew I had to have office space and laboratory and clinic space in order to get the Upjohn going again but it was abundantly clear that suitable space was not available at NYU After my dinner at Arthur Localio's, I spoke with him and asked him what Dr. Thomas had thought of my proposal. Arthur said that Dr. Thomas told him that "Mike Lepore had made an excellent impression—but feared that he might turn out to be another Howard Rusk!" I admired Dr. Rusk greatly and took this as the compliment it was not intended to be. The timing of Dr. Grace's interview was ideal, for I could now see a possible solution to my space problems. This was to accept the position at St. Vincent's as chief of gastroenterology, have my academic appointment at NYU and attending positions with admitting privileges at NY University Hospital, Bellevue, and St. Vincent's Hospital.

I saw the potential for this arrangement to provide me and the Upjohn Service with the best of two worlds. If my patients objected to being in a Catholic hospital, they had the option of being admitted to a modern air-conditioned, brand-new non-sectarian hospital, the newest in the city. I sensed also that I would be freer to innovate and advance clinical gastroenterology at St. Vincent's Hospital, where the need for a section of gastroenterology had already been recognized and implemented. My impression was that at the time NYU, with the possible exception of cardiology, was simply not committed to the subspecialties in medicine. For these reasons, I accepted the offer from St. Vincent's Hospital.

In 1966 I started my work at that institution. I had kept Mrs. Stearns apprised of my negotiations and had her encouragement and approval to proceed with the necessary arrangements.

My first major mission at St. Vincent's Hospital was to find space for a suite for gastrointestinal endoscopy. This was not easy but I finally succeeded due largely to the cooperation of Sister Marian Catherine Muldoon, who was the head of the St. Vincent's Hospital School of Nursing. She had control of a large room in the Seton ward building that housed four to six patients and had originally been a classroom for the nursing school. Funds for equipping an endoscopy unit had been donated to me by the Borea family, from New Jersey, whose mother had been spared from an unnecessary operation for a bleeding ulcer by my intervention as a consultant. The Borea family was becoming impatient because we had accepted the donation but had not yet built the room. I explained all of this to Sister Catherine, who recognized the position I was in and decided to let me have the room for this purpose. Sister Anthony Marie Fitzmaurice, the chief administrator, was happy that the room was in the ward building where it would serve the poor as well as those better-off. No mention was ever made by the administration that they would be losing the income from four to six patients each day by converting the room to an endoscopy suite. A subcontractor was hired to implement our plans under the eagle eye of Miss Martha Swensson, who could make a dollar go a long way and who had a flare for redesigning and architecture.

When the subcontractor asked, in his smart-alecky way, whether we wanted a Cadillac or Chevrolet type of room, our answer was that we wanted good sturdy materials without any frills. We were able to get volunteers to donate time and skills for developing several innovative devices we were installing for cleaning and storing our expensive endoscopes. The room was also equipped with x-ray viewing boxes and other audiovisual equipment for showing movies of the endoscopic procedures. The room was large enough to accommodate small classes of students, house staff, nurses, and attending staff, and it was nicely air-conditioned, making it attractive for staff and interns. This room proved to be a key resource for our teaching and training program in gastroenterology and was well worth the investment made in it.

I inherited the existing staff members in gastroenterology at St. Vincent's Hospital and provided them with every opportunity to advance themselves and to improve their skills in endoscopy and GI diagnosis. It did not take me long to find that I had a rising star in GI endoscopy in the person of Dr. Charles Bonanno of our attending staff, and I encouraged him because it was evident that he had excellent endoscopic skills. I saw, early on, that GI bleeding merited a vigorous around-the-clock diagnostic approach. For this, I quickly organized a GI bleeding team on twenty-four-hour call. This was also a great way to teach endoscopy to our Upjohn fellows. The attendings all volunteered to provide their services on the GI bleeding team without charge. While I realized that there would be substantial financial rewards from endoscopic procedures, I turned this special area over to other members of my staff while I was free to pursue puzzling diagnoses, the enigmas of inflammatory bowel disease, diseases of the pancreas, immunologic disorders, vascular malformations, and diseases of malabsorption, including sprue and celiac disease. Later, fulminant liver failure, viral hepatitis, cirrhosis, and the clinical application of plasmapheresis would attract my attention. My research was patient- and case-oriented, responding to the challenges posed by diseases threatening life and previously believed to be untreatable. My teaching at the bedside remains to this day the essence of my performance as a medical educator in the Oslerian tradition.

I would like to be remembered as a clinician who brought his students to the bedside in an era when this Oslerian form of teaching was becoming unpopular and being neglected in many large academic centers. The GI bleeding team proved to be a major contribution to the management of severe GI bleeding at this medical center. We were among the first to subject all patients with major GI hemorrhage to emergency endoscopy. By our definition, this was endoscopy as soon as the patient's general condition had been stabilized, not twenty-four or forty-eight hours later. The most serious condition with the highest mortality in our series was bleeding due to esophageal varices in patients with cirrhosis of the liver and portal hypertension. It would be many years before methods using sclerosing agents, lasers, or electrocoagulation were developed to successfully control variceal bleeding and reduce the mortality. Localizing the source of bleeding was a definite aid in decision-making by surgeons who were usually in charge of the management of these patients. It was at St. Vincent's Hospital where I found a considerable interest in solving the problem of GI bleeding in the person of Dr. Louis W. Rousselot, the chief surgeon, who was a great expert and pioneer in performing portacaval shunts. One of his protégés, Dr. Francis Ruzicka, director of radiology, was an early pioneer in New York in the application of selective visceral angiography to localizing more distal sites of bleeding in the small and large bowel. He had on his staff a young radiologist with great skills in performing visceral angiography, Dr. Plinio Rossi, who is now a renowned specialist in interventional radiology, working in Rome, Italy. With these energetic and skillful men, our GI service was soon able to detect previously undiagnosed neoplasms, vascular mal- formations, and other lesions of the small bowel and large bowel. If surgery were needed for GI bleeding, it would no longer be a blind date with an undetermined source. Many lives were saved because of these advances.

The program in gastroenterology at St. Vincent's Hospital rapidly became one of its major strengths. The GI bleeding team and our aggressive diagnostic approach to major bleeding from the digestive tract served to bring together the medical and surgical services and attracted patients from far and near. I have always felt that the patient is best served when medical specialists and surgeons work as a team, and I have never understood why in so many major institutions the two services may act as if they were mortal enemies rather than col- laborators. Ignorance of their respective techniques and a lack of communication are responsible for most of this attitude, which is clearly not in the best interest of our patients. Part of the difficulty is that many medical men and women seldom enter an operating room to observe what is being done to their patients. In the early days of surgery, the operating room was in a large amphitheater with students and referring physicians in the audience. With time and the ever-pres- ent fear of cross-infection, the operating theaters gradually dimin- ished in importance and finally, in most places, disappeared entirely. My friend, Owen Wangensteen, described this phenomenon in con- siderable detail in his superb chapter on "The Surgical Amphitheater" in his monograph, *The Rise of Surgery*,[1] describing the decline in facili- ties for observing operations in modern hospitals that provide piano music in their lobbies and flower shops and snack bars and fail to pro- vide adequate space for teaching and educational activities.

As a non-surgeon, I believe I have spent more time in operating rooms observing operations than some surgeons. How does one account for the decline and, in fact, disappearance of viewing facili- ties in the operating rooms of our modern hospitals. Wangensteen says it occurred because the doctors ceased to attend, leaving the gal- leries empty. I have always felt that, whenever possible, the attending

---

1. Owen H. Wangensteen and Sara D. Wangensteen, *The Rise of Surgery: From Empiric Craft to Scientific Discipline* (Minneapolis: University Minnesota Press, 1978), pp. 453–473.

physician who recommends an operation should make every effort to be present in person for at least part of the surgery being performed on his patient. This is the best way to keep abreast of the skill of the surgeon, the anesthesiologist, the resident staff, and the demeanor in the operating room. Here it is that you see whether it is the resident or the attending surgeon who does the operation. What are the pitfalls that may convert a fairly simple procedure into a life-threatening disaster? Where else can the referring doctor see whether the surgeon is in full command or perhaps beginning to lose his skills?

Are hemostasis and gentle handling of tissues up to par or neglected, leading to unnecessary blood transfusions and complications? Above all, most doctors who advise patients to have surgical procedures should witness their performance to keep abreast of developments and to see and never forget what their patients are going through. My plea, based upon my experience of more than fifty-five years in medical practice, is to restore the viewing areas in the operating rooms, albeit on a limited scale, with ease of access, without requiring disrobing to gain access, and with modern audiovisual facilities and precautions to prevent contamination of the operating room. I would go a point farther. In this day and era of modern communications technology, every teaching hospital should have the capacity to televise operations and other procedures on closed circuit to classrooms and selected private offices in the hospital. With a flick of the remote control, the referring doctor and others can have a view of the action in the operating room similar to that of a professional football or baseball game and at no great expense. My wish is that the next time on Teaching Rounds when I ask a medical intern or resident a favorite question, "When were you last in the operating room?," the answer will be "This morning." There is at least one caveat. When Dr. Louis M. Rousselot, the dynamic master surgeon-in-chief at St. Vincent's Hospital and Medical Center, installed a closed-circuit television in 1960 into one of the tenth-floor operating rooms, in the Smith-Raskob Pavilion with an outlet in his first floor office, he was accused by some members of his staff of spying upon them while they were operating, leading him to soft-pedal this innovation.

My teaching program in gastroenterology at St. Vincent's Hospital stressed Osler's "natural method" of teaching at the bedside on daily rounds. The weekly GI Conference held each Tuesday at noon in the Cronin 10 Auditorium was by far the most popular and best-attended medical conference in the medical center. The format was centered about two case presentations by the house staff and Upjohn fellows selected from current patients on the wards, private and semiprivate services of the hospital. These were never didactic lectures from a book. They were live, spontaneous presentations with ample opportunity for questions and answers from those attending.

Participation by radiologists, pathologists, and even surgeons was sought and welcomed. The medical students, chiefly from NYU, were welcome and seemed most eager to learn more about gastroenterology. In addition to our main weekly conference, I started a weekly combined GI Pathology Conference to review the current biopsies and surgical pathology of the week. Once monthly a distinguished visiting professor was invited to lecture on a topic of current interest. The support for this was provided by funds made available to me through private philanthropy. In retrospect, the list of visiting lecturers looks like a Who's Who in American Gastroenterology and Medicine. A sample of the participants is presented to demonstrate their high caliber and diverse interests: Dr. René Dubos, Dr. Saul J. Farber, Dr. Thomas Hendrix, Dr. Thomas B. Tomasi, Jr., Dr. Nicholas C. Hightower, Dr. Carroll M. Leevey, Dr. Thomas Chalmers. I was asked to conduct rounds in surgery and was appointed an attending in the surgical service in addition to my assignments on the medical service. Dr. Rousselot used to say that I was an internist who should have been a surgeon and I in turn, said he was a surgeon worthy of being a physician. One of the saddest and most touching experiences of my life was to participate in the 1974 memorial service of "Pete" Rousselot after his sudden and unexpected death. The memorial mass in the Hospital Chapel was beautifully conducted. The music by the Musica Sacra was provided by Dr. Eduardo Gonzalez, dear friend and former resident of Dr. Rousselot. The mass was filled to capacity with Pete's colleagues, friends and admirers from all walks of life and all of the major hospitals of New York. The Columbia-Presbyterian contingent was especially prominent. The Sisters of Charity, headed by our beloved Mother Loretto Bernard, were well represented. Many of Dr. Rousselot's residents and former students attended. A poignant eulogy was delivered by General Leonard D. Heaton the Surgeon General, United States Army and a close friend who praised Dr. Rousselot and announced how pleased he was that one of Pete's last great accomplishments was in succeeding, with Congressman Hebert, in establishing a new medical school for the Armed Forces. I had the pleasure of saying a few words of praise for the life of Dr. Rousselot and presented a beautiful custom-designed leather-bound complete set of "Pete's" published papers to Mrs. Rousselot as a gift from the Lepore Memorial Fund of St. Vincent's Hospital and Medical Center. Dr. Rousselot was not only a master surgeon, he was a devout practicing Roman Catholic whose ambition it was to make St. Vincent's a great Catholic Medical Center worthy of being the Flagship of Fleet of the Archdiocesan Hospital System of New York. May he rest in Peace!

Word of my vigorous and innovative program in gastroenterology was soon common knowledge at the New York University School of Medicine and at the other New York schools. Medical students came to us for electives and it was not long before further recognition came to us. In 1966 Dr. Saul J. Farber succeeded Dr. Lewis Thomas as chairman of the department of medicine at NYU. He appointed me associate professor of clinical medicine and associate attending in medicine at University Hospital and Bellevue and in 1968 promoted me to professor of clinical medicine and full attending at University Hospital and Bellevue. Dr. Localio continued to encourage my teaching and research, and together we revitalized the teaching program in gastroenterology at University Hospital through a biweekly combined Surgical and Medical Conference in Gastroenterology. In addition, I was admitting some very interesting patients to University Hospital, where I was able to enlist Dr. Localio's expert skills and experience in abdominal surgery for the benefit of my patients.

One of the most interesting patients I shared with Dr. Localio was a seventy-two-year-old Greenwich Village dowager that I first saw in consultation on 30 April 1975 in St. Vincent's Hospital at the request of her physician because of uncontrollable nocturnal and daytime profuse foul watery diarrhea that became progressively worse, necessitating admission to Roosevelt Hospital where she underwent many studies that failed to identify the cause of her illness. Shortly after her admission to St. Vincent's Hospital in 1975 by one of her physicians, Dr. Robert R. Morgan, I was called to see her. One of my cardinal tenets is that nocturnal diarrhea is always significant and cannot be of psychogenic origin. This sustained me in relentlessly pursuing this woman's problem. She was a very demanding and rather imperious woman of some wealth and considerable independence and had, over the years, seen many doctors for a variety of ailments. A four-pack-a-day smoker, and a reformed alcoholic, she could be charming at times and irritating at others. I have seldom seen a patient with severe diarrhea that I could not diagnose, especially one with nocturnal diarrhea. I instituted a thorough and intensive workup that I was able to persuade the patient to accept. We quickly ruled out the usual causes for severe diarrhea. Her stool volumes were enormous, exceeding 2.4 liters per 24 hours, containing a slight excess of fat and marked increases in potassium and sodium. No enteric pathogens were found and no evidence of inflammatory bowel disease seen. A small-bowel endoscopically obtained biopsy failed to show any evidence of sprue. Her serum potassium levels were repeatedly low, giving the first real clue to the diagnosis. I became convinced that she might have a pancreatic non-beta cell tumor, a Vipoma, secreting a vasoactive peptide capable of causing pancreatic cholera. We proceeded with selective visceral angiography, a procedure done with great skill at St. Vincent's Hospital, where I believe we have, over the years, had the best teams in the city in this field. They demonstrated a definite 1.5–2 cm blush in the tail of the pancreas consistent with a tumor.

At that time, the polypeptide-producing tumors of the pancreas were poorly understood and tests for them were virtually nonexistent. No one in New York City was working in this field, but I located an investigator, Dr. Sami I. Said of the Veterans' Administration Hospital in Dallas, Texas, who had developed a blood test for Vipoma. He agreed to perform this if I could send him frozen blood specimens from the patient. This I did and he reported that the values for VIP were elevated. With this documentation I called Dr. Localio and requested that he admit the patient to University Hospital where we could see her together. There was quite a delay before a bed could be obtained. The waiting list at University Hospital was very long, making it extremely difficult to cope with the demands of my active practice. Without the ease of access to beds at St. Vincent's, I would have been at a loss to maintain the high standards of medical practice demanded by my wonderful patients. Eventually the patient was admitted to Dr. Localio's service where I also saw her every day. Again, a problem arose because of the long waiting list for operating time at University Hospital. They chose to repeat the arteriogram at University Hospital, where the radiologist was uncertain whether the blush in the tail of the pancreas was significant. This irritated me because I knew that our arteriograms were better than those at University and our radiologist James Chang was better qualified than the one at University.

Days went by awaiting an opening in the operating-room schedule, but in the meantime our dowager patient was becoming impatient. She was always asking questions and expected doctors to spend a good deal of time with her. Dr. Localio, a very busy surgeon, made rounds early in the morning with his team before heading for the operating room, waking some patients up well before breakfast. One morning I received a telephone call from my patient saying she must see me right away for she was planning to leave the hospital. I hurried over and found her quite agitated and upset. Apparently she had voiced a number of complaints about the long wait for the operating room and unsatisfactory nursing care, and she had upset Dr. Localio, who suggested that perhaps she should go elsewhere for her operation. That really hit the fan and led to the patient's telephone call to me. I hurried over and quieted her down, explaining that we were all upset by the long delay in getting to the operating room. Later, I discussed the matter with Dr. Localio and suggested that he pass up his sunrise visits for his afternoon rounds until we could get her to the operating room. Arthur then said, "I'll bet one thousand dollars that I will give to our medical school (Rochester) alumni fund that she doesn't have a Vipoma." My instant reply was, "You're on." You can bet your bottom dollar that I was in the operating room when our patient was scheduled. So were the radiologist and the chief surgical pathologist, Dr. Fred Gorstein. Dr. Localio quickly searched the area of the pancreas and said he could not feel anything abnormal. He explored it further and said he still could not feel a tumor. He then looked at the arteriogram films of the pancreas and again questioned the radiologist, who seemed quite nervous and uncertain about the diagnosis. Arthur, who was playing cat and mouse, then turned to me asking what he should do. I said my understanding was that small Vipomas can be very soft and not palpable, resembling insulinomas. "Then, you think I ought to resect the tail of pancreas?" "Yes, because I believe the radiologic signs are clear and accompanied by high levels of VIP in the plasma, hypokalemia and symptoms of a pancreatic cholera." Of course this is what my friend had long before decided. He proceeded with his usual skill to complete the operation of distal pancreatectomy.

Soon the specimen was out and handed to Dr. Fred Gorstein, the pathologist, who palpated it and could not feel any mass. He then sliced the specimen and sure enough there were two discrete small tumor nodules in the tail, consistent with the diagnosis of a Vipoma. The operation was successful and the patient was quite well until September 1975, when she again developed diarrhea and hypokalemia with markedly elevated plasma levels of VIP. Arteriography demonstrated a 1 cm area of increased vascularity in the head of the pancreas. Her general condition precluded the performance of total pancreatectomy and it was decided to administer chemotherapy that included a course of streptozoticin and 5-FU. She responded well and she remained in remission for the rest of her life, dying in 1981 of causes unrelated to the Vipoma. I believe this was the first Vipoma documented in New York City by positive blood levels of the hormone as well as pancreatic arteriography. Dr. Localio kept his promise by sending his check for one thousand dollars to the University of Rochester Medical Alumni Fund that I requested be added to the Edward F. Adolph Medal Fund for the top medical student of each year in physiology.

One of the most interesting and challenging patients I have ever seen was referred to me on 10 September 1976. She was an attractive single, white, thirty-eight-year-old executive secretary complaining of weight loss of 34 pounds since February 1976, heartburn since May, plus rather severe pain below the left scapula and medial to it, and also epigastric distress and left-upper-quadrant discomfort appearing one hour after meals, unrelieved by antacids. She had developed sitophobia because of distress that followed eating even a small meal. She consulted an internist in early June and a gastrointestinal series and a gallbladder x-ray study were done with normal findings. She was told she was anemic and was prescribed an iron supplement which she stopped after one week because of constipation. In July she was admitted to St. Vincent's Hospital for further study. Stool guaiac tests were persistently negative. Gastric analysis with maximal histalog stimulation revealed a normal capacity for secreting hydrochloric acid. An ERCP (Endoscopic Retrograde Cholangio-Pancreatogram) was done by an expert who demonstrated a normal pancreatogram and reported multiple lesser curvature superficial erosions with surrounding gastritis. One serum gastrin level was high but subsequent ones were within normal limits. Because of her continued weight loss and abdominal pain, her doctors advised her to undergo surgery, a partial gastrectomy. It was at this point that the patient's employer insisted on further consultation and this is when I became involved. The key findings on my examination were marked cachexia in a tall, asthenic woman who was very keen and alert and clearly not a hypochondriac or bulimirexic. The most startling finding was a blowing prolonged systolic bruit localized to the epigastrium. I felt at first sight that this might be due to arterial encasement by carcinoma, primary in the pancreas, but hoped it would be a benign process causing celiac axis compression. I admitted her to my service at St. Vincent's Hospital and proceeded with appropriate studies, including a CAT scan of the pancreas and an ultrasonogram, which were negative. Selective visceral arteriography provided me with the answer, the findings being those of obstruction of the main celiac axis and narrowing of the inferior mesenteric and superior mesenteric arteries. Our radiologist assured me that the stenosis was not due to encasement by tumor but was due to other causes. There was no evidence of atherosclerosis, the aorta being quite normal. There was no evidence or history of periarteritis nodosa, vasculitis, or systemic lupus erythematosus. Repeat gastroscopy showed no erosions or ulcers and was deemed to be within normal limits. My diagnosis was that this patient was suffering with the classical picture of abdominal ischemia secondary to celiac artery compression. I recommended that she be operated upon by a surgeon with considerable experience in this field. Several names were mentioned and the patient selected an excellent one on the Columbia-Presbyterian staff. Arrangements were made to admit her there for the operation. As sometimes happens with surgeons, but should not, this one failed to send me a report and continued to follow the patient without getting in touch with me. My impression was that she was making an excellent recovery from her operation of 27 September 1976, a celiac artery decompression, and had returned to her office duties. I sent a letter to the surgeon at Columbia-Presbyterian on 24 January 1977 formally requesting his operative report. It was not until 27 June 1977 that he sent me his report with an apology for the "unconscionable delay." My next contact with the patient was on 4 May 1977 when I was asked to see her in consultation at Harkness Pavilion, where she had undergone a series of tests, including selective visceral angiography, gastroscopy, GI series, and gastric analysis. She had been told that they had been unable to find anything wrong and recommended that she have psychiatric advice. The patient became quite upset and demanded that they get in touch with me and request me to come in consultation. I responded promptly and spent much time reviewing the entire problem. The epigastric bruit was just as loud and impressive as it had been before the operation. She had failed to gain any weight and looked frail and emaciated at 93 pounds and her recurrent abdominal pain persisted as did her sitophobia. I had my doubts about their angiograms but decided to put this on the back burner for the moment. My interpretation was that the operation had failed to help her and some day she would have to face up to this but not at this point in time. She badly needed good medical follow-up and care with a definite program to improve her nutrition. She did not need a psychiatrist. She needed a solid, supportive friend. To paraphrase Gene Stead of Duke, what this patient needed was a good old-fashioned doctor. I started her on a schedule of frequent small feedings, including a good supplement and vitamins, and I saw her at regular intervals to monitor her progress or lack of it. After several months had gone by, with the pain and bruit no better, I broached the question of getting another opinion from a superb vascular surgeon at University Hospital, Dr. Anthony Imparato. This was arranged and he agreed with me that re-operation was indicated.

She was admitted to University Hospital, where she underwent an extensive abdominal operation on 24 October 1977, which I witnessed. The findings at operation were described by Dr. Imparato as follows:

The splenic artery was stenotic at its origin and the celiac axis artery was extremely thin-walled between the origin of the left gastric and hepatic arteries. There was a dense white structure which surrounded the celiac axis artery, passed over the origin of the left gastric artery, and covered the celiac axis for a distance of one inch which on frozen section study and by gross inspection was thought to represent celiac ganglion. This appeared to be producing stenosis of the celiac axis artery. Right crural fibers of the diaphragm were identified passing approximately ¼-inch below the true origin of the celiac axis artery which was obscured by the celiac ganglion. Pressure measurements in the aorta and celiac axis artery following removal of the celiac ganglion revealed a 5 mm mercury or less pressure gradient. There was a 50 mm pressure gradient across the area of stenosis in the splenic artery. Following completion of the operative reconstructive procedure, there was no pressure gradient, between the aorta and splenic artery. Measurements of pressure gradients in the superior mesenteric artery revealed identical pressure in the aorta and in the superior mesenteric artery.

NAME OF OPERATION (Oct. 24, 1977)

(1) Exploration of celiac axis, superior mesenteric and splenic and hepatic arteries (2) Resection of celiac ganglion (3) Autologous saphenous vein roof-patch angioplasty of celiac axis and splenic arteries across the ostium of the hepatic artery (4) Reversed autologous saphenous vein graft replacing segment of distal celiac axis artery (5) Intraoperative angiograms x2 (6) "EXCISION OF BOTH SAPHENOUS VEINS FROM GROIN."

This operation was a success. Her symptoms improved slowly but the epigastric bruit was unchanged. She began to gain weight and returned to full-time work. By January 1978 she had gained ten pounds. By the following year she had gained another ten pounds. By April 1981 she had gained another ten pounds reaching the level that she had before her illness, 122½ pounds. The epigastric bruit was audible but not as prominent as before the operation. She remained in a remission of her GI tract symptoms until mid-September 1983 when she said in a visit to me in October 1983. "I was feeling fine until mid-September and since then I have had a recurrence of my original illness, when I began to experience recurrent epigastric and left upper quadrant distress radiating to the back and scapula. The discomfort is dull, steady and seems worse 1–1½ hours after eating. I vomited twice last week, once at bedtime, clear colorless and very bitter fluid. Another episode of vomiting occurred in the morning." She added that the epigastric pain awakened her from sleep twice during the past week.

No dark stools; bowel movements were regular. Ten days ago she started Tagamet three times daily and Maalox but they failed to help. She began to lose weight, going from 125 lbs to 118 lbs during the past ten days. Her vital signs were normal and the general examination was normal except for definite epigastric and left upper quadrant tenderness. The epigastric bruit was present and of significant grade. Her routine blood tests were negative and serum amylase was normal. I discussed having a GI series done but she objected that they never had been helpful in the past. I then recommended gastroscopy which she agreed to have. I insisted that she try Zantac QID, continue with Maalox 30 cc q2h and a bland diet in frequent small feedings plus Ensure. Gastroscopy on 24 October 1983, revealed a small 3 mm gastric ulcer in the fundus blow the C.E. junction, esophagitis and hypersecretion of highly acid (Ph 1) gastric juice. She failed to respond to this program and lost weight steadily. The bruit remained the same. A CAT scan of the abdomen on 17 November 1983 revealed fullness in the anterior para-aortic region just below the level of the celiac axis. Arteriography was recommended but the patient preferred to wait. Finally after some persuasion, the patient agreed to enter the hospital on 7 December 1983 for further studies. On 8 December 1983, celiac angiography was performed by Dr. James Chang, who demonstrated complete occlusion of the celiac artery at its origin. An 80 mm drop in systolic pressure across the superior mesenteric artery was noted. All major branches of the celiac artery filled via the pancreaticoduodenal arcade and gastroduodenal arteries retrogradely from the superior mesenteric artery. Because of the clinical picture of recurrent abdominal pain; failure to respond to a bland diet, antacids, and H2 acceptor blockers; significant weight loss; and the positive angiographic findings, operation was recommended. Dr. Imparato saw the patient and agreed. An approving second opinion was obtained from Dr. Foster Conklin in compliance with requirements of the patient's insurance policy. My belief was that neurofibromas had re-encased the celiac artery and were responsible for her relapse. Less likely was intrinsic arterial disease in a young woman with no evidence of systemic vascular disease. In my notes on the hospital chart I listed a reference to a patient at the Mayo Clinic who had a similar condition that responded well to reconstructive surgery.[2]

On 9 January 1984 at University Hospital, I watched as Dr. Imparato operated upon the patient. He confirmed the angiographic findings of a markedly stenosed celiac axis artery with a significant pressure gradient between the aorta and the distal celiac axis artery, while the hepatic and splenic were widely patent as was the superior mesenteric. There was marked hypertrophy of the inferior mesenteric artery. Dr. Imparato decided that an aorto-celiac axis bypass was indicated, and he performed this with 8 mm knitted Dacron. The superior mesenteric artery, the aorta above the celiac axis artery, the celiac axis artery, splenic and hepatic arteries were dissected free. The celiac ganglion was resected. The tissue from the aorta close to the celiac axis was resected but there was no recognizable neural tissue. Pressure gradients were monitored. The patient had a smooth postoperative course. For the first time since my initial diagnosis of her condition in 1976, the abdominal bruit had disappeared following her third operation. She slowly but steadily regained her weight and strength and appetite. Except for several bouts of acute sigmoid diverticulitis and some orthopedic ailments, she has enjoyed good health for the eleven years since her last operation, an excellent response to the brilliant vascular reconstructive surgery performed by Dr. Anthony Imparato.

The GI program at St. Vincent's Hospital continued to grow steadily and continued to be strongly clinically oriented and attractive to the residents, fellows, house staff, medical students, and attending staff. When we first came to St. Vincent's, the funds for supporting the GI unit were supplied as needed by Mrs. Janet Upjohn Stearns. Mr. John Horn, a seasoned and well-informed vice president of the Morgan Guarantee Bank, had charge of the Upjohn funds and their management. Mr. Horn proved to be a warm friend and supporter of my work. He knew how to make the money set aside for us work for a maximal return.

The initial Upjohn gift was for at least one million dollars and substantially exceeded this before the final payment was made. I was learning a great deal by managing this generous fund, including many things I never learned in medical school. I learned early on that control over the money was of prime importance for achieving our goals. This responsibility should never be in the hands of administrators or others who had nothing to do with raising the money and were often ignorant as to the purpose of the fund. My agreement with St. Vincent's Hospital and Medical Center was never written. It was then

---

2. Alan J. Cameron, Peter C. Pairolero, Anthony W. Stanson, Herschel A. Carpenter, "Abdominal Angina and Neurofibromatosis," *Mayo Clinic Proc.* 57 (1982), pp. 125–128.

and remains to this day on a handshake basis. This is not to infer that we had no problems. In a day when indirect costs of the institution were deleted from any NIH or Foundation grant, I insisted that my fund was not a government grant but provided by private philanthropy for education and research that the institution should be willing to support, to enhance its image and the quality of patient care, education, and research at the medical center. The Sisters of Charity and the trustees of St. Vincent's Hospital understood this and gave permission for this policy to be followed. Periodically, I was called upon to defend this position. As an example of the kind of shenanigans that can occur when it comes to money, I divulge this experience. Mrs. Stearns decided to give me a check for $500,000 to continue supporting our program in gastroenterology at St. Vincent's Hospital. The check was sent to me by Mr. James Dolan, the attorney for the Upjohn Funds and Foundation, a member of the prestigious law firm of Davis, Polk and Wardwell. Jim told me that he could write a tough contract for me to ensure the achievement of my goals, but this wise counselor said, "Contracts can be restrictive and end up by tying you up as well as the institution. Show them the check so they can see it is real but don't give it to them until they agree to your terms of gift." I proceeded with this and ran into some unexpected resistance from the director of medicine, Dr. William J. Grace, the same one who had persuaded me to come to St. Vincent's Hospital by saying he was not interested in the Upjohn money. He now took the position that the check should be deposited in the department of medicine's account.

"Whenever you need the money, just send me a note and it will be forthcoming." My reply was that it was my money to control and not the department of medicine's. He then bounced me off to Mr. Albert Samis, the number-two administrator of the hospital. He was in alliance with Dr. Grace and backed up his position. I was yo-yo'd back and forth on this issue and the check remained in my pocket for six weeks while he and the administrator talked it over. Finally, exasperated and frustrated by this attitude, I decided to take this matter to Sister Anthony Marie Fitzmaurice, the president of the hospital. She could see that I was angry at being batted back and forth. I explained why I must control the fund in order to achieve the goals that the donor and I had set. Sister Anthony listened to me and said, "I don't understand why there has been any question whatsoever over the control of the Upjohn fund. You have earned it and are entitled to administer it. I want you to know how much we are indebted to you for the spirit and leadership you have brought to St. Vincent's Hospital. I thought doctors like you had died out. You have brought us your brilliant skills in diagnosis and treatment, attracting patients from far and wide to St. Vincent's Hospital, adding to its reputation. This has cost us nothing, for you serve without pay from hospital funds. Our full-time doctors collect salaries and wait for patients who would come here anyway for reasons of convenience and proximity to their homes." Then she said to me, "I have a problem. My chief administrative aide and chief of medicine will have to be overruled." She then proceeded to make several telephone calls in my presence. She then turned to me and said, "Dr. Lepore, you have my authorization to completely control the Upjohn funds without any interference by administration or other members of the professional staff." St. Vincent's has honored this commitment for the more than thirty years since it was made with only an occasional unsuccessful challenge from new arrivals on the scene.

Chapter 30

~✦~

Helicobacter Pylori and Peptic Ulcer: A Revolution in Gastroenterology

I N THE CURRENT ERA OF BIG-MONEY RESEARCH with multimillion-dollar grants, impressive buildings, laboratories, institutes, elaborate and highly sophisticated equipment, and teams of collaborating scientists, we tend to forget that an individual, in a remote area using simple facilities, may sometimes make an extraordinary discovery that has eluded those in leadership levels of research. Such a discovery, was announced in 1983 in Brussels at a meeting of infectious-disease authorities. The author was Barry Marshall, an unknown, brash young resident in medicine from Perth, Australia, who announced that he and his pathologist-collaborator, Dr. J. Robin Warren, had evidence that peptic ulcers were caused by a bacterial organism, Campylobacter Pylori (later called Helicobacter Pylori). Quoting from a superb essay entitled "Marshall's Hunch: The Unprecedented and Very Unorthodox Findings of an Unknown Doctor Point Toward Cures for Stomach Diseases That Afflict Millions" in the *New Yorker*, 20 September 1993 by Terence Monmaney.

> The way it looked to Marshall, people infected by the bug first developed stomach inflammation, and then some fraction of those went on to develop chronic indigestion or peptic ulcer. (Later, he even began to think that the bug might cause cancer.) And as far as he could tell, the bug itself wasn't some new pathogen that had sprung out of the rain forest and into the belly of humanity; he thought that his older patients had probably been infected for decades. When Marshall finished speaking, an audience member stood up and gently inquired, "Dr. Marshall what causes peptic ulcers in people who don't have the bacteria?" "If you don't have the bacteria, you don't have a peptic ulcer" Marshall said. He might as well have said he knew the secret of cold fusion. The scientists chuckled and murmured and shook their heads a little embarrassed for a junior colleague whose debut was such a disaster. Dr. Martin Blaser, the director of the Division of Infection Diseases at the Vanderbilt University School of Medicine, was in the audience. Marshall's talk struck him then as "the most preposterous thing I ever heard" he says.

"I thought, this guy is a madman." But far from simply dismissing Marshall's ideas, dozens of scientists more or less independently paid him the highest tribute their profession could bestow; they set out to prove him wrong. Dr. David T. Graham, a distinguished gastroenterology researcher at the Veterans Affairs Medical Center in Houston, recalls his first impression of Marshall's work, "Here's some crazy guy saying crazy things. It seemed that he was going to set the field back years. But the virtue of his idea was that it was testable—it wouldn't be hard to find out if it was true. Marshall tried to produce the disease in animals. This was delayed because he had been unable to grow the bug in vitro. When he succeeded, he injected the bacteria into the peritoneal cavity of rats without success and then into young pigs with no success. He finally came to the conclusion that he would try the bacteria culture on himself. In preparation for this, he was endoscoped with biopsies, all of them normal, and then swallowed the bacterial culture. He was perfectly well until the eighth day when he vomited and developed a foul breath. "In the middle of the experiment's second week, Marshall again underwent endoscopy and biopsy." But now, the physician who performed the biopsy noted that Marshall's stomach lining was inflamed, shiny, and punky as an old mushroom. Microscopic analysis of the biopsied material revealed a festering infection—swarms of bacilli seeming to hover around inflamed stomach cells. A third biopsy, performed four days later, revealed no infection; gone. Marshall's immune system had evidently managed to fight off the invasion, and he felt fine. Describing the ordeal in the April 15, 1985 issue of the *Medical Journal of Australia*, Marshall and his coworkers pointed out that his bug was no benign colonizer.

I became a Marshall believer soon after reading his papers in *Lancet* in 1983 and advised our endoscopists at St. Vincent's Hospital to pursue this important lead. This was never pursued as aggressively as I thought it should have been.

In 1986 one of my grateful patients, a renowned C.E.O. of a Fortune 500 Company and a generous philanthropist who had been cured by me of a Helicobacter Pylori—induced gastritis and papillitis of the papilla of Vater, made a substantial gift of a scintillation counter for doing Carbon 14 breath tests for the diagnosis of Helicobacter infection, making it possible for us to do non-invasive and low-cost testing for this organism. This equipment was not aggressively put to work by the endoscopists at St. Vincent's Hospital, with some of them fearing that the screening breath test might reduce the number of endoscopic procedures and, not incidentally, the income from gastroscopy. I persisted in utilizing the breath test for the diagnosis and also for non-invasive follow up of the patients that had undergone antibiotic therapy for their ailment.

In October 1987 my interest in what was then called Campylobacter Pylori paid off some interesting dividends in a patient with Menetrier's disease of the stomach that led to the submission of the following report to *The Lancet*.

"CAMPYLOBACTER IN A PATIENT WITH MENETRIER'S DISEASE CAUSAL, COMMENSAL, OPPORTUNISTIC OR COINCIDENTAL"

Nearly one hundred years ago P. Menetrier (1859-1935), a Parisian pathologist, published his report on giant hypertrophic gastritis that earned him an eponym and permanent fame. The condition is rare, a review in 1977 describing only 120 patients in the world literature with only a few individuals having the oportunity to study and follow such patients. The etiology of the disease remains an enigma that has eluded explanation despite advances in diagnostic techniques including fiberoptic gastroscopy with directed biopsy and the demonstration that a cardinal feature of the syndrome is protein-losing gastroenteropathy with hypoalbuminemia and edema. The senior author of this report (M.J.L.) has treated a woman now 63 years old with Menetrier's disease since 1965 when she was referred to him as a diagnostic problem because of severe pitting edema of both thighs and legs. She had a history of "bleeding duodenal ulcer" and large gastric rugae seen on x-ray without gastroscopy in 1964 during two hospital admissions in New Jersey. She was admitted to the Upjohn Gastrointestinal service, Roosevelt Hospital, N.Y.C. on 2-9-65 where a series of tests revealed hypoproteinemia (3.5 gm total protein per dl) and hypoalbuminemia (2.07 gm per dl) without albuminuria or evidence of renal or cardiac disease. Two studies with Chromium-tagged albumin injected intravenously showed substantial losses of albumin into the gastrointestinal tract lumen via the stomach. On radiologic examination of the stomach, giant hypertrophied rugae were seen without an ulcer or neoplasm. Gastroscopic examination with biopsy confirmed the clinical impression of Menetrier's disease. She responded well to a bland high protein diet, antacids, a protein supplement and diuretics, the edema clearing as the serum albumin gradually rose to normal values. During the past 22 years she has had a series of ailments and operations unrelated to the Menetrier's disease, including a modified radical mastectomy for carcinoma in January 1982 but despite this she has functioned effectively as a housewife and part-time bookkeeper.

Over the years she has had 5 hospital admissions for Menetrier's disease with the complaint of abdominal pain and dyspepsia without the recurrence of edema except for the admission of 1970. On another occasion she experienced severe melena.

During October 1987 while under considerable personal stress, she developed severe nausea and intermittent epigastric and right upper quadrant pain relieved temporarily by antacids only to recur. She could not tolerate any of the currently available H2 receptor-antagonists saying they seemied to make her worse.

Gastroscopy confirmed exacerbation of the Menetrier's disease. A startling finding in the biopsy specimens was the presence of a large number of Campylobacter-like organisms seen with hematoxylin and eosin stains, confirmed by Acridine-Orange fluorescent microscopy. This led us to review all of the available previous gastric biopsies in this patient with the following results:

Date	Mucosa Type	Histology	CLO**	Serum Albumin
1965	Body	Severe ACG* "foveolar hyperplasia	4+	2.07 gm/dl
1970	Body	Mild ACG	1+	2.23 gm/dl
1979	Body	Mod. ACG	2+	3.60 gm/dl
1985	Antrum	Severe ACG	4+	
	Body (x2)	Mod. ACG	4+	3.70 gm/dl
1987	Antrum	Severe ACG	1+	
	Body (x3)	Moderate to Severe ACG	2+	3.20 gm/dl

Table 1.—Gastroscopic Biopsy Findings

*ACG   = Active Chronic Gastritis
**CLO = Campylobacter-like organisms detected on acridine-orange stained biopsy sections examined with fluorescence microscopy, semi-quantitative score (1+ = less that 10 organisms entire section, 4+ = heavy colonization of entire or majority of surface epithelium, foveolar lumen by continuous layer of CLO's)

The pioneering observations and follow-up studies of Warren and Marshall on Campylobacter as a cause of gastritis are revolutionizing the understanding of this puzzling disorder and have focused attention on the elimination of Campylobacter with antibiotics and bismuth. Our patient appears to be responding to these agents but longer follow up is needed.

Are we seeing in the Menetrier's disease saga a phenomenon similar to that of Whipple's disease in which organisms originally described by Dr. George H. Whipple in 1907 were ignored for sixty years before they were proven to cause that disease, now a curable ailment responding to long-term antibiotic therapy? Our purpose in reporting these findings is to alert others to review their Menetrier's disease material looking for Campylobacter in an attempt to determine whether the relationship is commensal, opportunistic, coincidental or causal. The findings in our patient with Menetrier's disease of Campylobacter-like organisms in all of the gastric biopsies over the past 22 years, including the original ones of 1965, leads us to suspect a causal role.

> Michael J. Lepore, M.D.
> Fred B. Smith, M.D.
> Charles A. Bonnano, M.D.

The submitted manuscript was reviewed by *The Lancet* editor who quickly replied:

> Dear Dr. Lepore,
>
> With your letter of Dec. 15 you sent us a fascinating case of a potential association between Campylobacter-like organisms and Menetrier's disease. We see this as a Letter to the Editor and wondered if you would like us to proceed along these lines, showing you a proof before publication.
>
> Yours sincerely,
>
> David Sharp, MA.

The final word on Menetrier's disease and Helicobacter is still in question. The disease is rare and it is not given to many to have a large series under observation. A substantial series from the Mayo Clinic, based on specimens obtained at surgery have failed to show a significant evidence of Helicobacter. Recently, othes have reported a very high incidence of Helicobacter infection in a large series of patients with hypertrophic gastritis and Menetrier's disease. I have continued using the Carbon 14 breath test for Helicobacter Pylori performed on the scintillation counter as an inexpensive, non-invasive, and reliable method for screening purposes and follow-up of patients who have been given antibiotic therapy. This non-invasive and inexpensive test should be available in all major centers dealing with gastrointestinal ailments.

In closing this chapter, my comment is that Dr. Marshall and Dr. Warren have achieved an outstanding goal, a great discovery of a pathogen that is responsible for serious costly illness and loss of life. If the relationship to gastric carcinoma and gastric lymphoma hold up it will cause a revolution in oncology. Most of all, the beginning of this revolution was at the light microscope of two dedicated and iconoclastic physicians, one of them at the time a resident in medicine in a hospital in Perth, Australia. I believe Dr. Marshall and Dr. Warren have earned a Nobel Prize.

Chapter 31

∿

Plasmapheresis for Hepatic Coma at St. Vincent's Hospital

> "Diseases desperate grown by desperate appliances are relieved or not at all."
>
> (*Hamlet* IV:3)

THE STORY OF THE IMPORTANT VIRAL HEPATITIS RESEARCH conducted at St. Vincent's Hospital and Medical Center in New York City warrants a chapter of its own. My interest in viral hepatitis was whetted in 1942, when I volunteered for military duty in WW II and was awaiting my appointment as a captain in the Medical Corps of the Army of the United States and the call to active duty. At the time I was on the teaching staff of the Columbia University College of Physicians and Surgeons and in the private practice of general internal medicine and also director of the personnel medical department of the Columbia-Presbyterian Medical Center. Dr. Fred Soper of the Rockefeller Foundation, a renowned expert and investigator in yellow fever, came to the Medical Center to lecture on an epidemic of jaundice that had struck thousands of newly mobilized recruits in military service. I sat on the edge of my seat in the amphitheater as Dr. Soper regaled us with the tantalizing mystery of this ailment and its cause. He had been called in as a consultant because most of the cases had appeared in men who had received yellow fever vaccine injections. Was it a variant of yellow fever or was it something else? Fortunately, the illness was usually mild. Needle liver biopsies were not feasible at the time and routine biochemical studies were primitive and not very helpful. Of some value were the autopsy findings in a few soldiers who had been vaccinated against yellow fever and had died in military-training accidents. These showed no evidence of yellow fever but were positive for a mild form of hepatitis. Soon it was determined that only certain batches of the yellow fever vaccine caused the hepatitis. This research project was facilitated by the fact that the only organization authorized to manufacture the vaccine was the International Health Division of the Rockefeller Foundation. Each vial or lot of vaccine was numbered and the military kept records of each lot and persons vaccinated. By the late fall of 1941, the surgeon general and his advisors, in anticipation of the spread of WW II to areas where yellow fever was endemic, had recommended and started full-scale military use of the vaccine.

By March 1942 a disease characterized by jaundice was epidemic in the US Army, In March 1942, Dr. Karl F. Meyer of the Hooper Foundation in California claimed that the yellow fever vaccine injections were responsible for the jaundice. Others soon joined with him. Soon it was found that only certain lots of the vaccine were "icterogenic." They were identified as lots #331, 334, 335, 338, 367, 368, and 369. Since the epidemic of jaundice had appeared shortly after the mass production of the yellow-fever vaccine to meet with urgent military needs, investigators proceeded to re-check the methods of manufacture that were used:

> A number of changes in the technique of the manufacture of the vaccine were introduced in the course of the large-scale production between 1940 and 1942—the history of the seed virus used is complicated and will not be reviewed here, but the addition of *human normal serum* was a crucial point in the procedure. During the four years of in-vitro cultivation before final adoption for human immunization, the 17D strain of yellow fever virus originally derived from the unmodified Asibi strain was used. It was grown in a medium of chick-embryo tissue and Tyrode's solution containing 10 percent normal monkey or human serums. The reason for including human serum in the vaccine was to insure its efficacy as an immunizing agent. The virus of yellow fever is said to be one of the most labile viruses, and the addition of serum to it delays its inactivation process greatly. For large-scale manufacture of the yellow fever vaccine, therefore, large quantities of human serum were needed for the tissue cultures. This was usually obtained from professional blood donors, but in 1941 it became necessary to arrange for additional sources of serum, which was required at the rate of 8 or 10 liters per week. This additional source of serum was obtained through the School of Hygiene and Public Health, Johns Hopkins University, Baltimore, Maryland, where it was secured from volunteers in that city. The donors consisted largely of medical students, interns, nurses, and laboratory technicians, all presumably healthy. In retrospect it would seem that it was this "innocent" lot of serum which gave rise to contamination of the vaccine with an icterogenic agent, an accident which could hardly have been predicted at that time.[1]

There was also a flaw in the preparation of the vaccine by the manufacturers. Paul and Gardner state that reliance was placed on heating the serum at a temperature of 56° and 57°C for one hour.

"Whereas there is now abundant evidence that this temperature is insufficient to kill the virus of either infectious hepatitis or serum hepatitis."[2]

When human serum was eliminated from the manufacture of yellow-fever vaccine, the epidemic of serum jaundice that had incapacitated thousands of troops was stopped dead in it tracks. It should be noted that in 1940 most physicians knew little or nothing about hepatitis, which was then called "catarrhal jaundice." In my 1942 copy of Cecil's *Textbook of Medicine*[3] there is no mention of viral hepatitis but a thorough discussion of "catarrhal jaundice" by Cecil J. Watson (pp. 881–883), which includes the following:

> Catarrhal cholangitis is one type of so-called catarrhal jaundice. It was formerly believed that the latter condition was due only to a low grade, catarrhal inflammation of the common duct and ampulla of Vater, with obstructive jaundice. Much evidence has accumulated, however, which indicates that the majority of cases are instances of parenchymal or hepatocellular damage, more closely akin to acute and subacute atrophy, and to cirrhosis of the liver. Nevertheless there can be no doubt that a minority of catarrhal jaundice cases are due to cholangitis. Relatively little is known of the pathology of this disease due to the fact that recovery nearly always occurs. Eppinger[4] had some opportunity to study the anatomic changes in soldiers with mild catarrhal jaundice who remained on active duty and died of wounds received in action. Reference has already been made to the probable existence of three types of catarrhal jaundice; (1) hepatocellular, (2) pericholangitis, (3) choledochitic. The cause of the various forms is unknown. Eppinger includes the hepatocellular, or common form, among the "serous" inflammations, designating it as "serous hepatitis" . . . Microscopically, this form exhibits what Eppinger terms "dissociation" of liver cords. This is particularly marked toward the center of the dissociation lobules where there is considerable edema; the liver cells exhibit a vary-

---

1. John R. Paul and Horace T. Gardner, "Viral Hepatitis," in *Preventive Medicine in World War II, Vol. V: Communicable Diseases*, edited by Colonel John Boyd Coates, Jr. (Washington, D.C.: Office of the Surgeon General, Department of the Army, 1960), pp. 423–425.

2. Ibid., p. 424.

3. R. L. and A. B. Cecil, eds., *A Textbook of Medicine by American Authors* (Philadelphia and London: W. B.Saunders Company, 1942).

4. H. Eppinger, *Die Leberkrankheiten*. (Vienna: J. Springer, 1937).

ing degree of degeneration of outspoken necrosis with the result that the continuity of the liver cords is often broken or irregular. The edema is due to accumulation of fluid in the widened spaces between the liver cells and the "sinusoids."

This is a pretty good description of what we now call viral hepatitis. This section, written by Dr. Cecil J. Watson of Minnesota, represented the state of the art for 1942.

No wonder we sat on the edge of our seats in the auditorium at P&S as Dr. Soper methodically described this research and the marvelous detective work involved in pinning down the cause of the epidemic of hepatitis that struck the army in 1942.

Those of us awaiting military orders to active duty were happy to know that the flaw in the yellow-fever vaccine had been detected and corrective action taken to eliminate the risk. Little did we know that a second virus, one with a short incubation period, would soon become epidemic in the military, the two agents accounting for at least 200,000 cases of hepatitis in the armed forces during WW II. Little did I know that I would soon be seeing and treating hundreds of soldiers with hepatitis incurred in all of the far-flung theaters of war, including north Africa, the Pacific, the CBI theatre, and southern Italy, the Mid-East, and others. On Saipan alone, I was destined to diagnose and treat hundreds of soldiers with hepatitis, sending most of them home for convalescence. I learned much about the natural course of viral hepatitis, as did my colleagues, but in spite of all of our clinical work we ended our military careers without really pinning down the cause of viral hepatitis. This would remain for army-sponsored and civilian research to solve. It was not easy and it was not quick. Eliminating human serum from the yellow-fever vaccine solved one problem for the military but another remained, the appearance of another form of hepatitis, this one with a short incubation period, called infectious hepatitis as opposed to serum hepatitis with its long incubation period. Clinical evidence for the existence of a second virus came, in part, from observation that some soldiers who had recovered from homologous serum hepatitis developed infectious hepatitis when exposed to the second virus. When I completed my tour of military duty in 1946, the state-of-the-art position on viral hepatitis was that there were two forms and two different filterable viruses were causative factors but they had never been isolated or grown. The two diseases accounted for at least 200,000 cases in the army in World War II and constituted a major cause of disability or hospitalization, each case averaging twenty-five to fifty days of time lost from active duty.

The lessons of WW II were apparently forgotten in the Korean War (1950–1953) when pooled human plasma was used on a large scale, leading to yet another "epidemic" of hepatitis among our wounded.

My next major adventure with viral hepatitis occurred in August 1967 during my tenure as chief of gastroenterology at St. Vincent's Hospital and president of the Upjohn Gastrointestinal Foundation. One day I was asked by one of my best Upjohn fellows, Dr. Anthony J. Martel to see a very sick thirty-one-year-old white man who had been picked up, nameless, and brought to the emergency room of our hospital by ambulance, diagnosed as having "impending delirium tremens." He developed grand-mal seizures, became comatose, and was admitted to the neurological service. There he was found to be deeply jaundiced, with biochemical and clinical signs of severe hepatic failure. The question of treating him with exchange transfusions of whole blood had been raised on rounds prompted by recent reports that exchange transfusions had been successful in patients with fulminant hepatic failure. I examined the patient, who was in Stage IV coma, and agreed with the diagnosis of severe hepatic failure. Exchange transfusions with whole blood were out of the question, for his blood group was rare B Rh negative. It was August, the season when blood donors are scarce in New York City and our blood bank could not supply the amount of blood needed for even one exchange. Dr. Martel was appalled that a young person was going to die without a heroic effort to help him. The next day, Dr. Martel asked me whether I had any further thoughts about the care of Mr. No Name on St. Joseph's ward. I said there was another option, plasmapheresis, a procedure that involved removing the patient's whole blood, 500 cc at a time, centrifuging to separate the red cells from the plasma, discarding the plasma and returning the patient's own red cells to him. This would place no extra burden on the blood bank.

I explained to Dr. Martel that the procedure had been developed in 1914 by Professor John J. Abel of Johns Hopkins School of Medicine. I had learned about it as a student fellow in physiology in 1930 at the University of Rochester School of Medicine when I was doing research on the Starling hypothesis of fluid exchange. There I had plasmapheresed dogs to reduce their plasma-protein levels to produce edema. I had never used this procedure on a human being but I could see no reason why it could not be tried in the desperate situation with which we were confronted in the case of Mr. No Name. My hypothesis was that if it is true that hemodialysis and peritoneal dialysis are ineffectual in hepatic coma and exchange transfusions or cross circulation are beneficial, non-dialyzable, probably protein-bound, factors might be responsible for the coma. Were this the case, it would seem logical to subject the patient to plasmapheresis, returning to him his own red blood cells and adding pooled plasma to replace his plasma proteins, fibrinogen, and clotting factors. At the time, we did not have any special equipment for this procedure. It meant that it would all have to be done by hand, removing blood, centrifuging it, siphoning off the plasma, and returning the cells to the patient. It was very labor intensive and the laborer was going to be Dr. Anthony J. Martel. He was more than equal to the task, exchanging 5000 cc of the patient's blood within a twenty-four-hour period. The response was dramatic, the patient's coma clearing and his tests for coma improving remarkably to the point that he sat up to read the papers. We reported this experience in *The Lancet* with the following comment: "In the future it is planned to perform continuous plasmapheresis at the bedside, using apparatus designed to simplify the technique further and to speed up the rate of plasma exchange. We believe this procedure should be given a trial in acute hepatic failure with coma as a less cumbersome and more practicable alternative to the more drastic and demanding exchange transfusion, cross circulation, or bypass techniques."[5] Shortly after my experience with Mr. No Name, St. Vincent's Hospital, situated in Greenwich Village with its large population of homosexuals, aberrant lifestyles, and active intravenous drug culture, became the center of a serious epidemic of viral hepatitis.

Whereas the viral hepatitis of the 1950s and 60s had usually been mild to moderate, the new form of the disease was more aggressive, and young people in the Village and in the metropolitan area were dying in considerable numbers with an acute fulminant hepatitis with coma. At that time we were certain it was due to a virus but we had no specific diagnostic blood test for it. The virus had never been cultured or identified and there was no animal model of the disease. We were baffled as to how to treat the patients and sought advice from various experts. They were unable to offer any major therapeutic advice except to use every available supportive measure to attempt to carry our young patients through the acute phase of this lethal form of the disease. The death rate in these young patients was almost one

---

5. Michael J. Lepore and Anthony J. Martel, *The Lancet*, October 7, 1967, pp. 771–772.

hundred percent for those in Stage IV hepatic coma. In many ways, this severe form of viral hepatitis presented to those of us on the firing line with many of the features we would encounter later on in the 1980s when the AIDS epidemic struck in Greenwich Village. There were similarities in the demography of both diseases. The patients were young, previously healthy adults, a mysterious virus that had not been isolated or grown was responsible, and most of the patients would die, the chief difference from AIDS being the long duration of that illness, compared to the fulminant quickly lethal course of our patients with viral hepatitis. The form of viral hepatitis we were seeing differed markedly from the relatively mild disease most physicians had encountered. It was not unusual for one of our patients to walk into the hospital and within twenty-four hours collapse into Stage IV coma or go into cardiorespiratory arrest, necessitating emergency CPR and intubation or tracheostomy. Most of our patients were not I.V. drug users. Two were physicians, who became ill following a fingerstick and died despite all of our efforts, martyrs to their profession.

When we started our study there was no test to determine what type of hepatitis virus had affected our patients. Several years later I was asked by my preceptor in physiology, Dr. Edward F. Adolph of the University of Rochester, how I happened to get involved in hepatitis research and treatment of so many critically ill patients at an age when few would undertake so heavy a responsibility. I was then fifty-seven years of age. My answer to Dr. Adolph was that I simply could not merely stand by without doing something to attempt to save the lives of these young people. I was convinced that the current methods of treatment were ineffectual and grossly inadequate. My feeling was that the experts of the day knew nothing more and perhaps less than I did about the disease. My qualifications were chiefly clinical and my motivation was to try to save some lives and, in the process, to learn more about the disease and its causes and management.

In a way, I felt like Dr. Frederick Banting, the inexperienced young Canadian orthopedic surgeon, who was impelled to search for insulin because he hated to see children dying of diabetes mellitus. Despite many obstacles and the scorn of academicians, this young man with no previous research experience succeeded in solving the riddle that had stymied experienced scientists for many decades. I mention this because the belief held in some quarters is that only the thoroughly trained and duly anointed scientist in his laboratory is capable of producing any significant research. I believe it is still possible for important clinical investigation to be done by qualified clinicians whose stimulus is the challenge of curing the sick who seek their personal care. Some have called these individuals Triple Threat men and women, and concluded that in the present era this breed is extinct. Furthermore, many believe that it is impossible to be a Triple Threater—scientist, teacher, and clinician—in this era of massive information explosion. I refuse to accept this and will continue to demand that our educational and training systems be radically modified in the hope that the breed of the so-called Renaissance men and women will once again flourish in our academic centers and among the practicing physicians of the day. It is my belief that the really outstanding physician should be a clinician who is on the front line, laying hands upon his patients, suffering with them, and rejoicing when a victory is achieved. This is the stimulus that the laboratory scientist seldom has to spur him along the path to fame and recognition, and in this respect the practicing clinician has him at a disadvantage if he will only listen to the call for help from those with serious and complex diseases and be willing to make heavy sacrifices in order to pursue this path. While on this theme, I quote John Bunyan (1628–1688), the English preacher celebrated for his *Pilgrim's Progress,* the allegorical tale of Christian's journey from the City of Destruction to the Celestial City:

> Physicians get neither name or fame by pricking of wheals, or picking out at thistles, or by laying of plaisters to the scratch of a pin; every old woman can do this. But if they would have a name and fame—if they will have it quickly, they must as, I said, do some great and desperate cures. Let them fetch one to life that was dead; let them recover one to his wits that was mad; let them make one that was born blind to see; or let them give ripe wits to a fool; these are notable cures; and he that can do thus first, he shall have the name and fame he desires; he may lie abed till noon.

> John Bunyan (1628–1688)[6]

My motivation in medicine has never been to seek "name and fame" or "lie abed till noon." I have simply sought to live by the golden rule, giving to every one of my patients the best of modern medicine wrapped in the book jacket of the past. For those who are seriously ill, I have let nothing deter me from seeing that all is done to

---

6. M. B. Strauss, ed. *"The Jerusalem Sinner Saved: Or Good News for the Vilest of Men." Familiar Medical Quotations* (Boston: Little, Brown and Company, 1968), p. 74.

achieve a cure or failing that, to give my patients comfort, compassion, and the assurance that serving their interest is my main purpose and goal. The challenge for me in attacking viral hepatitis was its lethality; the youth of its victims; the doctor-patients and nurse-patients, martyrs to their profession; and above all the failure of anyone to come up with a new form of therapy based on sound physiological and biochemical principles. Even more impelling was my desire to put to practical use the years of basic research in physiology that I had spent at Rochester, Duke, and Yale in the 1930s. I wanted to repay my sponsors and teachers the debt I owed them for teaching me the lessons from the laboratory, the basic sciences, especially physiology and applying this knowledge at the bedside to the care of the seriously ill.

I felt that my medical school, my teachers, and the American College of Physicians had invested a great deal in my future and now, after some years, including four years of service in WW II, I was ready to pay back some dividends on their investments in my career. This is why I embarked on my work with viral hepatitis, knowing full well that it would not be a simple task. An additional factor was that this challenge came at a time in my life when I was in control of an important service in a fine hospital and responsible for the application of a magnificent gift from a member of the Upjohn family to advance the understanding and treatment of persons with gastrointestinal ailments.

I sat down with my staff and aroused their interest in this project and sought their active participation. I knew there would be risks, but I felt confident that if we observed good technique and great care, the danger of cross-infection was small, or I at least thought so. Fortunately, there was no liver guru at St. Vincent's who could compete with me. The liver belonged to my service and I was the chief and I had the resources to tackle the project with vigor and financial support. In addition to two or three Upjohn fellows, I had a large staff of competent attending physicians who were young, idealistic, and willing to serve without pay. My administrative staff was superb, headed by Miss Martha Swensson, who handled most of the administrative details of the project. A biochemist, Dr. Bo Prytz, and laboratory space were made available to me by Dr. Louis M. Rousselot, director of surgery. Dr. Leonard Stutman, a talented Rochester graduate, joined our team in charge of blood coagulation studies. The microbiologist-in-chief, Dr. Pearl Ma, worked effectively with clinicians. We met regularly to discuss our progress and communicated with each other daily. There was a collegial atmosphere that included dealing with house staff as colleagues in an important but novel and risky attempt to save lives. Ultimately a great many others were on what was called the Plasmapheresis Team, reaching a total of well over thirty individuals. Only one house staff, a young surgical resident, refused to participate in the plasmapheresis project, because he had a great fear of sticking his fingers and contracting hepatitis. All of the others participated willingly. I was especially pleased by the fearless and professional performance of our St. Vincent's nurses who accepted the risks and gave far and beyond the call of duty. I shall never forget them. Fortunately, none of the staff who participated in the plasmapheresis project contracted the disease they were treating, a tribute to their skill, professionalism, and a measure of good luck.

Before embarking on this project, I hand-searched the *Index Medicus* with the assistance of Miss Martha Swensson, gathering the literature on hepatitis, fulminant hepatic failure, and the various forms of therapy then in vogue. From this search and my extensive clinical experience with infectious hepatitis, I developed a hypothesis that plasmapheresis with plasma exchange was worthy of a trial in this disease. Since we were dealing with a form of the disease that was almost 100 percent fatal, we did not believe that randomization was justifiable, defensible, or ethical in patients in Stage IV coma. Our line of reasoning was as follows: Recent anecdotal reports that had received considerable publicity were to the effect that a few patients with acute fulminant hepatic failure and deep coma had recovered when subjected to whole-blood exchange transfusion or cross-circulation, whereas similarly ill patients subjected to hemodialysis or peritoneal dialysis had failed to respond, suggesting that a protein-bound factor or factors might be involved. My hypothesis was that if the factor were protein-bound, there was no need to subject the patient to whole-blood exchange, with its inherent hazards for the patient and increased demands upon the blood bank. Instead, I proposed that the patient be subjected to plasmapheresis with plasma exchange, returning the patient's own red blood cells, and replacing the plasma with easily available fresh-frozen human plasma. In chapter five, I discussed plasmapheresis, removal of plasma, a procedure developed by Dr. John Abel of Johns Hopkins in 1914, and described my use of this technique in dog experiments in 1930 at Rochester, testing the Starling's hypothesis of fluid exchange and edema formation. My experiments were confined to dogs and I had never plasmapheresed a patient, but I could not see any reason to doubt that it could be applied to human subjects.

I decided to modify the Abel method by replacing the patient's plasma with fresh frozen human plasma rather than the Locke's solution used by Abel in his dog experiments. By using fresh frozen plasma I would be giving the patient ample amounts of plasma protein to maintain positive nitrogen balance, essential coagulation factors, perhaps, immune antibodies against the hepatitis virus, adding to the supplement essential vitamins, minerals, electrolytes, and glucose to make an ideal intravenous feeding and support regimen to sustain the comatose patient until hepatocyte regeneration might occur. By removing the patient's plasma we might also be getting rid of bilirubin, ammonia, cryoglobulins, and other toxic and noxious substances of an unknown nature. To the best of my knowledge this technique had never before been used to treat severe illness in the human. Many questions would arise during the course of the study. I did not know how long the treatment would have to be continued or how many units should be exchanged. Should it be done around the clock? What equipment should we use? Where would this patient be admitted and housed?

After a few adverse experiences, we insisted that these patients be isolated in a single room in the intensive-care unit. In 1967, St. Vincent's was one of the first hospitals in New York to have an intensive-care unit in its new air-conditioned Cronin Building. Matters that we take for granted nowadays had to be resolved in a pioneering setting, leaving much room for innovation. We looked at various kinds of equipment for performing plasmapheresis and decided that the simplest and most practical equipment available at that time was the Dade Monofuge. This was well before the current fantastic plasmapheresis machines were being invented or marketed. A small, efficient, and quiet centrifuge (Monofuge)[7] was placed at the bedside. The patient was bled into 500 ml bottles containing citric acid dextrose (ACD) solution. When the bottle was full, it was inverted and placed into the centrifuge, where it was automatically centrifuged at 3300 RPM for 6 minutes and then allowed to decelerate for 12 minutes. The packed red cells were then reinfused from the same bottle into the patient, and the supernatant plasma sent to the laboratory or discarded. This system was closed, virtually foolproof, and could be used with safety by house staff after minimal instruction. We had no problems with sterility or air embolism. The main criticism was that it

---

7. Michael J. Lepore and Anthony J. Martel, "Plasmapheresis with Plasma Exchange in Hepatic Coma. Methods and Results in Five Patients with Acute Fulminant Hepatic Necrosis," *Ann Int Med* 72, no. 2 (February 2, 1970), pp. 165–174.

was labor intensive, an objection that would be resolved when better equipment was developed.

Since large amounts of freshly frozen plasma would be needed for this project, I met with key members of the New York Blood Center, Dr. Aaron Kellner, Dr. Arthur M. Prince, and Dr. Benjamin Alexander, who welcomed our study for several reasons, not the least of which was that if it succeeded it would reduce the demand on the Blood Center for whole blood. When the news spread that my group at St. Vincent's was performing plasmapheresis with plasma exchange for patients with severe fulminant hepatic failure, we were flooded with requests to accept patients from other medical centers in the metropolitan area as well as some in New Jersey. One of our early patients nearly broke our spirits when emerging from Stage IV coma, after six days of around-the-clock vigorous plasmapheresis with plasma exchange, she developed widespread antibiotic-resistant bronchopneumonia and died of cardiac arrest seventeen days after the initiation of plasmapheresis. What was especially disturbing for us was that she was a thirty-year-old physician, a native of the Philippines, who had been referred to us on 29 May 1968 from Riverdell Hospital, New Jersey, where she was a resident physician. Her illness began as a grippe-like syndrome on 20 May. Four days later she was noticeably jaundiced but mentally clear; on 27 May she became disoriented, required sedation and restraints, and told her colleagues that she was going to die of viral hepatitis. She was treated vigorously with the usual measures of that day for hepatic failure. Despite these measures she was in Stage IV coma by the following morning, when arrangements were made to transfer her to my service at St. Vincent's Hospital. The past medical history was essentially negative. There was no history of exposure to toxic agents, medications, ethanol, drugs, raw clams, transfusions, injections, or to patients with viral hepatitis. Later it was learned from one of her colleagues that four months before her illness she had pricked her finger while starting an infusion. The patient was gravely ill and deeply comatose on admission and responded only with movements of decerebrate rigidity. She became apneic and required endoral tracheal intubation and mechanical ventilatory assistance. Her blood chemical values were diagnostic of severe hepatic failure with serum bilirubin of 12.2 mg per ml., serum glutamic oxalacetic transaminase (SGOT) 2600, and blood ammonia 480 mg per ml. Blood coagulation factors were a markedly impaired prothrombin time, 56 seconds, fibrinogen less than 50 mg per 100 ml, partial thromboplastin time, prolonged, Factor X not present, Factors V and VI markedly diminished, platelet count 88,000. Plasmapheresis with plasma exchange was started on 29 May 1968 and vigorously pursued round the clock.

By the 30th of May, biochemical improvement was evident in an improved prothrombin time, reduced serum bilirubin and SGOT. The blood ammonia level was now normal. Hyponatremia had been corrected, blood pressure was well maintained, and urine output was adequate. The patient was tolerating vigorous around-the-clock plasmapheresis with plasma exchange without any adverse reaction, but she remained in coma. By the 31st of May, the patient's coma appeared lighter with loss of decerebrate rigidity and the return of pupillary reflexes. Seventy-eight units of whole blood had been removed. The liver was not palpable and appeared to be shrinking. Metabolic alkalosis and hypokalemia were treated energetically. On the 2nd of June, the sixth day of almost continuous plasmapheresis, she was emerging from coma and there was further biochemical improvement. By 6 June steady progress had continued. By that time the patient was able to answer questions by nodding her head and was showing signs of increasing alertness. She was able to move all extremities on command. On that day she developed fever (101°F) and a chest x-ray showed bilateral pneumonic infiltrates. Broad-spectrum antibiotics were given. The patient continued to improve steadily and was able to communicate with her family and attending personnel. She was clearly out of coma and appeared to be recovering. Plasmapheresis was discontinued on day 12, a total of 167 units of blood having been exchanged during the first 9 days. On day 12 the patient suddenly developed acute pulmonary edema with severe respiratory distress. Multiple pulmonary emboli were suspected. Despite intensive supportive therapy, the patient suffered cardiac arrest on 13 June and died. At autopsy pulmonary emboli were not found, but there was severe bilateral hemorrhagic bronchopneumonia. The liver weighed 900 gm and the autopsy reported noted the following histologic changes:

> The hepatic architecture is grossly distorted. There are small and large islands of regenerated liver cells separated one from another by small and large areas of stromal collapse with hemorrhage. The regenerated lobules display irregular arrangement of the cell cords. There is extensive canalicular bile stasis. Several large regenerating nodules are undergoing irregular subdivision by frond-like projections of collapsed stroma. The central to portal zone relationships are completely distorted in all liver sections examined. The collapsed stroma displays approximation of the reticular network, extensive hemorrhage, chronic and acute

inflammation, bile duct proliferation, necrosis of trapped hepatocytes and pigment-laden scavenger cells. Impression: the findings are those of acute viral hepatitis with necrosis, with beginning and established regeneration of hepatocytes.

It was apparent that the liver disease was in a recovery phase and that
death was caused by the severe bronchopneumonia.

What a blow this was for me and my team! Despite our heroic
efforts, with victory within our grasp, we lost the battle to save the life
of a fine young woman, a martyr to our profession. Chagrined and
saddened as we were, we knew we had come close to a victory. Her
valiant struggle and the clearing of her coma served to stimulate us to
persist in our efforts and to improve our management and understanding of the disease. The more I thought about it, the more I felt
that viral hepatitis was more than a liver disease; it simply had to be a
systemic disease affecting multiple organs. To prove this we needed
some sort of label to identify the responsible virus.

It was at this point in our work that I became acquainted with the
research studies of Dr. Baruch S. Blumberg, one of our former students at Columbia University College of Physicians and Surgeons
Class of 1951, who won a Nobel Prize in 1976 for the discovery of
the causative agent of Hepatitis B. In an interview in 1974 published
in *Modern Medicine*,[8] Dr. Blumberg said he had taken a three-month
elective in his junior year at P&S to travel to Surinam to study malaria and filariasis in several different population groups. "Since my first
field trip in 1950, my associates and I have done additional field work
around the world, including every continent except Antarctica,"
relates Dr. Blumberg. "In each place, we collaborated with local health
groups, usually obtaining numerous blood samples for analysis." A
large part of his early field work focused on the study of inherited
variation of serum proteins. These studies on inherited variation in
serum proteins led to some further speculations. Dr Blumberg says,
"For example, a patient who had received multiple transfusions would
be likely to receive a foreign blood constituent which he himself had
not inherited or acquired and to which he might develop antibodies."

In 1960 Dr. Blumberg and his associates began systematically
evaluating serum samples from transfused patients. Using a double-
diffusion agar gel technique that would detect both antigens and
antibodies, he and Dr. Anthony C. Allison and others were able to

---

8. M. L. N. Luy, "Investigative Coup: Discovery of the Australia Antigen — An
Interview with Dr. Baruch S. Blumberg," *Modern Medicine*, March 4, 1974.

report a complex system involving inherited antigens on low-density beta lipoproteins, which they called the Ag system. Once the Ag system was discovered, the investigators continued this on the presumption that if one type of antigen could be found, perhaps others existed as well.

And shortly thereafter they detected a second precipitating antibody. Its antigen appeared in the serum of an Australian aborigine, one sample among an array of twenty-four drawn from many different populations. The antibody was found in the serum of a transfused hemophilia patient. Dr. Blumberg and his group called this the Australia antigen and pursued this lead by testing various population groups. They found that the antigen was rare, 0.1 percent in normal Americans. Americans who had received multiple transfusions had a significantly higher incidence of the Australia antigen as did patients with lymphocytic leukemia. Since patients with Down's disease are more prone to develop leukemia, they too, were tested and found to have a high incidence of the antigen if they were living in an institution. Those living in homes with their parents had a lower incidence. These findings caused Blumberg and his group to explore several blind alleys, including the possibility that the Australia antigen might be a cause of leukemia. Serendipity as well as scientific talent had led to the initial discovery but the tale was still evolving. Dr. Blumberg's group had tested a patient with Down's disease and found his blood test for Australia antigen to be negative. When retested several months later, the test was positive, much to their surprise. They hospitalized the patient and performed liver function tests that revealed he had contracted viral hepatitis at some time after the initial examination. In the interview Dr. Blumberg said, "So in 1966 we found that Australia antigen was associated with hepatitis."

I remember discussing Dr. Blumberg's findings and conclusions with Dr. Hans Popper, the great liver pathologist, who expressed some skepticism as to the validity of Blumberg's conclusions. I decided to invite Dr. Blumberg to spend a day with us at St. Vincent's Hospital and New York University School of Medicine, making rounds, meeting my staff, and giving a lecture on Australia antigen. He agreed to come and his visit with us was the highlight of that year. I was convinced that he had put his finger on a marker for viral hepatitis and I told him that I believed he would win a Nobel Prize for the discovery. I was also virtually certain that Dr. Alfred M. Prince of the New York Blood Center later had rediscovered the same antigen but had a different name for it. I was also persuaded by the work of Dr. David Gocke, then of Columbia-Presbyterian, that all blood submitted for transfusions should be tested for Australia antigen.

I fired off a letter to the executive committee of the medical board at St. Vincent's Hospital, recommending that all blood for transfusion be screened with this test. It was quickly adopted, the second medical center in New York to do this screening. When I made the same recommendation at NYU at one of the Lepore-Localio GI conferences, the head of laboratories at Bellevue got up and said it would be too expensive to do the test. Dr. Localio rose and in his inimitable style said, "I have a patient in University Hospital whose colon cancer I cured six months ago but he is now dying of homologous serum hepatitis from blood given by us. Don't tell me that the test is too expensive! Let's start doing it."

During Dr. Blumberg's visit to St. Vincent's Hospital, he observed one of our deeply comatose patients, a sixteen-year-old girl undergoing plasmapheresis with plasma exchange with little prospect of recovery. Her blood Australian antigen was positive, her serum bilirubin 36.6 mg per 100 ml, prothrombin time prolonged to 32 seconds, coagulation factors II, V, VIII, and X markedly diminished. With vigorous plasmapheresis and plasma exchange, the bilirubin level was reduced to 6 mg per 100 ml, the circulating Australia antigen test became negative, the prothrombin time improved to 16.4 seconds and the coagulation factors improved markedly. She appeared to be doing well during the second day of plasmapheresis and exchange when, without warning she suffered cardiorespiratory arrest that responded to CPR and insertion of an endotracheal tube and institution of mechanical respiration. A chest x-ray revealed collapse of the upper lobe of the right lung and bilateral infiltrates. Two days later, she was oliguric and her blood pressure had fallen below 90 mm. Hg systolic. Serum amylase that had been normal on admission had risen to 1182 units per ml. Abdominal examination revealed a striking change consisting of spasm and rigidity of the abdominal muscles with percussion dullness in both flanks. There was no Grey-Turner's or Cullen sign. Hemorrhagic pancreatitis was suspected and confirmed by the finding of bloody peritoneal fluid that contained amylase, 680 units per 100 ml. Peritoneal lavage and dialysis were instituted and plasmapheresis and exchange were terminated. The patient's course was progressively downhill. She died at 8:30 P.M. on 13 November 1969, six days after admission to St. Vincent's Hospital.

During Dr. Blumberg's visit I had discussed this patient's problem in considerable detail, with especial reference to the multiple systems involved in her illness suggesting to me that her hepatitis virus was not confined to the liver, but was systemic and involving the pancreas, the lungs, the kidneys, the heart, and the brain. In 1969 the conventional thinking was that the virus selectively struck the liver parenchyma and failed to invade other organs. Any changes seen in other organs were attributed to sepsis or toxic effects of substances secreted or not detoxified by the injured liver. I suggested to Dr. Blumberg that an attempt should be made to detect Australia antigen in the tissue of all of the body organs as well as the liver using immunofluorescence techniques. He thought it was a good idea and he agreed to perform the tests in his laboratory if we would send the samples to him for examination. He suggested that in the event of our patient's demise, an autopsy should be started within twenty minutes of her death and specimens obtained from all organs and placed immediately on dry ice and dispatched by courier to his laboratory in Fox Chase, Philadelphia. This seemed to be a logical and practical thing to do and we did not foresee any problems in putting the plan into action.

I discussed the patient's poor prognosis with her family and as her condition began to deteriorate, I tried to prepare them for the end and advised them to remain on the floor with us while we continued to administer to her needs. When she was nearly terminal, I requested the family's permission for an autopsy for which they quickly signed saying that they were so grateful for the care she had been receiving. I pronounced the patient dead and notified the nurse in charge and also told her that we had permission to do an autopsy as soon as possible. The nurse then told me that time had to be allowed for the patient's spirit or soul to leave the body. I knew of no such rule and paged the administrator on call. He advised me to proceed with my plan and to disregard any advice to the contrary. The pathologist on call came in quickly because he was interested in our work, but he had only recently joined our staff and at his other hospital there was always a diener who would open the skull to extract the brain. My Upjohn fellows, Dr. James Robilotti, Jr. and Dr. Anthony J. Martel, knew the experienced chief technician who usually did this portion of the postmortem. We located him at home and promised him taxicab fare back and forth plus a twenty-dollar bill. He almost flew into the hospital.

Then we discovered there was no dry ice in the hospital. Jim Robilotti knew how to get some as a special favor from Sutter's, the famous nearby ice cream parlor in the Village. In short order we had several ice-cream buckets full of dry ice. The buckets were sturdy and ideally suited to hold the dry ice and the specimens. The autopsy revealed the following conditions (1) Acute fulminant viral hepatitis with acute liver atrophy (liver weighed 460 gm), (2) Acute hemorrhagic pancreatitis with extensive fat necrosis, (3) acute bronchopneumonia, (4) marked cerebral edema and softening attributed to ischemia.

<u>Microscopic Diagnosis:</u>

<u>Myocardium</u>: epicardial and endocardial hemorrhage

<u>Lungs</u>: hemorrhagic bronchopneumonia, acute tracheobronchitis

<u>Pancreas</u>: extensive acute hemorrhagic necrosis involving the entire organ

<u>Liver</u>: acute submassive necrotic hepatitis consistent with viral hepatitis

<u>Brain</u>: diffuse and severe ischemic changes

<u>Kidneys</u>: congestion, tubules showed osmotic nephrosis with hyaline droplet formation, several tubules with bile cast.

Specimens were obtained and placed in the dry-ice buckets and Dr. James G. Robilotti was the courier who drove to Philadelphia and delivered them to Dr. Blumberg at Fox Chase. We waited patiently for Dr. Blumberg's report. In the meantime, Dr. Patrick J. McKenna, a superb immunologist, hematologist, and head of our blood bank, had joined our team and had made it possible for us to test blood for Australia antigen and antibody before any of the kits and other techniques were commercially available. He was also experimenting with immunofluorescent techniques for demonstrating Australia antigen in fixed tissues. Using these techniques, he showed very clearly that it was present in all of the organ samples from our patient. Its location was in the nuclei of the affected cells. We had clearly demonstrated that fulminant viral hepatitis is a systemic disease and not confined to the liver. I prepared a paper on this topic for presentation before the Section on Gastroenterology at the 119th annual convention of the American Medical Association on 20 June 1970 in Chicago, Illinois. The title was "Plasmapheresis with Plasma Exchange in Hepatic Coma-Fulminant Viral Hepatitis as a Systemic Disease." We waited for Dr. Blumberg's report on the specimens from our patient. Many months went by without an answer. We were told they were having some difficulty with their methods of demonstrating the Australia antigen with immunofluorescent techniques. The deadline for my paper was approaching and still no report from Philadelphia. By this time, I had done enough work with Dr. McKenna to appreciate his excellent capabilities and I knew that he was a topflight investigator. So, I decided to rely on his reports and prepared my paper for the Chicago meeting. Still no word from Philadelphia. The day of the AMA meeting, minutes before I was scheduled to make my presentation, I discovered that Dr. Blumberg was giving a talk in an adjacent room. I managed to find him and questioned him about my patient. He then told me, much to my relief, that he had confirmed what we already knew thanks to Dr. McKenna, viral hepatitis is a systemic disease. Australia antigen had invaded all organs and systems.

Our first efforts with plasmapheresis and plasma exchange in fulminant viral hepatitis failed to save any lives but there were several near-successes that encouraged us to persist in pursuing the project.

In 1970 we published our first major paper on "Plasmapheresis with Plasma Exchange in Hepatic Coma," reporting on the first five patients treated by this technique. Our conclusions were as follows:

> Five patients with acute fulminant hepatic necrosis with coma were subjected to vigorous, massive and prolonged plasmapheresis with plasma exchange on the theory that removal of the patient's plasma would eliminate or reduce circulating noxious protein-bound factors responsible for coma and that replacement of the patient's plasma with fresh frozen human plasma would support the patient through the critical period required for hepatocyte regeneration. One of the five patients emerged from Stage IV coma on day 6 and another on day 8 of vigorous plasmapheresis and appeared to be recovering until severe and relentless bronchopneumonia led to their deaths. The technique can be conducted in humans without undue risk and is more practicable and more in keeping with the pathology of hepatic necrosis than pig liver bypass, human cadaver liver bypass or cross-circulation with humans, baboons or chimpanzees.

Although there were no survivors in the group of seriously ill patients, we did not harm any of them and we learned a great deal about the effects of plasmapheresis with plasma exchange in this condition. We knew we could quickly reduce serum bilirubin levels to normal, replace clotting factors, including prothrombin and platelets, and remove blood ammonia and probably other noxious materials owing to massive hepatic failure due to necrosis of hepatocytes. Serum electrolytes, serum proteins, blood glucose, and creatinine and BUN were maintained at normal levels.

In addition, it was hoped that immunoglobulins from normal donor plasma might contain anti-viral antibodies. We learned to intervene quickly to combat cardiac and respiratory arrest and maintain excellent cardiorespiratory function with appropriate monitoring and use of mechanical ventilatory assistance. Superior and personal nursing care was supplied by dedicated and topflight nursing staff. As we became accustomed to the techniques, our confidence grew that one day in the not too distant future one of our patients in Stage IV coma would overcome the disease and walk out of our hospital to resume a normal life.

Our discovery that severe viral hepatitis is a systemic disease affecting all organ systems suggested to me that perhaps this was why our patients were dying and caused me to theorize that perhaps some lives might be saved if we included in our therapy the intravenous administration of high titre Australia antibody plasma obtained from hemophiliac donors, many of whom had received multiple blood transfusions as well as clotting factors inadvertently contaminated with Australia antigen, causing them to be a rich source of Australia antibody. I discussed this matter with Dr. Joseph P. McKenna, our immunologist and he thought it was a good concept. I also discussed it with Dr. Leonard Stutman, our blood-coagulation specialist and he agreed that we should give it a trial. The only problem was that the supply of antibody-rich plasma was quite limited. In fact, Dr. Stutman had only one hemophiliac patient who could act as a donor. In preparation for a trial of our theory, Dr. Stutman collected three or four units of this patient's plasma and kept it frozen. Its titre was very high, making it ideal for the trial we were contemplating. We discussed the possible dangers that immune complexes might be formed when the high-antibody titre plasma was administered. Dr. McKenna believed there was little danger of this if we administered a high titre plasma that would overwhelm the patient's capacity to form immune complexes. Others had some reservations. There was talk of some severe reactions to high antibody titre serum administered in the therapy of other viral diseases.

It was not long before we had to make the decision to use or not to use the high Australia antibody titre plasma we had been hoarding. The patient who permitted us to test our hypothesis was a twenty-year-old black woman who developed Australia antigen positive hepatitis in the sixth month of her pregnancy and was admitted to St. Vincent's Hospital and Medical Center. She denied drug use but her consort, a known heroin user, had been ill with hepatitis three months before the onset of the patient's illness. Except for scleral icterus, slight hepatomegaly, and an enlarged uterus, physical examination was within normal limits. Her blood chemical studies were as follows: serum bilirubin 7 mg per 100 ml, direct bilirubin 4.5 mg per 100 ml, SGOT 520 units. serum total protein 6.4 gm per 100 ml, albumin 2.4 gm per 100 ml, alkaline phosphatase 13.9 K.A. units, BUN 4.9 mg per ml, amylase 65 units, sodium 135.2 mmEq/L, potassium 3.6 mmEq/L. Prothrombin time 11.2 seconds with control of 12.6 seconds. Chest x-ray was negative. Electrocardiogram revealed a normal tracing. She responded well to bed rest and a regular diet and by the fourth hospital day, the SGOT had fallen from 520 units on admission to 263 units. The serum bilirubin had fallen from 7 mg per 100 ml to 2.5. One week later she developed anorexia, the SGOT rose to 730 units, jaundice reappeared and the liver size shrank. By the 18th hospital day, the total liver dullness to percussion in the right midclavicular line had diminished to only 4 cm, the SGOT was 2460 units and the serum bilirubin was 8.3 mg per 100 ml. On the 20th hospital day (6 September 1970) she spontaneously and prematurely delivered a male child weighing 1.9 kg. No anesthesia was necessary and there was only minimal blood loss. The umbilical cord blood was negative for Australia antigen as was the amniotic fluid and the baby's blood. The mother's blood remained strongly positive for Australia antigen. The baby was isolated from the mother, with her consent, and followed closely by our staff. He has developed normally and has not had Australia antigen in his blood or any evidence of hepatitis. Within 24 hours of the delivery, the patient became lethargic and confused, the SGOT rose to 3900 units and the prothrombin time to 36.5 seconds (control 13.5 seconds). Later that day (7 September) the patient became comatose and would respond only to painful stimuli. It was decided to proceed with plasmapheresis with plasma exchange. Before this could be initiated, she stopped breathing and required intubation followed later by tracheostomy. Supportive measures consisting of intravenous fluid, glucose, hydrocortisone, and vitamin K were instituted. Plasmapheresis with plasma exchange was started on 8 September. By the 20th exchange on 9 September, she began to intermittently open her eyes and to move her head from side to side. She did not respond to verbal stimuli. On the following day she was intermittently decerebrate and began to bleed from the tracheostomy site.

She developed hypofibrinogenemia and thrombocytopenia that responded to 4 gm of fibrinogen intravenously and eight units of platelets intravenously. Her general condition continued to improve and she responded to verbal stimuli. On 12 September, she was clearly out of coma and plasmapheresis was discontinued that day. She had undergone a total exchange of 57 units of blood and was given a total of 125 units of fresh frozen human plasma since initiation of plasmapheresis on 8 September. The Australia antigen blood test that had been positive repeatedly before plasmapheresis, became negative within 12 hours after starting plasmapheresis and remained negative during the four to five days of plasmapheresis. Two days after termination of plasmapheresis, she became febrile and developed leucocytosis (WBC 43,000) and the chest x-ray for the first time revealed pulmonary infiltrates consistent with pneumonia. She was alert and fully conscious. The Australia antigen test which had been negative on 9 September through 14 September once more became positive on 15 and 16 September. Antibiotics were changed from cephalothin to gentamycin but the pulmonary infiltrates increased and the febrile course persisted. Since 11 of our previously treated patients had died with pulmonary complications, it was felt that the time had come to intervene with a new form of therapy aimed at neutralizing the hepatitis virus. After much discussion and deliberation on possible hazards of producing immune complexes, we administered intravenously one unit (220–350 ml) of hyperimmune Australia-antibody-rich plasma over an eight-hour period each day for three days, starting on 17 September. This plasma had been obtained by plasmapheresing a hemophiliac donor who very generously donated his plasma. The patient's response was dramatic, the temperature falling to normal, leucocytosis diminishing, and the pulmonary infiltrates clearing rapidly. Following the administration of hyperimmune Australia-antibody-rich plasma, her blood test for Australia antigen became negative on counter immunoelectrophoresis. It is our interpretation that the Australia-antibody-rich plasma inactivated the Australia antigen in the patient's blood stream so that it was impossible to detect the antigen by the immunologic techniques that we employed. In addition, in-vitro testing was performed by mixing Australia-antigen-positive plasma with Australia-antibody-rich plasma, resulting in a negative test for Australia-antigen by counter immunoelectrophoreses. The patient made a steady and full recovery from her viral hepatitis and was the first one in our small series to walk out of the hospital and resume her usual activities. A liver biopsy on 20 July 1971 confirmed her complete recovery.

This patient's case report was first published in the *American Journal of Gastroenterology* 58:381–389, October 1972. It was selected for republication as a milestone report in *Plasma Therapy*, vol. 1, no. 1, March 1979.

Our experience with plasmapheresis with plasma exchange in the treatment of fulminant hepatic failure with coma satisfied us that it was worthy of further trial in this serious, often lethal disease. With proof that this form of hepatitis is a systemic disease, not confined to the liver, came the hypothesis that in those patients with Australia antigen causing it, hyperimmune Australia-antibody plasma might be effective therapy. Its dramatic effect in one of our patients served to spur us to pursue this lead. The practical question was how could we obtain enough of the Australia-antibody-rich plasma for a trial. An obvious source was hemophiliac patients.

I approached the National Hemophilia Foundation and met with an officer, hoping to enlist help in securing Australia-antibody-rich plasma for a trial. We were told that they had the donors but they would have to charge one dollar per cc. for the plasma because the Foundation needed the money to purchase supplies of Factor VIII for their constituents. They had no provision for research trials. I also learned from this source that plasmapheresis had become big business in the United States, especially in Texas, where Mexicans were sneaking across the border into cities like Nogales to sell their plasma, obtained by plasmapheresis at a plasma center, for three cents for each cc. The processed plasma was then sold to large companies for a handsome profit. The extent of this commercial enterprise, according to an article in *American Medical News* of 8 February 1987 is mind-boggling. "Traditionally the United States has been the major world supplier of plasma. In 1986, 11.3 million paid donors (in America) underwent the procedure (plasmapheresis) providing about a million liters of processed plasma"—which would be sold to large companies for fifty to sixty dollars per liter, by any account an enormously profitable business. I was also told that a doctor in Texas was hoarding Australia-antibody-rich plasma in the hope that he would make a killing by selling it at a high price. Confronted by what I deemed to be crass commercialization of plasmapheresis, no matter what the justification, I began to have some doubts about pursuing this line of therapy. It seemed to me that my team and I were exposing ourselves to serious risks without remuneration while others were in it just to make money. But, *c'est la guerre!*

In October 1970 a concise and accurate story on our plasmapheresis project appeared on the front page of the St. Vincent's Hospital and Medical Center of New York *News* under the title "Miracle on Eleventh Street," which included a photograph of our plasmapheresis team and a description of our successful treatment of the young mother who was the first of our patients with Stage IV hepatic coma to walk out of the hospital and go on to complete recovery. The article, written nearly a quarter of a century ago, concludes with the following statement:

> Dr. Lepore feels that this technique can be conducted in humans without undue risk and may sustain the patient's life until regeneration of liver cells occurs. It is more practical and more in keeping with the pathology of severe hepatic injury than previously suggested methods of treatment including whole blood exchange transfusion, pig liver bypass, human cadaver liver bypass, or cross-circulation with humans, baboons, or chimpanzees. The advantages of plasmapheresis with plasma exchange over whole blood exchange are many: 1) it can be conducted for periods as long as 9 to 12 days, far longer than whole-

blood exchanges, 2) it reduces the demands upon the blood bank for whole blood and is especially useful in patients with rare blood types whose blood may be in critically short supply, 3) use of the patient's own red cells reduces the occurrence of transfusion reactions, 4) it not only removes noxious metabolites and protein-bound substances but adds essential material produced by the normal liver and present in normal fresh frozen plasma. The success of this plasmapheresis procedure portends many beneficial results. Hopefully, it will help in future liver transplants to support the patient without liver function by doing for the liver what the artificial kidney does for the kidney. It may also lead to the eventual isolation of the virus or viruses causing hepatitis and to the development of a vaccine. Viral hepatitis is high on the list of enemies of public health. At least 50,000 to 60,000 cases are reported annually and for each reported case, there are probably ten or more unrecognized or unreported ones. It affects people in all age groups but is especially apt to strike persons in their most productive years. In New York, we are seeing an increasing incidence in drug users. However, hepatitis may affect persons in many walks of life, for example a person receiving a blood transfusion or a nurse, technician or doctor working on patients with hepatitis or on hemodialysis units and open heart teams or others handling human blood products in the course of their work. Fortunately most of the cases are mild to moderate and are followed by complete recovery.

Occasionally patients become severely ill and for them the disease is life-threatening. Here plasmapheresis with plasma exchange may be life-saving.

Our next patient with viral hepatitis, is etched in my memory forever. He was a very bright seventeen-year-old Phillips Exeter Academy graduate who was admitted to St. Vincent's Hospital by his family internist on 31 May 1976 because of the onset five days before of general malaise, nausea, slight fever, and epigastric distress accompanied by darkening urine and jaundice. There was no history of contact with hepatitis, prior liver disease, excessive alcohol ingestion, use of illicit drugs, raw shell fish ingestion, or exposure to toxic chemicals or transfusion, vaccinations, or injections or surgical procedures. His general physical examination on admission revealed no abnormalities except for jaundice, slight fever, and slight lethargy plus slight hepatomegaly. Neurological examination was normal.

Initial Laboratory Data:

Urinalysis

Color amber	Ketones negative	WBC 6–7
Sp grav 10.30	Blood negative	Urine was icto-test positive
Sugar negative	Protein negative	RBC 0

CBC 5/31/76	Electrolytes 5/31/76	Serum Protein
Hbg 15.7	Sodium 131	5/31/76
Hct 45.7	Potassium 4.2	Albumin 3.58 g/dl
WBC 12,7000	Chloride 92	Al glob 0.25 g/dl
Poly 36%	CO2 .35	A2 glob 0.39 g/dl
Lymph 42%	BUN 12	Gamma glob 0.88 g/dl
Mono 2%	Amylase 69	Total protein:
Bank 20%		5.4 g/dl
Atypical lymph 1%		
Platelets decreased		
MCV 85		
MCH 29		
MCHC 35		
Prothrombin time 33.4/10.5 seconds		
VDRL nonreactive.		

Electrocardiogram 6/1/76: Sinus tachycardia of 110 per minutes with nonspecific ST-T wave changes

INITIAL X-RAY REPORT: Chest 5/31/76: negative.

HOSPITAL COURSE

Within two hours after hospital admission, the patient was noted to become alternately lethargic and agitated. He became extremely uncooperative in answering questions and over the next several minutes became disoriented and lapsed into coma. He exhibited decerebrate posturing with widely dilated pupils that were equal and reactive to light. Patient was noted to have labored and irregular breathing and an endotracheal tube was placed after a 20-second apneic period. The patient was not triggering the respirator after intubation and on physical examination was completely unresponsive to verbal or painful stimuli. Pulse and blood pressure were maintained adequately. Examination of the fundi showed no papilledema. Pupils were dilated but reactive to light directly and consensually. Eye movements were random. Doll's reflexes were present. Hypertonic muscular tonicity of all four extremities were present as were both Babinski reflexes. Deep tendon reflexes were hyperactive, bilaterally. A lumbar puncture was performed without difficulty under sterile conditions with the needle inserted in the L-3, L-4 interspace. Approximately 5 cc of clear, sightly yellow fluid was withdrawn. Opening pressure was 220 mm. Results of the spinal fluid analysis showed no cells present, protein 40, glucose 141. Culture for bacteria and viruses were negative. The initial liver function studies obtained on 6/1/76 showed a bilirubin of 37 mg total with 35 mg direct bilirubin. SGOT 404, LDH 918 and CPK 273, Alk phos 233. In addition, total protein was 5.5, albumin 3.7, calcium 8.6 and phosphorus 2.0. Creatinine was 0.9. Uric acid 6.9. Serum ammonia level on 6/1/76 was 223 micrograms percent. Mono spot test on 6/1/76 was negative.

The patient was seen in consultation by Doctor Stutman of the Coagulation Laboratory because of his elevated prothrombin time of 33/11.8 seconds control. Doctor Stutman's laboratory found the APTT to be 83.0/30.8, fibrinogen to be 182, T.T. 23 and SDPS positive 1–20. Initial arterial blood gas on 6/1/76 showed the pH to be 7.52, PCO2 31, bicarb 25, PO2 108 with saturation of 98.3%. Of particular importance was the finding of a negative serum Australia antigen.

After transferring the patient to the Medical Intensive Care Unit, decision was made conjointly with Doctors Lepore, McKenna and Felder to begin exchange plasmapheresis as a treatment modality for acute hepatic encephalopathy secondary to fulminant hepatitis.

Exchange plasmapheresis with fresh frozen plasma was begun at 3 P.M. on 6/1/76 by Doctors Gualtieri, Webb and Flannery. Plasmapheresis exchange with access to the circulation was obtained via a cannula placed in the left iliac vein by Dr. Foster Conklin of Vascular Surgery. Over the next 16 hours under the conditions of reverse isolation, 14 units of blood were withdrawn at a rate of approximately 1 unit per hour, centrifuged and the red cells retransfused with fresh frozen plasma. The patient's own serum from each of these units was sent for study to Dr. Joseph McKenna's laboratory in the blood bank. Patient maintained adequate blood pressure and urine output and a total of 20 units of fresh frozen plasma were transfused. In addition he was given Vitamin K intramuscularly as well as calcium gluconate 2 amps IV q6h. Approximately 20 units of platelets were also transfused. Serum bilirubin after 14 units of plasmapheresis exchange dropped from 37 mg on 6/1/76 to 13.2 total on 6/2/76. SGOT on 6/2/76 was 516, an LDH of 668, CPK 250, alkaline phosphatase 114.

The patient remained in deep coma but began to trigger the respirator spontaneously and move his arms and shoulders with purposeless movements. Periods of muscular rigidity alternated with muscular flaccidity and the patient exhibited alternate periods of decerebrate posturing. Repeat studies by Doctor Stutman's Coagulation Laboratory showed improvement in coagulation profile with a prothrombin time of 19.6/12 seconds control. APTT 48/30.8 seconds control, Fibrinogen 174, platelets 90,000. White blood cell count had dropped to 2200. Hct. 33.

As of 6/3/76, the patient had received a total of 32 exchange plasmapheresis units with only slight improvement in mental status. In view of the falling hematocrit, leukopenia and thrombocytopenia present at that time, Doctor Lepore in conjunction with Dr. McKenna decided to begin whole blood exchange transfusion. A Scribner's shunt was inserted for vascular access into the right forearm by Dr. Foster Conklin on 6/3/76. On 6/5/76, 10 units of whole blood were exchanged and bilirubin remained at a level of 16.8 mg total with 13.6 direct. SGOT had dropped from 516 to 195. There was still no change in mental status. Positive blood cultures for Staph aureus were obtained on 6/3/76 and the patient was started on Ampicillin and Oxacillin IV therapy. On 6/7/76, 11 units of whole blood were exchange-transfused. At this time the patient maintained adequate vital signs and arterial blood gas with no significant change in mental status until 4 A.M. when the patient suddenly woke up, extubated himself and began to verbalize. He was able to follow simple commands and was able to verbalize his urge to urinate. Serum bilirubin at this time was 13.6 mg total over 13. direct with an SGOT of 87, LDH of 286 and a CPK of 365. Alpha feto-protein done on 6/7/76 was negative. Coagulation studies showed a prothrombin time of 12/12 seconds control with an APTT of 36.0/32.6 seconds control. Serum ammonia at this time was 325 micrograms percent.

When David emerged from his deep coma after six days of plasmapheresis and blood exchange, pandemonium cut loose on the ICU floor in celebration. When I arrived on the scene that Monday morning, my first move was to enter David's room. He was wide awake and able to motion to me and respond to my commands. I lack even now the capacity to describe how I felt to bear witness to this miracle of modern medicine and to realize that it was brought about by a new form of therapy that I had introduced into medicine. Even now, as I write this, there are tears as I recall the scene and the events. I thought then and now of the marvelous team I had brought together, the dedicated nurses, the house staff, technicians, and attending staff who risked their lives to bring about this marvelous result. What

I lack in words describing the event was more than compensated for by the eloquence of David's father, an eminent Harvard Law graduate who threw his arms about me and thanked me for having brought David back to life. In a letter to me, his father and mother warmed the cockles of my heart.

June 11, 1976

Dear Dr. Lepore:

David Rice Ecker, our son, won the Senior English Prize and graduated from Phillips Exeter Academy, Exeter, New Hampshire, on Sunday, May 30; on Monday, May 31, he was admitted to St. Vincent's Hospital just before noon; he became delirious in the afternoon, twice ripping out the IV connections; he went into a coma around midnight (observed by his night nurse to be unarousable); he entered your care on Tuesday morning, June 1.

David emerged from his coma on Monday, June 6, at 4 A.M.—six days later.

These six days were the longest in our memory. You made them seem shorter by your "take it day by day" approach—your constancy of care, concern and optimism—your organization and leadership of a truly remarkable team of doctors, nurses and technicians—your mobilizing and alternating of a variety of weapons (pheresis, exchange, steroids, antibiotics and others)—your clear, patient and candid reports to us, his parents.

Throughout, you never seemed to doubt that David would make it. It was almost as if you communicated that confidence to David across the great barrier of unconsciousness.

We looked and we looked into familiar but unseeing eyes. Then finally recognition lit them up, and we said "This is your mother, and I, your dad" and he answered "I know that." A great moment.

It is impossible for us to express our admiration and gratitude to you for what you have done. David was born in St. Vincent's on August 13, 1958. You have given us David again— and we are very glad to have him.

The achievement of your knowledge, your genius and your courage combined with the discipline and devotion of St. Vincent's medical, nursing and support staff is a medical miracle. We know that you will all receive well-merited recognition from your professional colleagues. (You already have that of our "regular" doctor, Dr. Seymour Felder, and of our brother-in-law, Dr. Arthur Ludwig).

But no one will ever out-thank us. We will never forget what you have done, and you will always be in our thoughts and prayers.

Sincerely yours,
Elizabeth and Allan Ecker

David continued to improve and became progressively more alert in the ensuing hours. Over the next day, his muscular strength and coordination improved. Corticosteroids which had been started for treatment of cerebral edema were decreased from Decadron 8 mg IV q6h over a gradually diminished schedule. Ampicillin and Oxacillin were continued for 10 days as treatment of septicemia with Staph aureus. The Scribner shunt was removed on 6/9/76 and the patient continued to show improvement in muscular strength and mental alertness. Cultures of urine and sputum grew Enterobacter and Klebsiella in significant numbers and the patient was treated with Keflin and Oxacillin. He was transferred off the ICU on 6/11/76 to a private room where reverse isolation procedures were maintained. His dietary protein was severely restricted and he was initially allowed only fresh frozen plasma IV as his only protein source. Regimen consisted of Neomycin 1 gr po q6h with Neomycin enemas evening and morning. Prednisolone 10 mg qid was also continued. Over the next several weeks, the patient showed continued improvement and dietary protein was increased to near normal levels. Bilirubin remained between 20 and 25 with SGOT's in the 200–300 range. At time of discharge on 7/18/76, the patient was afebrile, eating well, and able to walk without assistance. The liver edge was palpable 3 finger-breadths below the right costal margin.

His bilirubin at the time of discharge was 11.2 mg total with 6.7 direct. SGOT was 422. LDH 286. CPK 53. Alk phos 350. Blood sugar (fasting) 74. Repeat Australia antigen and antibodies were negative. Antigen for Type A hepatitis was also negative. The patient was discharged improved, to be cared for at home by his family on 7/18/76.

I shall never forget David and his wonderful family. I thank heaven for my research fellowship in physiology at Rochester in the 1930s when I developed the plasmapheresis technique on dogs, little knowing that one day I would apply it to saving human lives.

In 1975 I retired as chief of gastroenterology at St. Vincent's Hospital, planning to devote some time to writing a monograph on medical education and continuing with my personal practice of medicine. The unit I developed in gastroenterology at St. Vincent's hospital using the generous Upjohn gift as well as donations to the Lepore Memorial Fund was now well established as a strong division meriting support from the general funds of the hospital. With my retirement from the directorship, the hospital would now have to support the unit and its fellowships. It would take a while before adequate support was forthcoming but it finally did arrive. The plasmapheresis project fell by the wayside because of lack of funds for personnel and the expensive new equipment needed to keep up with modern technology.

Unfortunately from a pioneer in plasmapheresis or apheresis, St. Vincent's Hospital was among the last of the major hospitals in New York to acquire the sophisticated plasmapheresis equipment needed to pursue this new form of therapy. It was not until 1991 that St. Vincent's Hospital acquired one plasmapheresis machine, and this was primarily for plasmapheresis of neurological patients with the Guillain-Barré syndrome. During the intervening years since 1975, and especially starting in 1980, I had become concerned over the use of fresh frozen plasma as the replacement fluid in plasmapheresis with plasma exchange because of the hazard of transmission of a mysterious and lethal virus for which there was no diagnostic or screening test. That virus was eventually identified as HIV, the cause of AIDS. When a diagnostic screening test for this virus was developed and added to screening for Hepatitis A, B, and C, plasma once more became acceptable for use in plasmapheresis with plasma exchange.

Many of my predictions on plasmapheresis expressed in the previously quoted interview of 1970 have come true. The technique has been successfully employed to keep a patient alive until a suitable liver has become available for transplantation. The viruses causing hepatitis have been identified and an excellent and safe recombinant vaccine prepared against Hepatitis B by cloning into yeast a portion of the Hepatitis B virus gene coding for HBsAg. Surgeons, nurses, technicians, and children with high exposure to Hepatitis B are being vaccinated to prevent its occurrence and spread. Vaccines against other hepatitis viruses are on the planning board. Plasma therapy with high titre antibody for viral diseases is in its infancy. Elegant and superb equipment for performing plasmapheresis has made it a practical form of therapy for a wide variety of ailments. Refinement of the technique and equipment has made it possible to perform selective apheresis of many sorts, including leukophoresis and modification of T lymphocytes. Graft rejection has been successfully treated by this method. I believe that plasmapheresis and its modifications will be to modern medicine what the leech appliers and bleeders of the past were searching for. The concise two-volume monograph, *Therapeutic Hemapheresis*, by James L. McPherson and Duke O. Kasprisim,[9] describes the equipment and its applications. I also recommend the

---

9. Published in 1984 by CRC Press, Inc., Boca Raton, Florida 33431.

10. Published in 1979 by Eden Medical Resource, Inc., PO Box 51, St. Albans, Vermont 05478.

excellent short monograph, "Plasmapheresis and Plasma Exchange," by T. J. Hamblin.[10]

The Plasmapheresis Project at St. Vincent's Hospital taught us a number of lessons. First and foremost, there is still room for creative clinical investigation in almost any modern hospital with a strong professional staff, a sound teaching program, and an abundance of young people of idealistic temperament who will give more than they take out of medicine. Second, good clinical investigation is not and should not be confined to the academic ivory tower. Third, the stimulus that sustained us was the desire to develop an innovative approach to the treatment of a serious disease threatening and taking the lives of a group of young people. Fourth, our desire to learn more about the mysteries of liver disease, its treatment, and its prevention. Fifth, participation in the project taught several generations of our house staff the excitement of the chase inherent in participation in good clinical investigation destined to bring benefits to other patients seen and treated in our hospital. Years after the fact, members of our plasmapheresis team speak with gratitude for all they learned through their dedicated service in the program. Sixth, the stimulus for participating in the program was to save lives, the basic reason why many of our young people enter the profession of medicine. Seventh, the project brought forth the best efforts of our nursing and laboratory services and their personnel. The St. Vincent's nurses of that era were, to my mind, among the best in their profession at the bedside caring for sick patients. Dr. McKenna, our immunologist and blood bank chief was a tower of strength. He is a most unusual immunologist who worked effectively with clinicians and loved to help solve our problems.

Last but not least, I derived great satisfaction for pioneering in an exciting new venture through which I was repaying my illustrious teachers at Rochester, Duke, Yale, Columbia University, and New York University for their faith in me and their investment in my career as a clinician, teacher, and investigator.

Finally, medicine is replete with examples of serendipitous and innovative discoveries paving the way to new therapy and scientific concepts. While most of these emerge from highly sophisticated laboratories and the ivory towers of academe, there is still room for well-trained practicing clinicians in these modern times to make substantial contributions to new knowledge. These men and women on the firing line of personal practice, admittedly an endangered species, have as their inspiration the challenge of the patients they meet each day. Some, as they have in the past, will make significant contributions to the conquest of disease and the recognition of new entities. Where will the next Frederick Banting come from? Is the recently introduced Lorenzo's Oil a flash in the pan or will it emerge as a treatment for a dreadful, lethal hereditary disease, "Adrenoleukodystrophy" (ALD), through the efforts of the parents of an afflicted child named Lorenzo? Without any medical training these intelligent and well-educated people, Augusto and Michaela Odone, searched the scientific literature and spotted a report from a researcher, Dr. William B. Rizzo of the Medical College of Virginia in Richmond, that monounsaturated fatty acids could largely prevent cells from making long-chain fatty acids, the hallmark of adrenoleukodystrophy. Why not try it on their son?, asked the parents. It was not that simple, but by persistent and tireless effort they finally persuaded manufacturers to make and market an oil containing oleic acid and erucic acid. They named it for their son, Lorenzo. Their claim that the oil has arrested the course of the disease and prolonged his life is disputed by several respected scientists, but the Odones are convinced they are on the right track. The Odones's side of the argument is presented in a recent movie, *Lorenzo's Oil*, starring Nick Nolte and Susan Sarandon as Augusto and Michaela Odone, with Zack O'Malley Greenberg playing their son, Lorenzo.

Scientific caution is warranted when anecdotal support is the only "evidence."[11, 12] Even if this may be only a step in the direction of understanding more about ALD, perhaps one of the half-way technologies, using Lewis Thomas's phrase, the Odones have succeeded in graphically depicting and publicizing the tragedy of their son's illness in the hope that our scientists will focus on this admittedly rare disease and one day find the gene that is responsible. Where else but in America could this have come to pass?

---

11. W.B. Rizzo, "Lorenzo's Oil—Hope and Disappointment," New England J of Med 1993; 329: 801-802.

12. A. Odone, M. Odone, "More on Lorenzo's Oil," New England J of Med 1994; 330: 1904.

Epilogue

These are the researches of Herodotus of
Halicarnassus, which he publishes, in the
hope of thereby preserving from decay the
remembrance of what men have done...

The History of Herodotus,
The First Book, Titled
Clio

MICHAEL J. LEPORE, MD died on 2 September 2000. The year
of his birth, 1910, was marked by the publication of the now
famous Bulletin Number Four of the Carnegie Foundation
for the Advancement of Teaching, *Medical Education in the United States
and Canada,* by Abraham Flexner. The Flexner report would lead to
the closure of substandard proprietary medical schools, to the creation of University of Rochester School of Medicine which my father
would enter in 1929, and to emphasis "on medicine as a science, while
the practice of the art would be relegated to a secondary role."[1] The
year of his death brought forth completion of a working draft of the
DNA sequence of the human genome. This would delineate an estimated 90% of genes on every chromosome and "the first time in the
story of life on earth that a species has read its own recipe."[2] The years
1910 and 2000 bracket a time of great ferment and unimaginable
progress in the evolution of the field of applied biology known as
medicine. In these 90 years my father observed the dawn of the atomic age at close hand, was physician to patients from all walks of life,
including a President, made significant contributions to the treatment
of hepatic disease, and used the new technology of TV to educate

---

1. Michael J. Lepore, *Death of the Clinician.* Springfield, Charles C. Thomas,
1982, p. viii.
2. Matt Ridley, *Genome, The Autobiography of a Species in 23 Chapters.* New York,
Harper Collins, 2000, p. 2.

doctors. To my mind his life's work was emblematic of a heroic age of medicine which ended with the decline of the Oslerian clinician-scholar and the advent of the "corporatization" of American medicine.

As *Life of the Clinician* ends in 1976, the curtain has not yet been brought down on the embattled clinician-scholar and my father graphically communicates the excitement and hope surrounding the use of plasmapheresis to treat fulminant acute viral hepatitis—a malady regarded up until that time as invariably fatal. We are left with a snapshot of an indefatigable team of St. Vincent's Hospital physicians and nurses, a monofuge spinning off plasma, and a young man emerging from hepatic coma. The memoir concludes with my father at the bedside 104 blocks south of the flat in Harlem's little Italy where he had entered the world 66 years earlier. The preceding pages of the *Life of the Clinician* depict his journey "downtown" as a doctor passionately engaged in the exciting enterprise of 20th century American medicine, and the reader learns how (and more importantly, *why*) Dr. Lepore came to "bear witness to this miracle of modern medicine" in an ICU room in St. Vincent's Hospital.

My father's motivation was to give each of his patients "the best of modern medicine wrapped in a book jacket of the past" and "seeing that all is done to achieve a cure or failing that, to give my patients comfort, compassion, and the assurance that serving their interest is my main purpose and goal." To accomplish these ends he utilized the "Triple Threat" talents of scientist, teacher, and clinician. His arduous and successful pursuit of these three skills is the stuff of a modern *bildungsroman* in the guise of a memoir.

Born of the literary collaboration of Sinclair Lewis and the bacteriologist Paul de Kruif, *Arrowsmith* inspired my father (and his generation) with its vivid descriptions of the restless scientist-physician, Martin Arrowsmith, and a temple of the biomedical establishment, the Mc Gurk (a.k.a. Rockefeller) Institute. Fictional inspirations aside, among my father's scientific cynosures were his teachers George Hoyt Whipple, Nobelist and founding dean of the University of Rochester School of Medicine, Edward F. Adolph, Professor of Physiology at Rochester, and John P. Peters, Professor of Medicine at Yale. All were mentors during my father's medical school and fellowship years, and beyond. During his fellowships my father was able to further define the physiological role of the plasma proteins, and with this were sown the seeds of the therapeutic application of plasmapheresis for his patients with acute hepatic failure. My father viewed plasmapheresis in the context of the link between teachers and students: "Even more impelling was my desire to put to practical use the years of basic research in physiology that I had spent at Rochester, Duke, and Yale in the 1930's. I wanted to repay my sponsors and teachers the debt I owed them for teaching me the lessons from the laboratory, the basic sciences, especially physiology and applying this knowledge at the bedside to the care of the seriously ill." Implicit in my father's research was the tenet that scientific research should not become the exclusive province of the biomedical basic scientist. Trained in an era when a young surgeon, Frederick Banting, could discover insulin, my father believed that it was "still possible for important clinical investigation to be done by qualified clinicians whose stimulus is the challenge of curing the sick who seek their personal care."

My father's debt to his teachers was also repaid by his dedication to teaching. He often quoted James A. Garfield's assessment of the value of a true teacher, Mark Hopkins of Williams College: "Give me a log hut, with only a simple bench, Mark Hopkins at one end and I at the other, and you may have all the buildings, apparatus and libraries without him." My father could stimulate and excite housestaff and seasoned clinicians at his rounds and conferences in University Medical Centers, however, he was equally adept at creating a vigorous teaching program not in a "log hut," but in the Quonset huts of Saipan and Tinian during World War II.

Although my father was nine years old at the time of Sir William Osler's death, Osler's students such as Drs. McCann, Davison, and Hanes were my father's revered teachers, and Osler's proposed epitaph, "I taught medical students in the wards," was a guiding principle in my father's approach to teaching.[3] Michael J. Lepore's ability to discover an unnoticed but significant physical finding and not only relate it to the most current physiology but place it in the historical evolution of medical concepts made him an unrivalled teacher at the bedside. The resident presenting a case to my father might be asked, as Dr. Corner asked my father in 1929, "Who was Malphigi?" and he would learn about the discovery of capillaries—an achievement which eluded the great Harvey. The history of medicine was a dynamic and vibrant discipline which my father used adroitly and with contagious enthusiasm to delight and instruct his students and colleagues. The bedside was his lectern, and his teaching could captivate equally well the handful of housestaff, fellows, and nurses, attending his ward rounds or the "20,000 doctors in one evening on closed circuit television" for The Upjohn Grand Rounds. I recently reviewed

---

3. William B. Bean, *Osler Aphorisms*. Springfield, Charles C. Thomas, 1961, p. 155.

the kinescope entitled, "Diagnosis and Management of Acute Abdominal Problems" which aired on January 18, 1956. At that time my father was in his mid-forties; he stood 5 feet 5 inches tall with powerful shoulders developed from his youthful work as an iceman. His nose was aquiline, his jaw was square, and his hair was jet black (as it would remain until his 80's). Beyond these physical characteristics, which I have known my entire life, was the impression of immense energy and informed intelligence which transcended the flickering shadows of black and white film. To see the thrust and parry of my father's animated discourse with the distinguished Grand Rounds panel as they hammered out the correct diagnosis was a compelling exercise in the art of bedside teaching and the image will always remain with me.

Of the triad of scientist, teacher, and clinician, the vocation which mattered most to my father was "clinician." He practiced pure "Oslerian medicine, emphasizing careful history-taking, meticulous physical examination, and close observation of my patients. What the patient really gets when he is seen by me is an attentive human being using his five senses aided by that marvelous instrument developed by Laennec, the stethoscope, and making the most of some rather simple tests. I learned long ago that medicine is not a science but an art based on scientific principles. The essence of medicine is in the art of diagnosis." Nothing could compare to the marvelously cognitive, synthetic, and creative act of tracking down an elusive diagnosis or, as my father termed it, "hitting a home run." Among the factors in my decision to become a physician were my father's dramatic and exotic accounts of diagnosis in which an amyloid nodule of the tongue or a blue bleb rubber nevus on the sole of the foot solved the mystery of an ailment and blazed the way to successful therapy. I would be on the edge of my seat as he recounted tense moments in the operating room before the surgeon announced that he had found the Meckel's diverticulum which Dad had boldly predicted was the source of his patient's GI bleeding. As Osler knew, "to talk of diseases is a sort of Arabian Nights' entertainment," and my father's stories conveyed a sense of wonder and possibility which invigorated my nascent interest in medicine.[4]

My father never lost sight of the simple fact that correct diagnosis was a means (and not an end) of caring for the patient. The cor-

---

4. Ibid., p. 132.

rect diagnosis obtained at the autopsy table held no great attraction for him. Of clinicopathologic conferences he archly said, "Quite frankly I prefer to make the diagnosis in the living patient." He unfailingly followed Francis Peabody's dictum that the "secret of the care of the patient is in caring for the patient."[5] The importance of empathy in a physician was underscored in a story which my father would tell about Professor Robert Loeb who during a medical student case presentation at the patient's bedside was told that the diagnosis was gastric carcinoma. Dr. Loeb, Chairman of the Department of Medicine at Columbia "P&S" at the time, grimly ordered the student to go back to his room because "he was through." After what must have seemed like a lifetime, Loeb appeared at the student's room in Bard Hall where the aspiring doctor was packing his bags with the certainty that his medical career had abruptly ended in failure. Dr. Loeb told the student to unpack and resume his course of studies; the Professor had made the student believe that his short career was finished so that he might in some small way experience the hopelessness and despair of a patient who had first learned of his terminal diagnosis from the student's insensitive case presentation. This cautionary tale was my father's way of saying that the patient came first.

In the age of the "health care provider," we begin to forget that there was a time when medicine was truly regarded as a "higher calling" and my father sincerely believed that he "lived and served in the Golden Era of American Medicine" and that there would never be "an age so remarkable, exciting, and productive." His path was arduous, with detours to the Bronx ("the graveyard for specialists") and Saipan and Tinian during World War II, but he was always guided by his "north stars"—teachers like Whipple, McCann, Hanes, Palmer, Peters, Loeb, Fitz-Hugh, and Fulton. He nerve forgot them and they walk the wards again in the pages of this memoir.

To the end of his life my father remained intensively engaged with medicine. He published his first book, *Death of the Clinician*, and scientific correspondence in *The Lancet* in his eighth decade of life, and his office practice was active until his late 80's. When he became ill with right upper quadrant pain, his self-diagnosis of intermittent "ball-valve" obstruction of the common bile duct as described by Osler was both erudite and accurate. He never dodged the big issues of his era, and I will always treasure our ongoing discussions of full-

---

5. Francis W. Peabody, *The Care of the Patient*. Cambridge, Harvard University Press, 1928, p. 48.

time vs. private (or as he called it, "personal") practice, generalist vs. specialist, or the depredations of managed care. Although he was a perceptive critic, Michael J. Lepore was fundamentally an idealist and an optimist. He believed in America, his family, the decency of people, and "my teachers and role models" who were "almost all, pupils of Sir William Osler, the greatest physician of modern times." "To them," he acknowledges at the beginning of this memoir, "I owe a tremendous debt that I can never repay." By the end of *Life of the Clinician,* I hope that you will agree that Michael J. Lepore has settled his account.

Frederick E. Lepore, MD
Departments of Neurology & Ophthalmology
Robert Wood Johnson Medical School

Michael J. Lepore, M.D. (1910-2000) was an internist who helped to define the nascent specialty of gastroenterology in the 1930s, but first and foremost he was a clinician in the tradition of Sir William Osler. The first graduate of the University of Rochester School of Medicine and Dentistry to receive the degree of M.D. with Honors, Dr. Lepore went on to a distinguished career at the College of Physicians and Surgeons of Columbia University, New York University School of Medicine, and St. Vincent's Hospital and Medical Center of New York. The Italian-American experience in the early part of the Twentieth Century is seen through the eyes of Dr. Lepore, who counted Greta Garbo and President Herbert Hoover among his patients. His story ranges from the Island of Tinian and the launching of the Atomic Bomb to a hospital room in lower Manhattan where a young man's life was saved by the development of a new therapy called plasmapheresis. Along the way, Dr. Lepore incisively applauds the triumphs of medical science and mourns the passing of the "triple-threat" physician who could teach at the bedside, forge a powerful therapeutic alliance with patients, and carry on innovative research.

Michael Lepore was a member the class of 1934 of the University of Rochester School of Medicine and Dentistry, and a resident in Internal Medicine at Duke University School of Medicine (1934-37), and the American College of Physicians Research Fellow at Yale University (1935-36). In later years, he was the Director of the Upjohn Gastrointestinal Service at St. Vincent's Hospital and Medical Center in New York City and Professor of Clinical Medicine at New York University School of Medicine. Dr. Lepore was the author of *Death of the Clinician: Requiem or Reveille?* and numerous scientific publications.